Rand McNally
Retirement Places Rated

All you need to plan your retirement

Richard Boyer & David Savageau

Rand McNally & Company

Chicago • New York • San Francisco

Acknowledgments

Each time we produce a volume in the *Places Rated* series, we realize the book could not have been written but for the help given us by persons in government and with private organizations. Many of the improvements in this thoroughly updated, revised, and expanded version of our 1983 *Places Rated Retirement Guide* were suggested by them.

We particularly recognize our debt to Susan Betz-Keating and Jon M. Leverenz at Rand McNally for contributions every step of the way; to Calvin Beale of the U.S. Department of Agriculture for his vast knowledge of America's small places; to Gladys Bowles of Athens, Georgia, for her statistical insights; to Mark Kozak, M.D., of Baltimore for his recommendations on climate and comfort; to Charles Longino at the University of Miami for his intelligence on college towns and World War II veterans; to Edward Sherman, CPA, of Lynnfield, Massachusetts, for his insights on taxes; to the hundreds of retired persons who've shared with us their own perceptions of places, particularly Donald and Judy Dumont, formerly of Boston and now on a two-year tour of the country in search of their own ideal, and Rex and Elsie Stubblefield of Denver for their appreciation of the Ozarks and Ouachitas, the Pacific Northwest Cloud Belt, and the Rocky Mountains.

We also thank Dr. Thomas F. Bowman, Dr. George Giuliani, and Dr. M. Ronald Minge, for permission to adapt their "Prospering Test" to the subject of retirement relocation.

Finally, special thanks are due Woods & Poole Economics, Inc., of Washington, DC, for their population, employment, and income forecasts for each of the retirement places. The use of this information, and the conclusions drawn from it, are solely the responsibility of the authors.

Contents

Personal Safety: Violent and Property Crime Rates   **79**

Services: Health Care, Public Transportation, and Continuing Education   **97**

Housing: Market Values, Property Taxes, and Utility Bills   **130**

Preface

Readers will note the differences in the final rankings for the 85 places profiled in both the 1983 and 1987 editions. There are four reasons for this.

1. The interval effect. With 107 places in our 1983 edition and 131 places in this edition, the ranks of the 85 places common to both editions will necessarily change. For example, Yuma, in Arizona's south-western corner, has nearly the same personal safety score in this edition as it had in the crime chapter in the previous book, yet its rank for this factor slipped from 86 to 114. Yuma isn't getting more dangerous; it's just that 27 other places with better personal safety ratings have moved it to a lower ranking.

2. Time series data. Local population figures (for deriving per capita access to public golf, for example), prices (for measuring living costs), and personal incomes (for gauging how far Social Security benefits will stretch in a given place) have increased at varying rates since our previous edition was published. For example, Reno's current ranking in "Money Matters" shows a drop since 1983 partly because the Nevada retirement place has seen a rapid increase in average household income during a period when average Social Security benefits remained stable.

3. New scoring elements. For the first time, statistics for public transportation, continuing education, health care costs, and the acreage in state recreation areas are included. These are all significant factors in determining an area's appeal to a wide range of older adults. These additional considerations have influenced changes in the final rankings. For example, part of the reason that Cape Cod's score for Outdoor Assets increased 331 points was that 5,488 state park acres were added to the retirement place's 44,554 national park and wildlife acres.

4. New scoring methods. The scoring methods have been refined and improved in all six chapters.

MONEY MATTERS: The 1987 scoring method adjusts local household income for living costs, then calculates the extent to which U.S. average Social Security benefits can replace that income. Growth figures for income and jobs, though they are included in the Place Profiles, are no longer scoring elements because they may work to the advantage of some older adults and to the disadvantage of others.

CLIMATE: Rather than staying with the previous edition's six steps for determining climatic mildness, this edition adopts a vastly simplified and scientifically more valid method. Any monthly variation from a high of 80 degrees Fahrenheit and a low of 65 is subtracted from an ideal score of 1,000. Bioclimatologists have concluded that an outdoor air temperature of 65 generally marks the point below which people either increase their activity, put on extra clothing, or come indoors. An outdoor air temperature of 80 degrees generally marks the point where a person's body temperature rises. The discomfort felt by most older adults at temperatures above and below these norms reflects the stress put on the body as it attempts to keep its "core temperature" within a comfortable range. While an area's climate has not changed, this simplified scoring method (as well as the interval effect) results in rankings different from those in the previous edition.

PERSONAL SAFETY: Except for averaging crime rates over the last five years rather than the latest single year, the scoring method is identical to that of the 1983 edition. Five-year averages tend to level off "blips" that may occur — particularly in lower population areas — that may not be truly representative.

SERVICES: Though retaining the focus of the 1983 edition's "Health and Health Care" chapter, this chapter is now quite different because it also looks at the local supply of public transportation and continuing-education options at local colleges and universities. Both criteria have been found to be significant to large numbers of older adults.

HOUSING: Except for substituting median market prices for average prices, the scoring method in this edition is identical to that of the 1983 edition. Knowing that half the housing in an area falls above, and half below, a certain figure gives a potential resident a better picture of the likelihood of finding housing within a specific price range. Rank differences are due to varying rates of housing price inflation among regions.

LEISURE LIVING: Information on good restaurants and state park areas has been added. Like other segments of the population, older adults are dining out more often for both pleasure and convenience and participating in recreational activities more frequently.

Information on museums has been dropped from this edition, partly because of the difficulty of classifying museums in a way that is meaningful to older adults without giving too much weight to this single category.

The method of scoring the performing arts has also been changed. Feedback from both specialists and lay readers of the first edition helped to refine the technique in a way that makes this information more helpful to many readers.

As a result of the changes in scoring methods and criteria, the rankings better reflect what each retirement place has to offer older adults, thus making this a more useful and informative publication.

Introduction

"The best place to retire," says Dr. Robert Butler, former head of the National Institute on Aging, "is the neighborhood where you spent your life."

It's hard to disagree with that statement, so many are the reasons for staying put. You certainly have more practical knowledge and influence where you are now than you may ever have in a distant location. You've known your neighbors for years, your doctor knows you, you don't need to look up the movie theater's phone number, ask for the route to a discount hardware store, or spend time finding out the name of the one person in city hall who can get the sewer fixed.

Besides, if the seasons are good and your old friends are alive and healthy, if the neighborhood is safe and recreational opportunities are plentiful now that you've got the time to take advantage of them, relocation may be unthinkable. What you may ultimately want from retirement is R and R in familiar territory, not an agenda that requires high energy and risk just to sink new roots.

But there may be more to staying put than just convenience. The kind of sentiment that comes from launching children into the world, working at a job, and paying off a mortgage in one town may be missed in a new one. When you move, you certainly can take the philodendron, the oak blanket chest, the canoe, and the car, but you can't necessarily pack a deep sense of place.

If all this is true, by all means stay where you are. But perhaps—just perhaps—there is someplace in this country where you might thrive even more than you do now. And perhaps, too, it is a lack of objective information that keeps you from taking a look.

In 1983, the authors published *Places Rated Retirement Guide*, a book that offered objective information about 107 retirement places throughout the country. The response confirmed that people do indeed want reliable, practical information about places. This new edition, *Retirement Places Rated*, takes the same approach as its predecessor but has been thoroughly updated, revised, and expanded.

Like its predecessor, *Retirement Places Rated* is meant for those who are retired or are planning for retirement, and who may be weighing the pluses and minuses of moving or staying. It is a guide that offers a wealth of facts about 131 carefully chosen places, places that together attract a large number of retired persons who make interstate moves.

You won't find these facts in standard guidebooks or puff pieces from highly publicized resort-retirement spots. In what other single source, for instance, can you find where you'll encounter tougher driving examinations because of your age, where hurricanes repeatedly hit, where you might have trouble finding an apartment to rent, a public golf course, or a part-time job?

But *Retirement Places Rated* is more than a collection of odd, interesting, and useful information about places, because it also rates and ranks them on the basis of six factors greatly influencing the quality of retirement life: money matters, climate, services, housing, personal safety, and leisure living.

Retirement Places Rated might be considered a self-help book with a difference. Rather than describing retirement as the prime of one's life or a kind of second career, turning point, or transformation, the book simply gives you the facts you need to start evaluating other locations in this country where you might live. After using the book, your hunch that you've never had it so good might well be confirmed. On the other hand, you may be in for a surprise.

WHERE ARE THESE PLACES?

If you were suddenly asked, in a kind of geographic word-association test, to name seven states that spring to mind when you hear the word *retirement*, you might well say Arizona, California, Florida, New Mexico, North Carolina, South Carolina, and Texas.

You'd be right, of course.

These are key states of the Sun Belt. During the last half of the 1970s, they attracted half of all older adults who packed up and moved to another state. Several of their cities—Phoenix, San Diego, Albuquerque, Fort Myers, Asheville, Charleston, and McAllen—are as synonymous with retirement as any in the country.

But other states outside the Sun Belt also belong in retirement geography. Oregon and Washington draw

RETIREMENT REGIONS

In addition to the 131 retirement places, you'll also find references to 16 *regions* where these places are located. Few of these regions match the political boundaries you'll find in a road atlas; most of them embrace parts of more than one state, and some states are apportioned among more than one region. Southport, South Carolina, for example, is grouped with Fairhope–Gulf Shores, Alabama, and other South Atlantic and Gulf Shore spots because it has more in common with them than with such New Appalachia places as Asheville or the Mid-South area of Chapel Hill.

Big Ten Country
Ann Arbor, MI
Bloomington–Brown County, IN
Iowa City, IA
Madison, WI

Desert Southwest
Lake Havasu City–Kingman, AZ
Las Vegas, NV
Phoenix, AZ
Prescott, AZ
St. George–Zion, UT
Tucson, AZ
Yuma, AZ

Metropolitan South Florida
Bradenton, FL
Daytona Beach, FL
Fort Lauderdale–Hollywood–
   Pompano Beach, FL
Fort Myers–Cape Coral, FL
Lakeland–Winter Haven, FL
Melbourne–Titusville–Palm Bay, FL
Miami–Hialeah, FL
Naples, FL
Ocala, FL
Orlando, FL
St. Petersburg–Clearwater, FL
Sarasota, FL
West Palm Beach–Boca Raton–
   Delray Beach, FL

Mid-Atlantic Metro Belt
Canandaigua, NY
Cape May, NJ
Charlottesville, VA
Columbia County, NY
Easton–Chesapeake Bay, MD
Lancaster, PA
Monticello–Liberty, NY
New Paltz–Ulster County, NY
Ocean City–Assateague Island, MD
Ocean County, NJ
Rehoboth Bay–Indian River Bay, DE
State College, PA
Virginia Beach–Norfolk, VA

Mid-South
Athens, GA
Chapel Hill, NC
Crossville, TN
Franklin County, TN
Lexington, KY
Murray–Kentucky Lake, KY
Paris–Big Sandy, TN

New Appalachia
Asheville, NC
Blacksburg, VA
Clayton–Clarkesville, GA
Front Royal, VA
Gainesville–Lake Lanier, GA
Hendersonville–Brevard, NC
Winchester, VA

North Woods
Door County, WI
Eagle River, WI
Houghton Lake, MI
Oscoda–Huron Shore, MI
Petoskey–Straits of Mackinac, MI
Rhinelander, WI
Traverse City–
   Grand Traverse Bay, MI

Ozarks and Ouachitas
Branson–Cassville–
   Table Rock Lake, MO
Fayetteville, AR
Grand Lake–Lake Tenkiller, OK
Hot Springs–Lake Ouachita, AR
Mountain Home–Bull Shoals, AR
Springfield, MO

Pacific Beaches
Kauai, HI
Maui, HI
Salinas–Seaside–Monterey, CA
San Diego, CA
San Luis Obispo, CA
Santa Rosa–Petaluma, CA

Pacific Northwest Cloud Belt
Bellingham, WA
Bend, OR
Eugene–Springfield, OR
Friday Harbor–San Juan Islands, WA
Medford–Ashland, OR
Newport–Lincoln City, OR
Oak Harbor–Whidbey Island, WA
Olympia, WA
Port Angeles–Strait of
   Juan de Fuca, WA

Rio Grande Country
Albuquerque, NM
Brownsville–Harlingen, TX
Deming, NM
Las Cruces, NM
McAllen–Edinburg–Mission, TX
Roswell, NM
Santa Fe, NM

Rocky Mountains
Boise, ID
Coeur d'Alene, ID
Colorado Springs, CO
Flagstaff, AZ
Fort Collins–Loveland, CO
Grand Junction, CO
Hamilton–Bitterroot Valley, MT
Kalispell, MT
Missoula, MT

South Atlantic and Gulf Coast Shore
Biloxi–Gulfport, MS
Brunswick–Golden Isles, GA
Charleston, SC
Fairhope–Gulf Shores, AL
Fort Walton Beach, FL
Hilton Head–Beaufort, SC
Myrtle Beach, SC
Panama City, FL
Southport, NC

Tahoe Basin and the Other California
Carson City–Minden, NV
Chico–Paradise, CA
Clear Lake, CA
Grass Valley–Truckee, CA
Red Bluff–Sacramento Valley, CA
Redding, CA
Reno, NV
Twain Harte–Yosemite, CA

Texas Interior
Athens–Cedar Creek Lake, TX
Austin, TX
Burnet–Marble Falls–Llano. TX
Canton–Lake Tawakoni, TX
Fredericksburg, TX
Kerrville, TX
San Antonio, TX

Yankee Belt
Amherst–Northampton, MA
Bar Harbor–Frenchman Bay, ME
Bennington, VT
Burlington, VT
Camden–Penobscot Bay, ME
Cape Cod, MA
Hanover, NH
Keene, NH
Laconia–Lake Winnipesaukee, NH
Litchfield County, CT
North Conway–White Mountains, NH
Portsmouth–Dover–Durham, NH

thousands of midwesterners and Californians. The 160-mile stretch of New Jersey's sandy Atlantic coastline from Cape May up to Monmouth owes a good part of its economic rebound to older newcomers who hail from the densely settled Boston–Washington corridor. Maine and New Hampshire attract the retired, too— including a surprising number from California and Florida.

Despite press coverage devoted almost exclusively to the Sun Belt, it's no secret that one or more counties in practically every state have benefited from retirement settlement. There are 515 of these areas, according to a recent U.S. Department of Agriculture report. They are found along country roads within commuting distance of big cities, on the edges of forested federal lands, along rocky coastlines, in river valleys, around lakes, on mountain slopes, and in desert crossroads with striking distant vistas.

Based on the demographic evidence and the advice of experts, and the recommendations of many older adults, *Retirement Places Rated* presents 131 places in 38 states that reflect the preferences of many mobile retired persons. Although these places do not by any means include every desirable retirement destination, they do include many of the country's best, and they represent the kinds of places many people are choosing to retire to.

THE RETIREMENT PLACE-NAMES

The 131 places profiled in this guide aren't towns or cities. For good reason, they are counties.

Thanks to the automobile, the territory we cover every day has expanded tremendously since pre–World War II days when a "shopping center" was the corner store and the term *strip mall* wasn't even in the lexicon. Nowadays we typically live in one town, work in another town, visit friends in still another town, shop at a mall several miles away, and get away to the countryside—all within an easy drive. So when we consider the virtues of living in a particular place, we include not just the town but all the environs to which we have ready access.

It is no different in retirement places. Our definition of Phoenix, for example, takes in the Arizona capital plus Chandler, Scottsdale, Sun City, Tempe, and all other places in suburban Maricopa County including a vast area of open desert where new growth is taking place. A few places in this book embrace more than one county. San Antonio, for example, includes heavily urbanized Bexar County plus two suburban counties, Comal and Guadalupe.

Several counties described in this book have names that make them readily identifiable to most people. Kauai and Maui counties in Hawaii are two such places. Connecticut's Litchfield County is another. Other counties—Santa Fe in New Mexico, Bennington in Vermont, and San Luis Obispo on the southern

FINDING YOUR WAY IN THE CHAPTERS

Each of *Retirement Places Rated*'s first six chapters has five parts:

- **Introduction:** This section gives basic information on the chapter's topic, interspersed with facts and figures to help you evaluate the retirement places. We also include details of the system used to rate and rank the 131 retirement places for that particular concern.
- **Scoring:** This is an explanation of the method used in the chapter to arrive at the point scores for each retirement place. At the end of the section, several places are selected for detailed comparison to show you why one performs better than another in the ratings.
- **Rankings:** This part ranks the 131 retirement places. They are listed first in their rank order, from best to worst, along with their *Retirement Places Rated* score. An alphabetical list of the places follows, with their individual rankings, so that you can quickly find the ranks of specific places.
- **Place Profiles:** Arranged alphabetically by place, these capsule comparisons cover all the elements used to rate the retirement places for that chapter's topic; often the profiles provide additional data. Here you can see differences among the areas at a glance.
- **Et Cetera:** This section expands on topics mentioned in the Introduction and also contains information on related subjects. These encompass anything from state-by-state college tuition breaks for older adults to lists of the worst places for ragweed pollen to essays on such subjects as state tax breaks for older adults and tactics for avoiding property crime.

The final chapter, "Putting It All Together," adds up the ranks to identify America's best all-around retirement places and discusses the strengths and weaknesses of the top 25. We also weigh the pros and cons of city and countryside retirement living and profile the regions where these 131 places are found.

California coast, for example—have the same name as their well-known seats of government. In these instances, it's natural that the retirement place be called by its county name.

But county names aren't part of the common discourse as they were in the 19th century. Washington County, Arkansas, is one of 31 counties honoring the first president of the United States. The name draws a blank to persons from nearby Missouri or Oklahoma (states which have their *own* Washington County), and it may be only dimly familiar to a citizen of Little Rock. Fayetteville, the home of the University of Arkansas and the seat of Washington County, is better recognized by everyone. So in our list of places, you'll find

Population Size

LARGEST RETIREMENT PLACES

	1987 Population
San Diego, CA	2,191,700
Phoenix, AZ	1,877,700
Miami–Hialeah, FL	1,854,000
San Antonio, TX	1,300,200
Fort Lauderdale–Hollywood– Pompano Beach, FL	1,198,400
Orlando, FL	918,800
Virginia Beach–Norfolk, VA	884,400
St. Petersburg–Clearwater, FL	859,300
West Palm Beach–Boca Raton– Delray Beach, FL	794,000
Austin, TX	711,600

SMALLEST RETIREMENT PLACES

	1987 Population
Friday Harbor–San Juan Islands, WA	9,800
Deming, NM	15,700
Fredericksburg, TX	16,000
Eagle River, WI	17,000
Houghton Lake, MI	20,500
Front Royal, VA	23,000
Petoskey–Straits of Mackinac, MI	24,300
Hamilton–Bitterroot Valley, MT	25,900
Door County, WI	27,900
Oscoda–Huron Shore, MI	28,000

Source: Woods & Poole Economics, Inc., population forecasts.

that Fayetteville is the name given to the retirement place, although it actually includes all of Washington County, Arkansas.

A similar case is Barnstable County, Massachusetts, which embraces all of Cape Cod from Buzzards Bay out old U.S. 6 on the famous sandy spit of land to Provincetown. Long ago, the term Cape Cod elbowed Barnstable County aside in popular New England usage. Accordingly, Cape Cod is our name for the retirement place in Barnstable County.

Sometimes the name given a retirement place is that of the one or two biggest populations centers; thus New Mexico's Luna County becomes Deming, and Arizona's Mohave County becomes Lake Havasu City –Kingman. In other instances, the name of a town may be paired with a well-known natural feature: Hamilton –Bitterroot Valley is our name for Ravalli County,

The Last Move?

Most people move 11 times in their lifetime. The common reasons are job changes or job transfers, shifts out of rental housing into homeownership and moves up to larger homes. Is retirement yet another reason to move? For most people, not at all.

Each year, fewer than one-quarter million persons over 65 pack up and relocate to another state. Another million simply move out of a big house into smaller housing within the same city. Consider your own options. You might:

- Stay at your present address. Nine out of ten older adults do, according to the latest census statistics on geographic mobility.
- Stay close to town but sell or rent your home and move to another address, perhaps an apartment, condominium, or smaller home. One in 30 older adults takes this route.
- Move out of town to another part of the state—to occupy a vacation home year-round, perhaps. Just one in every 86 older adults does this.
- Move to another state. For every 123 older adults, only 1 of them takes this course.

In retirement, hometown turf clearly wins out over the distant Eden. Even if you aren't thrilled with your present environment, you still have to decide whether moving is the key to future happiness. A University of Miami study of where older adults moved during the late 1970s showed the surprising number of adults who moved to another state and subsequently either moved to still another state or returned home within a decade.

It's axiomatic that "destination pull" must be much stronger than "origin push" for relocation to succeed. The whole process involves time, energy, money, and risk; it shouldn't be attempted without careful planning and investigation.

Montana; likewise, New Hampshire's Carroll County becomes North Conway–White Mountains.

The list that follows provides the county definitions of the retirement places as they are used throughout this edition of *Retirement Places Rated*.

The Places We Rate: 131 Retirement Places

Retirement Places and Component Counties	1980 Population	1987 Population	Growth, 1980–1987
Albuquerque, NM Bernalillo County	419,700	486,200	15.84%
Amherst–Northampton, MA Hampshire County	138,813	139,900	0.78
Ann Arbor, MI Washtenaw County	264,748	272,000	2.74
Asheville, NC Buncombe County	160,934	168,100	4.45

Retirement Places and Component Counties	1980 Population	1987 Population	Growth, 1980–1987
Athens, GA Clarke County	74,498	76,800	3.09
Athens–Cedar Creek Lake, TX Henderson County	42,606	52,900	24.16
Austin, TX Hays, Travis, and Williamson counties	536,688	711,600	32.59

Retirement Places and Component Counties	1980 Population	1987 Population	Growth, 1980–1987
Bar Harbor–Frenchman Bay, ME Hancock County	41,781	45,000	7.70
Bellingham, WA Whatcom County	106,701	116,700	9.37
Bend, OR Deschutes County	62,142	70,600	13.61
Bennington, VT Bennington County	33,345	35,600	6.76
Biloxi–Gulfport, MS Hancock and Harrison counties	182,202	204,200	12.07
Blacksburg, VA Montgomery County	63,284	71,100	12.35
Bloomington–Brown County, IN Brown and Monroe counties	111,162	120,200	8.13
Boise, ID Ada County	173,036	198,400	14.66
Bradenton, FL Manatee County	148,442	178,100	19.98
Branson–Cassville–Table Rock Lake, MO Barry, Stone and Taney counties	60,462	70,900	17.26
Brownsville–Harlingen, TX Cameron County	209,727	260,000	23.97
Brunswick–Golden Isles, GA Glynn County	54,981	59,900	8.95
Burlington, VT Chittenden and Grand Isle counties	120,147	136,300	13.44

Population Growth

FASTEST-GROWING RETIREMENT PLACES	Population Increase 1980–1987
Ocala, FL	49%
St. George–Zion, UT	42
Grass Valley–Truckee, CA	39
Naples, FL	39
West Palm Beach–Boca Raton–Delray Beach, FL	39
Fort Myers–Cape Coral, FL	38
Kerrville, TX	35
Lake Havasu City–Kingman, AZ	35
Prescott, AZ	35
Yuma, AZ	34

SLOWEST-GROWING RETIREMENT PLACES	Population Increase 1980–1987
Eugene–Springfield, OR	– 1%
Monticello–Liberty, NY	– 1
Oscoda–Huron Shore, MI	– 1
Amherst–Northampton, MA	1
Columbia County, NY	1
Deming, NM	1
Grand Junction, CO	1
Missoula, MT	2
Murray–Kentucky Lake, KY	2
Ann Arbor, MI	3

Source: Woods & Poole Economics, Inc., population forecasts.

The nation's population increased 8 percent between 1980 and 1987; among the 131 retirement places, population grew 18 percent.

Retirement Places and Component Counties	1980 Population	1987 Population	Growth, 1980–1987
Burnet–Marble Falls–Llano, TX Burnet and Llano counties	27,947	36,300	29.89
Camden–Penobscot Bay, ME Knox County	32,941	35,100	6.55
Canandaigua, NY Ontario County	88,909	95,100	6.96
Canton–Lake Tawakoni, TX Van Zandt County	31,426	36,900	17.42
Cape Cod, MA Barnstable County	147,925	171,000	15.60
Cape May, NJ Cape May County	82,266	88,300	7.33
Carson City–Minden, NV Carson City and Douglas county	51,443	62,500	21.49
Chapel Hill, NC Orange County	77,055	85,700	11.22
Charleston, SC Charleston County	276,974	302,400	9.18
Charlottesville, VA Charlottesville city; Albemarle, Fluvanna, and Greene counties	113,568	125,000	10.07
Chico–Paradise, CA Butte County	143,851	166,800	15.95
Clayton–Clarkesville, GA Habersham and Rabun counties	35,486	38,200	7.65
Clear Lake, CA Lake County	36,366	48,500	33.37
Coeur d'Alene, ID Kootenai County	59,770	70,800	18.45
Colorado Springs, CO El Paso County	309,424	368,700	19.16
Columbia County, NY Columbia County	59,487	60,200	1.20
Crossville, TN Cumberland County	28,676	31,900	11.24
Daytona Beach, FL Volusia County	258,762	303,600	17.33
Deming, NM Luna County	15,585	15,700	0.74
Door County, WI Door County	25,029	27,900	11.47
Eagle River, WI Vilas County	16,535	17,000	2.81
Easton–Chesapeake Bay, MD Talbot County	25,604	28,900	12.87
Eugene–Springfield, OR Lane County	275,266	271,500	– 1.37
Fairhope–Gulf Shores, AL Baldwin County	78,556	92,200	17.37
Fayetteville, AR Washington County	100,494	107,000	6.47
Flagstaff, AZ Coconino County	75,008	87,900	17.19
Fort Collins–Loveland, CO Larimer County	149,184	182,500	22.33

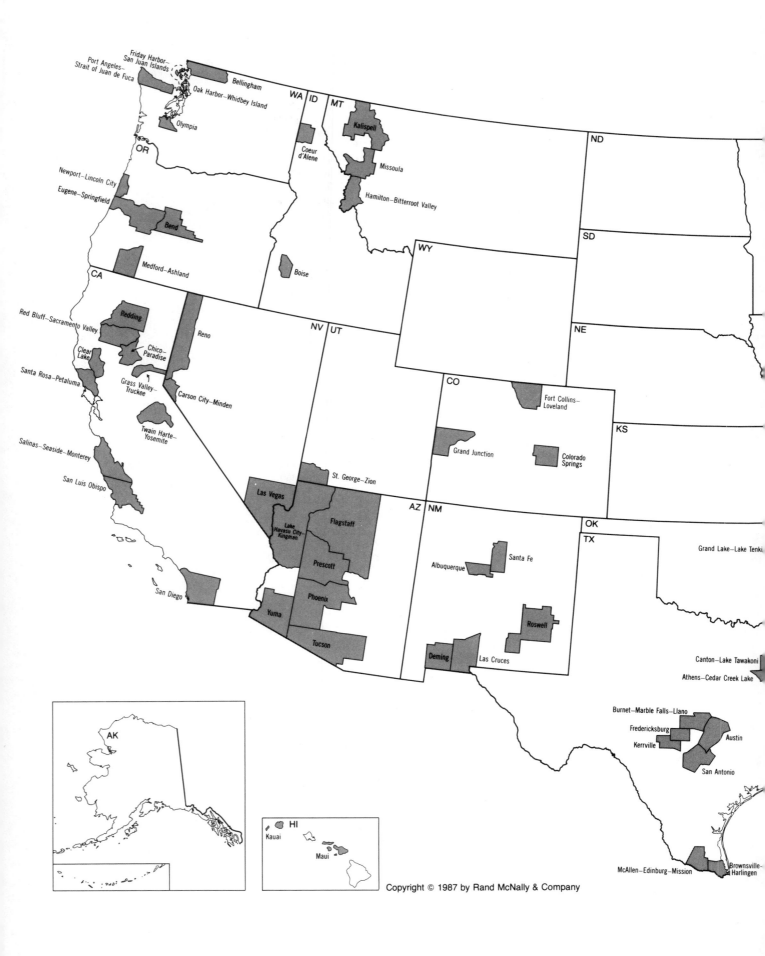

Friday Harbor–
San Juan Islands
Port Angeles–
Strait of Juan de Fuca
Bellingham
Oak Harbor–Whidbey Island
Olympia

WA | ID | MT

Coeur
d'Alene

Kalispell

Missoula

Hamilton–Bitterroot Valley

ND

SD

OR

Newport–Lincoln City
Eugene–Springfield
Bend
Medford–Ashland

Boise

WY

NV | UT

CA

Red Bluff–Sacramento Valley
Redding
Clear
Lake
Santa Rosa–Petaluma
Chico–
Paradise
Grass Valley–
Truckee
Reno
Carson City–Minden
Twain Harte–
Yosemite
Salinas–Seaside–Monterey
San Luis Obispo

NE

CO

Fort Collins–
Loveland

KS

Grand Junction

Colorado
Springs

St. George–Zion

Las Vegas
Lake
Havasu City–
Kingman
Flagstaff

AZ | NM

Prescott

Phoenix

Yuma
San Diego

Tucson

Deming

Las Cruces

Albuquerque

Santa Fe

Roswell

OK

Grand Lake–Lake Tenki

TX

Canton–Lake Tawakoni
Athens–Cedar Creek Lake

Burnet–Marble Falls–Llano
Fredericksburg
Kerrville
Austin
San Antonio

AK

HI
Kauai
Maui

McAllen–Edinburg–Mission
Brownsville–
Harlingen

Copyright © 1987 by Rand McNally & Company

Retirement Places

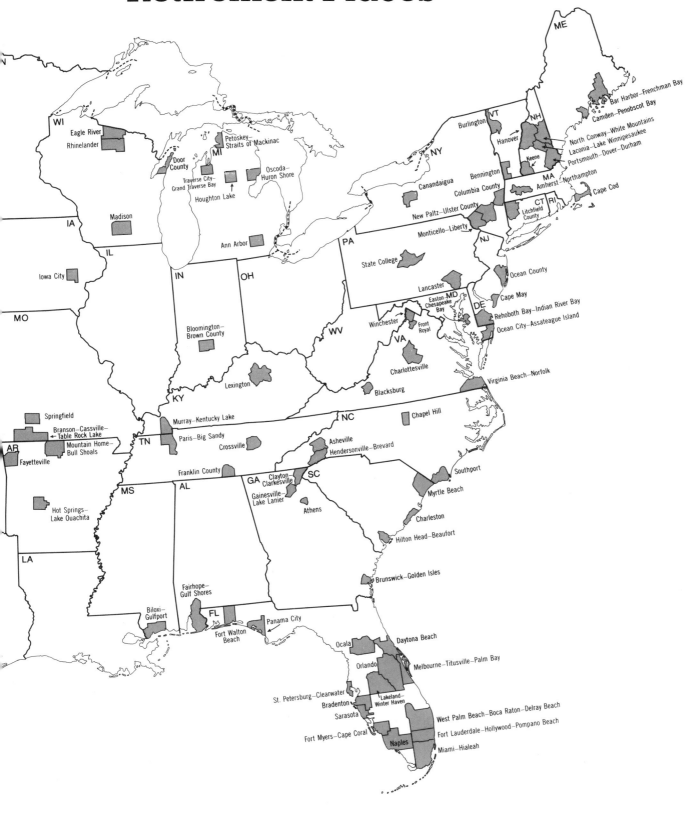

Retirement Places and Component Counties	1980 Population	1987 Population	Growth, 1980–1987
Fort Lauderdale–Hollywood–Pompano Beach, FL Broward County	1,014,043	1,198,400	18.18
Fort Myers–Cape Coral, FL Lee County	205,266	283,900	38.31
Fort Walton Beach, FL Okaloosa County	109,920	134,600	22.45
Franklin County, TN Franklin County	31,983	33,000	3.18
Fredericksburg, TX Gillespie County	13,532	16,000	18.24
Friday Harbor–San Juan Islands, WA San Juan County	7,838	9,800	25.03
Front Royal, VA Warren County	21,200	23,000	8.49
Gainesville–Lake Lanier, GA Hall County	75,649	81,000	7.07
Grand Junction, CO Mesa County	102,755	104,100	1.31
Grand Lake–Lake Tenkiller, OK Cherokee and Delaware counties	54,630	63,300	15.87
Grass Valley–Truckee, CA Nevada County	51,645	71,800	39.03
Hamilton–Bitterroot Valley, MT Ravalli County	22,493	25,900	15.15
Hanover, NH Grafton County	65,806	70,900	7.74
Hendersonville–Brevard, NC Henderson and Transylvania counties	81,997	94,000	14.64
Hilton Head–Beaufort, SC Beaufort County	65,364	81,300	24.38
Hot Springs–Lake Ouachita, AR Garland County	69,916	78,000	11.56
Houghton Lake, MI Roscommon County	16,374	20,500	25.20
Iowa City, IA Johnson County	81,717	86,600	5.98
Kalispell, MT Flathead County	51,966	56,000	7.76
Kauai, HI Kauai County	39,082	45,900	17.45
Keene, NH Cheshire County	62,116	66,000	6.25
Kerrville, TX Kerr County	28,780	38,900	35.16
Laconia–Lake Winnipesaukee, NH Belknap County	42,884	45,800	6.80
Lake Havasu City–Kingman, AZ Mohave County	55,693	75,400	35.39
Lakeland–Winter Haven, FL Polk County	321,652	358,100	11.33

Retirement Places and Component Counties	1980 Population	1987 Population	Growth, 1980–1987
Lancaster, PA Lancaster County	362,346	387,600	6.97
Las Cruces, NM Dona Ana County	96,340	106,200	10.23
Las Vegas, NV Clark County	461,816	593,700	28.56
Lexington, KY Bourbon, Clark, Fayette, Jessamine, Scott, and Woodford counties	317,629	342,200	7.74
Litchfield County, CT Litchfield County	156,769	165,000	5.25
Madison, WI Dane County	323,545	353,600	9.29
Maui, HI Maui and Kalawao counties	70,847	94,200	32.96
McAllen–Edinburg–Mission, TX Hidalgo County	283,229	359,900	27.07
Medford–Ashland, OR Jackson County	132,456	141,300	6.68
Melbourne–Titusville–Palm Bay, FL Brevard County	272,959	319,300	16.98
Miami–Hialeah, FL Dade County	1,625,979	1,854,000	14.02
Missoula, MT Missoula County	76,016	77,300	1.69
Monticello–Liberty, NY Sullivan County	65,155	64,500	−1.01
Mountain Home–Bull Shoals, AR Baxter and Marion counties	38,743	45,300	16.92
Murray–Kentucky Lake, KY Calloway and Marshall counties	55,668	57,000	2.39
Myrtle Beach, SC Horry County	101,419	126,100	24.34
Naples, FL Collier County	85,971	119,400	38.88
New Paltz–Ulster County, NY Ulster County	158,158	167,400	5.84
Newport–Lincoln City, OR Lincoln County	35,264	39,600	12.30
North Conway–White Mountains, NH Carroll County	27,931	32,200	15.28
Oak Harbor–Whidbey Island, WA Island County	44,048	46,800	6.25
Ocala, FL Marion County	122,488	183,000	49.40
Ocean City–Assateague Island, MD Worcester County	30,889	34,600	12.01
Ocean County, NJ Ocean County	346,038	379,300	9.61
Olympia, WA Thurston County	124,264	153,900	23.85
Orlando, FL Orange, Osceola, and Seminole counties	700,699	918,800	31.13

Retirement Places and Component Counties	1980 Population	1987 Population	Growth, 1980–1987
Oscoda–Huron Shore, MI Iosco County	28,349	28,000	−1.23
Panama City, FL Bay County	97,740	110,600	13.16
Paris–Big Sandy, TN Benton and Henry counties	43,557	45,800	5.15
Petoskey–Straits of Mackinac, MI Emmet County	22,992	24,300	5.69
Phoenix, AZ Maricopa County	1,508,030	1,877,700	24.51
Port Angeles–Strait of Juan de Fuca, WA Clallam County	51,648	53,300	3.20
Portsmouth–Dover– Durham, NH Rockingham and Strafford counties	275,753	325,900	18.19
Prescott, AZ Yavapai County	68,145	91,800	34.71
Red Bluff–Sacramento Valley, CA Tehama County	38,888	45,800	17.77
Redding, CA Shasta County	115,715	138,000	19.26
Rehoboth Bay–Indian River Bay, DE Sussex County	98,004	109,600	11.83
Reno, NV Washoe County	193,623	235,300	21.52
Rhinelander, WI Oneida County	31,216	32,600	4.43
Roswell, NM Chaves County	51,103	61,500	20.35
St. George–Zion, UT Washington County	26,065	37,100	42.34
St. Petersburg– Clearwater, FL Pinellas County	728,531	859,300	17.95
Salinas–Seaside– Monterey, CA Monterey County	290,444	319,700	10.07

Retirement Places and Component Counties	1980 Population	1987 Population	Growth, 1980–1987
San Antonio, TX Bexar, Comal, and Guadalupe counties	1,071,954	1,300,200	21.29
San Diego, CA San Diego County	1,861,846	2,191,700	17.72
San Luis Obispo, CA San Luis Obispo County	155,345	196,500	26.49
Santa Fe, NM Santa Fe County	75,306	96,500	28.14
Santa Rosa–Petaluma, CA Sonoma County	299,681	359,500	19.96
Sarasota, FL Sarasota County	202,251	257,800	27.47
Southport, NC Brunswick County	35,777	47,200	31.93
Springfield, MO Greene County	185,302	201,300	8.63
State College, PA Centre County	112,760	120,100	6.51
Traverse City– Grand Traverse Bay, MI Grand Traverse County	54,899	59,300	8.02
Tucson, AZ Pima County	531,263	630,700	18.72
Twain Harte–Yosemite, CA Tuolumne County	33,920	42,600	25.59
Virginia Beach–Norfolk, VA Chesapeake, Norfolk, Portsmouth, Suffolk, and Virginia Beach cities	795,862	884,400	11.12
West Palm Beach– Boca Raton–Delray Beach, FL Palm Beach County	573,125	794,000	38.54
Winchester, VA Winchester city and Frederick County	54,367	60,100	10.54
Yuma, AZ Yuma County	77,997	104,700	34.24

Source: U.S. Bureau of the Census, *1980 Census of Population,* and Woods & Poole Economics, Inc., population forecasts.

Decisions, Decisions

There are three basic viewpoints when it comes to rating quality of life in different places. The first says that you can't do it with total fairness, so don't do it at all. The second says you can but you shouldn't because ratings make places unwilling competitors of one another and often lead to wrong conclusions. The third says you can, as long as you make clear what your statistical yardsticks are and go on to use them consistently.

Although the first and second theories may be valid, *Retirement Places Rated* subscribes to the third.

RATING PLACES: A CONTINUING AMERICAN TRADITION

It may seem the height of effrontery to judge places with statistics. Yet *numeracy* is almost as strong a national character trait as *literacy* is. When it comes to choosing where to live, we've been using numbers for a long, long time.

To entice settlers to pick Maryland over Virginia, 17th-century promoters assembled figures showing heavier turkeys, more plentiful deer, and fewer deaths from foul summer diseases and Indian massacres, all yours if you settled in the northern reaches of Chesapeake Bay. *California for Health, Wealth, and Residence,* just one volume in a library of post–Civil War guides touting the West's superior quality of life, compiled data to show the climate along the southern Pacific coast to be the best in the world.

In our own century, the statistical nets were flung even wider. "There are plenty of Americans who regard Kansas as almost barbaric," noted H. L. Mencken back in 1931, "just as there are other Americans who shudder whenever they think of Arkansas, Ohio, Indiana, Oklahoma, Texas, or California." Mencken wrote these words in his *American Mercury* magazine to introduce his formula for statistically measuring the progress of civilization in each of the states. He mixed the numbers of Boy Scouts and *Atlantic Monthly* subscribers with those of lynching targets and pellagra victims, added a dash of *Who's Who* listings along with rates for divorce and murder, threw in figures for rainfall and gasoline consumption, and found that,

hands down, Mississippi was the worst American state. Few were surprised by this finding, since Mencken didn't like the rural South anyway. Massachusetts, a state he admired, came out best.

But the Bay State got a demotion of sorts in 1978, when it was rated the worst state for retirement by the consulting firm of Chase Econometrics. And the best state for retirement according to the Chase forecasters? Utah.

Rating Retirement Places: One Way

Retirement Places Rated, we believe, is more useful than any system that just looks at each state as a whole. Statewide averages hide local realities. For some persons, there may be a world of difference between Las Cruces and Santa Fe in New Mexico, and these differences may be more important in retirement than the differences between California and Florida.

Certainly this book is more objective than the hearsay opinions that travelers may share at a rest stop on the interstate highway. Each of the 131 places is

---

This Edition's Special Features

These features make it easier for you to do your own independent research on places, rate the places in this book by your own standards, and locate cities and towns within them.

Preference Inventory. Given the infinite range of human needs and concerns, each of the 131 places featured in this book can be regarded as best under certain conditions. To find *your* best place, a simple assessment in the "Decisions, Decisions" section following this introduction helps you identify what your needs and concerns might be.

Relocation Resources. Doing your own research on retirement places can be enlightening. Each chapter has a "Relocation Resources" box detailing published sources, addresses, and telephone contacts the authors have found useful for obtaining basic, objective information at long distance.

rated by six factors that most persons planning for retirement deem highly important.

- **Money Matters** looks at the cost of living, the part-time job market, and the outlook for job and income growth in each place between now and 1995.
- **Climate** is rated on mildness; that is, where outdoor temperatures remain closest to a low of 65 degrees Fahrenheit and a high of 80 degrees throughout the year.
- **Personal Safety** is measured by the annual number of local violent and property crimes per 100,000 people in each of the retirement places.
- **Services** are evaluated on the relative supply of health care, public transportation, and continuing-education amenities in each place.
- **Housing** is rated simply on how much it costs. We look at local market values, property taxes, and utility bills, and we note the availability of single homes, condominiums, and mobile homes. We also consider the rental option, since one out of five retired persons who move between states starts out renting in his or her destination.
- **Leisure Living** compares recreational and cultural assets such as golf courses, libraries, orchestras and opera companies, and lakes and national parks.

Some readers may fault *Retirement Places Rated*'s choice of criteria. Admittedly, our measurements for health care, public transportation, continuing education, and the performing arts favor big places over small ones. On the other hand, our methods for rating personal safety and costs of living favor small places over big ones. Our standards for warm, occasionally hot climates and outdoor recreation assets are certainly not everyone's. But they have nothing to do with population size.

We have tried to gather the most up-to-date data for all 131 retirement places. In most instances, the information is current as of late 1986. Our sources, which we document throughout this book, come from federal and state agencies and a variety of private organizations.

Retirement Places Rated is a snapshot of a moving target; retirement places are dynamic and won't always sit still for their statistical portraits. An oil spill on the Gulf Coast can ruin a Texas barrier island's stretch of beach for years to come, just as a few hurricanes may later multiply a Florida condo's hazard-insurance payments beyond belief. With so much in life that is unpredictable, it's necessary to supplement *Retirement Places Rated* with your own independent verification.

Rating Retirement Places: Your Way

At the end of this book, in "Putting It All Together,"

RELOCATION RESOURCES

There are two basic impressions about places you can form at long distance: how they present themselves to the outside world, and what's important every day of the year to persons who actually live in these places.

Writing to chambers of commerce for their "newcomer's pack" produces a collection of promotional brochures, maps, business statistics, cost-of-living information, and events calendars. The annual *World Wide Chamber of Commerce Directory* lists the chamber of commerce name, address, and telephone number, plus the name of the chamber's executive or other contact person, population of the area served, and the names of members for over 4,000 locations in the United States. It is available in libraries, or order it for $18.25 (price includes handling and shipping) from

> World Wide Chamber of Commerce Directory
> P.O. Box 1029
> Loveland, CO 80539
> (303) 663-3231

An invaluable supplement to the chamber's picture is a short-term subscription to the local newspaper. After reading a month's worth, you can get an excellent idea of consumer prices, political issues, and other matters on the minds of residents. For the name, address, telephone number, monthly price, special features, and politics (typically independent) of each of the country's 1,651 daily newspapers, the best source is Editor & Publisher's *International Yearbook*. For similar information on 6,857 weekly newspapers (often the only publication in small places), the *IMS Directory of Publications* is the best source.

---

money matters, climate, personal safety, services, housing, and leisure living are given equal weight to identify the best all-around retirement places.

You may not agree with this scoring system. You may give more weight to personal safety than to good fishing spots. For you, a place where fixed incomes go further might be more important than an abundance of physicians, an ocean coastline, or a busy performing arts calendar. To identify which factors are more important and which factors are less, you might want to take stock of your preferences.

YOUR PREFERENCE INVENTORY

The following Preference Inventory has 45 pairs of statements. For each pair, decide which statement is more important to you when judging a place for retirement. Even if both statements are equally important or neither is important, select one anyway. If you can't decide quickly, pass up the item but return to it after you complete the rest of the inventory.

Don't worry about being consistent. The paired statements aren't repeated. There are no right or wrong answers, only those that are best for you. There is no time limit, although the inventory takes about 15 minutes to finish. Before you start, you might want to photocopy the inventory and ask your spouse or a friend to take it independently. Comparing your preference inventory with another person's can be a very interesting exercise.

Directions

For each item, decide which of two statements is more important to you when choosing a retirement place. Mark the box next to that statement. Be sure to make a choice for all items.

1. A. ☐ The local cost of living,
   or
   B. ☐ How cold the winters are.

2. C. ☐ The local supply of public transportation,
   or
   D. ☐ The median sales price of housing.

3. E. ☐ The local rates for burglary and robbery,
   or
   F. ☐ Performing arts bookings at local civic auditoriums.

4. A. ☐ Local taxes and health care costs,
   or
   C. ☐ Opportunities for taking courses at a local college.

5. B. ☐ Seasonal temperature variation,
   or
   D. ☐ Typical costs for owning a home.

6. C. ☐ Accredited short-term, acute care hospitals,
   or
   E. ☐ The number of burglaries and thefts in an area.

7. D. ☐ The cost of natural gas and electricity for the home,
   or
   F. ☐ Golf, movies, bowling, libraries, and good restaurants.

8. B. ☐ The number of months when the thermometer drops below 32 degrees Fahrenheit,
   or
   C. ☐ The number of family practitioners and medical specialists.

9. E. ☐ The local murder, rape, and robbery rates,
   or
   B. ☐ How hot the summer months are.

10. E. ☐ The annual property crime rate,
    or
    A. ☐ The cost of health care in an area.

11. C. ☐ Continuing-education opportunities,
    or
    F. ☐ Local performing arts bookings.

12. A. ☐ How far Social Security benefits will stretch in an area,
    or
    D. ☐ Local market values of housing.

13. F. ☐ Public golf holes and tenpin bowling lanes per capita,
    or
    A. ☐ Local household incomes.

14. D. ☐ The annual cost of home utilities,
    or
    E. ☐ The annual violent crime rate in an area.

15. F. ☐ Nearby national parks, forests, and wildlife refuges,
    or
    B. ☐ The average monthly temperature ranges throughout the year.

16. B. ☐ Mild daily temperatures year-round,
    or
    A. ☐ The bite state taxes take from household income.

17. D. ☐ Taxes on residential property,
    or
    C. ☐ Physicians and accredited hospitals in an area.

18. F. ☐ Ocean coastlines and inland lakes,
    or
    E. ☐ The raw odds of encountering violent crime.

19. C. ☐ Academic programs at local colleges and universities,
    or
    A. ☐ Where the living is inexpensive.

20. D. ☐ Property taxes on homes in an area,
    or
    B. ☐ A stable pattern of warm days and cool nights all year.

21. E. ☐ Local homicides, burglaries, and holdups,
    or
    C. ☐ Accredited hospitals, public transit, and colleges in an area.

22. F. ☐ Symphony orchestras and opera companies,
    or
    D. ☐ Annual mortgage costs, property taxes, and utility bills.

23. C. ☐ The number of buses and the length of their routes,
    or
    B. ☐ Where the winter months are mild.

24. B. ☐ Seasonal temperature variation,
    or
    E. ☐ The raw odds of being a victim of property crime.

25. A. ☐ Low state and local taxes,
    or
    E. ☐ Violent and property crime rates throughout the year.

26. F. ☐ Opportunities for camping, fishing, and hiking,
    or
    C. ☐ Public transportation alternatives to driving a car.

27. D. ☐ The local market values of housing,
    or
    A. ☐ Places where fixed incomes go further.

28. A. ☐ Tax bites and health care costs in an area,
    or
    F. ☐ Local symphony and opera seasons.

29. E. ☐ The local auto thefts and burglaries,
    or
    D. ☐ The average property taxes in an area.

30. B. ☐ The number of months when the thermometer exceeds 80 degrees Fahrenheit,
    or
    F. ☐ Public golf courses, good restaurants, and movie theaters.

31. A. ☐ The local cost-of-living index,
    or
    B. ☐ The duration of the winter.

32. D. ☐ Local property taxes as a percentage of housing values in an area,
    or
    C. ☐ The supply of doctors and accredited hospitals.

33. F. ☐ The area's fine arts calendar,
    or
    E. ☐ How free an area is from criminal activity.

34. C. ☐ Accessibility of public transportation,
    or
    A. ☐ Where physician fees are low.

35. D. ☐ Home heating and air conditioning costs in an area,
    or
    B. ☐ Mild summers.

36. E. ☐ Auto thefts, robberies, and burglaries in an area,
    or
    C. ☐ Short-term, acute-care hospitals and medical specialists.

37. F. ☐ Libraries, good restaurants, and movie theaters,
    or
    D. ☐ The local median sales price of homes.

38. C. ☐ Local public colleges and universities in an area,
    or
    B. ☐ Pleasant springs and autumns.

39. E. ☐ The amount of criminal activity in an area,
    or
    B. ☐ Annual temperature extremes.

40. E. ☐ The local crime rate,
    or
    A. ☐ Where a fixed income will stretch further.

41. F. ☐ Opportunities for boating, fishing, and swimming,
    or
    C. ☐ Health care and public transportation services.

42. D. ☐ Housing affordability,
    or
    A. ☐ Local household incomes adjusted for living costs.

43. F. ☐ The local performing arts calendar,
    or
    A. ☐ Taxes and other costs of living in an area.

44. E. ☐ The chances of being mugged,
    or
    D. ☐ Typical costs for owning a home.

45. F. ☐ Access to the great outdoors,
    or
    B. ☐ The months when the thermometer tops 90 degrees Fahrenheit.

Source: Adapted from "The Prospering Test," courtesy Thomas F. Bowman, Ph.D; George Giuliani, Ph.D; and M. Ronald Minge, Ph.D.

Plotting Your Preference Profile

It is important that you make a choice for each of the 45 items. Have you left any unchecked? If not, you're ready to draw your Preference Profile.

First Step. Count all the marks you've made in the boxes next to the letter A. Then enter the number of "A" statements at the top of your Preference Profile. In the same way, count the number of "B" statements, "C" statements, "D" statements, and "E" statements. Enter their totals in their respective places at the top of your Preference Profile.

Second Step. Now plot your totals on the blank chart. Place a dot on the appropriate line for each of the numbers and connect the dots to form a line graph of your results. A sample Preference Profile is provided.

Analyzing Your Preference Profile

Each of the factors in your Preference Profile—money matters, climate, personal safety, services, housing, and leisure living—is not only a major retirement concern, it also has a special chapter in this book. The purpose of the Preference Inventory is to help you determine the relative importance of each of the chapters to you personally.

If your scores are high for one or two of these

factors, you may want to give extra attention to the chapters devoted to them. Likewise, if your scores are low for any of the six, you may not need to give as much consideration to them as you would the ones with high scores. Bear in mind that the inventory *orders* your preferences in a hierarchy, that each of the factors has some importance for you, and that none should be completely ignored.

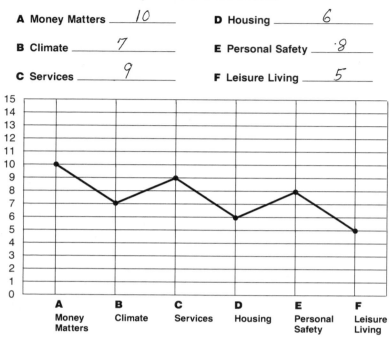

Sample Preference Profile

A Money Matters _____10_____   **D** Housing _____6_____

B Climate _____7_____   **E** Personal Safety _____·8_____

C Services _____9_____   **F** Leisure Living _____5_____

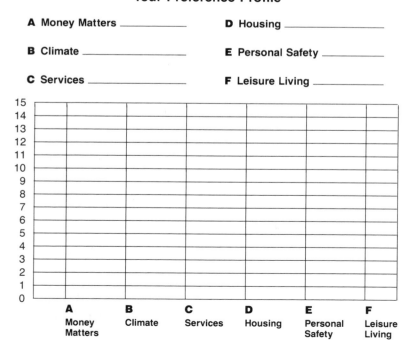

Your Preference Profile

A Money Matters _____   **D** Housing _____

B Climate _____   **E** Personal Safety _____

C Services _____   **F** Leisure Living _____

Money Matters:

Costs of Living, Jobs, and Future Growth

INTRODUCTION: Money Matters

In the dispassionate view of classical economics, we humans are living resources constantly relocating to wherever our cash value is highest.

This certainly can't mean everyone, however. When a younger person quits one state for another, and he or she isn't simply returning home, the odds are good that the person is tracking down a better job or being transferred by an employer. But retired adults just may not have the same motivations.

A few years ago, demographers at the University of Wisconsin wondered just what it was that caused retired people to move from one state to another. After looking at migration patterns between 1950 and 1980, the researchers decided that the mobile retired, less vulnerable to the ups and downs of business cycles than their sons and daughters, passed up boomtowns for places that offered lifestyle.

So what else is new? Because of the windowed envelopes that regularly show up in the mailbox—interest, dividends, annuities, pensions, and Social Security checks—you aren't necessarily rooted in the place where you've lived and worked for so many years. The best economic reason you'll ever need for leaving your hometown is the chance for enjoying a dramatically lower cost of living someplace else during the final quarter of your life.

If you choose the right place, it can make the difference between thriving comfortably or existing precariously, between paying high taxes or paying no taxes at all, and between landing a part-time job or getting used to the idea of never working again even if you want to.

MONEY IN RETIREMENT: GETTING IT

"Money's no problem," any accountant will tell you.

"Lack of money . . . now *that's* a problem." Can you afford to retire? More to the point, can you swing retirement where you're living now—or might there be somewhere else where you can do it more easily?

Lack of enough money to retire on causes many people to cling to unsatisfactory jobs. For those of you who do retire, it crimps plans for travel or for year-round living in a warm, sunny, clean-air place where the bass fishing is good. It indefinitely defers the dream of a small part-time business or the book you've been meaning to write. And it works hardships on your family.

A simple approach for deciding whether you can stop working and settle in another part of the country is to (1) look at how your own circumstances stack up against typical persons who've retired recently and (2) weigh your own income and spending habits against typical incomes and living costs in other places.

For older adults, there isn't just one source of income but many. Apart from Social Security, there is a multitude of annuities, Individual Retirement Accounts (IRAs) and Keogh Plans, some 6,000 government-employee plans (federal civil service, military, state, and municipal) and one-half million private pension plans, each of which has different rules for age of eligibility, years of service required, amounts to be paid, and how spouses are covered.

For a typical husband and wife just embarking on retirement, the main income sources—ranked in descending dollar amounts—are Social Security benefits, earnings from a job or self-employment, private pensions, and asset income.

Social Security

Social Security is money paid out by the federal government at the end of each month to retired

Where the Money Comes From		
Of every 100 newly retired couples in the United States . . .	**receive a median income of . . .**	**annually from . . .**
84	$2,160	Interest, dividends, rents, and royalties
50	$10,056	Social Security, when both spouses are eligible
47	$6,048	Social Security, when just the husband is eligible
46	$5,652	Husband's private pension
17	$5,016	Earnings, when only the husband works
17	$7,992	Earnings, when only the wife works
10	$12,648	Earnings, when both work
7	$9,084	Private pensions for both spouses
3	$2,568	Wife's private pension
1	$3,648	Social Security, when just the wife is eligible

Source: Social Security Bulletin, January, 1985.

Preretirement and Postretirement Income Equivalents

A standard rule knocking about in folk wisdom is the one which states: "If your retirement income is 66 to 75 percent of what it was when you were working, you'll never notice a change in your standard of living." Actually, higher-income people need a lower percentage because their preretirement income was dramatically reduced by the federal income tax bite. Here are the most recent estimates:*

To keep your preretirement standard of living,		
you'll need roughly . . .	**or . . .**	**of a gross preretirement income of . . .**
$5,590	86%	$6,500
$7,800	78%	$10,000
$10,650	71%	$15,000
$13,200	66%	$20,000
$18,000	60%	$30,000
$27,500	55%	$50,000

Source: Preston C. Bassett, consulting actuary, White House Conference on Aging.

*Figures do not reflect the impact, if any, that the 1986 Tax Reform Law will have on these income equivalents.

workers who paid into the system during their working years. The amount is based on a worker's earning record and bears a mathematical relationship to the dollars made over many years. By the current formula, single workers who earned minimum wages before retiring will collect Social Security checks amounting to slightly more than half what they were making just before retirement, while those at the maximum wage level will receive less than one third. In 1986, the maximum monthly benefit was $739 for a single worker, $1,108 for a couple with one dependent spouse, and $1,478 for a couple when both spouses were eligible. The average amount mailed each month to a retired couple was $698, or $8,376 a year.

Earnings

Once you start collecting Social Security and private pension checks, there's almost nothing you can do to dramatically increase their amounts. If they aren't enough, the surest way of boosting your income is to get a job. The options run all the way from an 8-hour-a-day, 50-week-a-year new career to part-time or seasonal work.

Though savings, investment, and pension income don't affect the amount of your Social Security check, there is a ceiling on how much you can make on the job and still collect full Social Security benefits. In 1986 workers under 65 could earn up to $5,760 without losing benefits; those between 65 and 70 could earn $7,800 without penalty. If your income exceeds this amount, your benefits will be reduced by $1 for every $2 you're paid over the ceiling. After 1989, $1 in benefits will be lost for every $3 of excess earnings for persons who have reached full retirement age.

Private Pensions

Everyone working in government contributes to a pension. Just half of all workers in the private sector, however, are covered by an employer pension plan. And only half of these will ever see the money because of vesting requirements. Unlike the Social Security system, to which workers contribute no matter how many different jobs they hold, private pensions are the equivalent of a corporate loyalty test—at least for the standard eight to ten years of service required before an employee is vested and shares in a pension fund. Unlike Social Security, too, most employer pension plans don't have a cost-of-living escalator clause.

In 1983 the median amount of income from a public or private pension was $5,880 for newly retired couples who were eligible for payments. While that amount isn't paltry, it isn't lavish. According to a recent study from the Social Security Administration, only 7 out of 100 retired people who collect pension checks from their old employer rely on them for at least half their income.

Assets

Dividends from blue-chip stock investments you've made over the years; rents from real estate you own; royalties from your invention, song, computer software, best-selling book, or oil well; and interest from IRAs, Keogh Plans, certificates of deposit, passbook savings accounts, and loans are all examples of asset income.

Like private pensions and earnings from a job, income from assets supplements Social Security for a more comfortable retirement. Nearly nine out of every ten couples who are newly retired count on money from these sources. In 1983, the median amount of asset income was $2,160 per year.

MONEY IN RETIREMENT: SPENDING IT

If a couple were to retire tomorrow, *and* each spouse received Social Security plus dividends and interest from their combined assets, money from the husband's or wife's pension, and earnings from either the husband's or the wife's self-employment or part-time job, *then* that couple would have a median income of around $25,000 a year. Could they survive? Definitely, if they didn't owe much. Those total dollars are really the equivalent of a preretirement joint income of $46,000. The difference that retirement makes is a marked reduction of income taxes, an elimination of daily commuting costs, dwindling clothing costs, and decreased personal insurance payments.

If this couple has relocation in mind, they might well consider how far their money will go in other places. Comparing personal incomes in different areas provides the first clue; adjusting personal incomes by local living costs completes the picture.

Scraping By on $29,754 a Year

Do local personal incomes reflect local living costs? For the most part, yes.

A recent Bureau of Labor Statistics study showed that two thirds of the difference in personal incomes between, say, residents of Orlando and Olympia reflects their different costs of living; the other third is due to different employers and worker skills and prevailing wages.

To estimate the income for a typical two-person household, *Retirement Places Rated* started with 1987 per capita income forecasts from the Washington, DC–based firm of Woods & Poole Economics, Inc. These incomes were doubled to estimate the income of a household composed of two persons. The national average is $29,754 a year. Among retirement places, incomes range from $38,764 in West Palm Beach–Boca

Average Income for Two, 1987

HIGHEST

West Palm Beach–Boca Raton–Delray Beach, FL	$38,764
Fort Lauderdale–Hollywood–Pompano Beach, FL	37,534
Easton–Chesapeake Bay, MD	37,036
Sarasota, FL	36,382
Reno, NV	35,162
Ann Arbor, MI	34,576
Cape Cod, MA	34,244
Portsmouth–Dover–Durham, NH	34,020
St. Petersburg–Clearwater, FL	33,777
Litchfield County, CT	33,647

LOWEST

McAllen–Edinburg–Mission, TX	$15,056
Grand Lake–Lake Tenkiller, OK	16,810
Brownsville–Harlingen, TX	16,893
Crossville, TN	17,438
Franklin County, TN	17,698
St. George–Zion, UT	18,165
Deming, NM	18,383
Athens–Cedar Creek Lake, TX	18,471
Hamilton–Bitterroot Valley, MT	18,642
Clayton–Clarkesville, GA	18,969

Source: Woods & Poole Economics, Inc., personal income forecasts.

The national average for income before taxes for a two-person household is $29,754; the national average Social Security replacement rate is 29 percent.

Raton–Delray Beach, Florida, to $15,056 in McAllen–Edinburg–Mission, Texas.

So much for two-person household incomes. Are they really helpful in estimating living costs for a retired couple? They are if you consider to what extent Social Security checks can replace the income of a two-person household in different retirement places. Read on.

Local Social Security "Replacement Rates"

You're not going to live comfortably on Social Security alone; these payments by themselves were never intended to completely support you and your spouse in retirement. If you are a $42,000-a-year employee retiring at 65 with maximum earnings in "covered employment" (a job in which wages are deducted for Social Security) each year since 1955, for example, you can expect a monthly check of $739. That's only $8,868 a year. If you have a dependent spouse over 65, this amount is boosted by $369, for a combined benefit of $1,108, or $13,296 a year. Even though Social Security payments do increase with the cost of living, the money comes way short of the dollars you were pulling down at work.

One useful indicator of how far your Social Security benefits will go is to consider the rate at which they would replace average personal incomes around the country. Throughout 1986, the average benefits for a retired couple were $8,376. That won't replace much of the income a typical New Yorker, Bostonian, or Chicagoan is accustomed to.

In certain retirement places in Rio Grande Country and in New Appalachia, however, Social Security checks go a lot further in replacing local household incomes. Small wonder that retired persons who've moved over the last 30 years have tended to quit richer areas with high living costs for poorer places with low personal incomes. They were in search of spots where their own fixed Social Security and pension benefits could be stretched; in short, where living costs were lower.

Local Living Costs

It's a "black hole," the *Wall Street Journal* commented recently on just what is meant by *cost of living*. So what if the Consumer Price Index has octupled since the start of World War II; what does all that have to do with the high price of getting by in San Diego as opposed to a small town in the Blue Ridge Mountains?

In 1980, a committee appointed by the U.S. Department of Labor to come up with better ways to measure living costs between places threw in the towel. Given the infinite range of consumer tastes and household tactics for saving a dollar, they reported, the only way to pin down why life in one place was more expensive than in another was to focus on the weather's effect on clothing costs and household utility bills. Then look at taxes.

Taxes certainly do make a difference. But clothing and home energy bills? Not that much. According to one national retailer, the cost difference between wardrobes in the double-knit Sun Belt and the down-filled Frost Belt amounts to less than 1 percent of a household's annual budget. As for the comparative costs of keeping warm in the North Woods winter and staying cool in Metropolitan South Florida, often the only difference is the season during which local residents pay most of their bill.

One firm that counsels transferred employees adopts an 80/20 rule. In its experience, 80 percent of the difference in living costs between where you've come from and where you're going comes down to two things: housing and direct taxes. The other 20 percent comes from prices for everything from frozen orange juice and soap flakes to a shampoo, trim, and blow-dry at a beauty salon.

To gauge the cost of living in each place, *Retirement Places Rated* looks at housing and taxes, too. But we also include health care. Together, these three items account for half of a typical retired couple's annual budget.

Housing. By *Retirement Places Rated* estimates, the national average costs for natural gas, electricity, and a 25-year, 10 percent mortgage on an $82,300 single-family house (after making a one-fifth down payment) are $8,290 a year, excluding property taxes. (For a detailed analysis of homeownership costs, see the chapter "Housing: Market Values, Property Taxes, and

Taxes. Though you've hung up the business suit, given a niece your battered briefcase, and bid goodbye to co-workers and commuting hassles, you aren't completely immune from paying taxes in spite of the many tax breaks coming on your 65th birthday.

Although your tax bracket will probably be a good deal lower after you retire, federal income taxes will hit you with the same force whether you surface in San Diego, Santa Fe, or San Antonio. But state and local taxes differ tremendously. To measure the tax bite in retirement areas, *Retirement Places Rated* focuses on the three most common levies: those on personal income, retail sales, and residential property.

Based on the two-person household income in a retirement place, state personal income taxes are estimated from the Census Bureau's latest *State Government Tax Collections*. The dollars spent in the store on local sales taxes are also based on the retirement place's income for a couple, using U.S. Internal Revenue Service tables of state sales taxes paid at that income level. Property taxes are estimated from effective state rates on the market value of typical housing in the retirement place. (For a detailed analysis of property taxes, see the chapter "Housing: Market Values, Property Taxes, and Utility Bills.")

All together, these three taxes take their biggest bites in Massachusetts, Michigan, New Jersey, and New York. In Florida, New Mexico, and Texas, the bite is smallest.

Housing Cost Index

LOWEST	Cost Index (U.S. Average = 100)
Brownsville–Harlingen, TX	50
McAllen–Edinburg–Mission, TX	50
Roswell, NM	50
Deming, NM	54
Canton–Lake Tawakoni, TX	55
Houghton Lake, MI	56
Paris–Big Sandy, TN	56
Crossville, TN	59
Oscoda–Huron Shore, MI	59
Clayton–Clarkesville, GA	61
Franklin County, TN	61

HIGHEST	Cost Index (U.S. Average = 100)
Maui, HI	164
Kauai, HI	137
Litchfield County, CT	137
Naples, FL	132
San Diego, CA	129
Cape Cod, MA	125
Burlington, VT	124
Santa Rosa–Petaluma, CA	123
Salinas–Seaside–Monterey, CA	121
Friday Harbor–San Juan Islands, WA	120

Source: Derived from *Retirement Places Rated* figures, based on average homeownership costs exclusive of residential property taxes. See the chapter "Housing: Market Values, Property Taxes, and Utility Bills."

The above figures are percentages of the U.S. average of 100. All figures are rounded.

State and Local Income, Sales, and Property Taxes

LOWEST TAXES	Tax Index (U.S. Average = 100)
McAllen–Edinburg–Mission, TX	34
Brownsville–Harlingen, TX	35
Deming, NM	35
Ocala, FL	36
Panama City, FL	36
Lakeland–Winter Haven, FL	37
Roswell, NM	38
Canton–Lake Tawakoni, TX	39
Daytona Beach, FL	40
Las Cruces, NM	41

HIGHEST TAXES	Tax Index (U.S. Average = 100)
Canandaigua, NY	191
Ann Arbor, MI	190
New Paltz–Ulster County, NY	186
Burlington, VT	181
Monticello–Liberty, NY	178
Columbia County, NY	176
Madison, WI	168
Ocean County, NJ	168
Cape Cod, MA	167
Cape May, NJ	165

Source: Derived from Advisory Commission on Intergovernmental Relations, *Significant Features of Fiscal Federalism*, 1986; U.S. Bureau of the Census, *State Tax Collections*, 1986; and U.S. Internal Revenue Service, *Your Individual Income Tax*, 1986.

The above figures are percentages of the U.S. average of 100. All figures are rounded

Utility Bills.") In Maui, Hawaii, housing costs are 164 percent of that figure, while in three places in Rio Grande Country, they are just 50 percent.

Health Care. Whether your health is poor or good, the cost of looking after it will require more and more of your income each year as you get older. True, basic

Medicare covers hospital bills after you turn 65 (you'll pay a $520 deductible, however), but it won't cover things like an outpatient diagnostic visit, a prescription painkiller, or a splint for a broken thumb. Most importantly, it doesn't cover physicians' fees.

Even if you buy supplementary Medicare to cover medicines and services outside the hospital, you still have to pay the first $75 of your yearly expenses under the program plus 20 percent of any expenses above that $75. Count on it—things like prescriptions and lab tests will cost you money, but most of what you'll spend on health care will go to physicians.

To measure health care costs in each place, *Retirement Places Rated* looks at the amounts Medicare permits five typical specialists to charge their older patients for specific services. These fees are then weighted by how frequently they are billed older adults across the country. The physicians and their selected services are:

- Family practitioner—one hour comprehensive consultation
- Internist—electrocardiogram and report
- Psychiatrist—one hour psychotherapy
- Orthopedic surgeon—open reduction of fracture
- Ophthalmologist—comprehensive eye examination

Health Care Cost Index

LOWEST	Cost Index (U.S. Average = 100)
Lexington, KY	76
Murray–Kentucky Lake, KY	76
Charleston, SC	77
Hilton Head–Beaufort, SC	77
Myrtle Beach, SC	77
Blacksburg, VA	80
Front Royal, VA	80
Winchester, VA	80
Biloxi–Gulfport, MS	82
Clayton–Clarkesville, GA	83
Fayetteville, AR	83
Hendersonville–Brevard, NC	83
Hot Springs–Lake Ouachita, AR	83
Mountain Home–Bull Shoals, AR	83
Southport, NC	83

HIGHEST	Cost Index (U.S. Average = 100)
Miami–Hialeah, FL	130
San Diego, CA	128
Clear Lake, CA	125
Santa Rosa–Petaluma, CA	124
Carson City–Minden, NV	123
Las Vegas, NV	123
Reno, NV	123
Salinas–Seaside–Monterey, CA	121
Twain Harte–Yosemite, CA	121
Chico–Paradise, CA	120
Red Bluff–Sacramento Valley, CA	120
Redding, CA	120

Source: Derived from Health Care Financing Administration, *Medicare Directory of Prevailing Charges,* 1984, and unpublished data, 1986.

The above figures are percentages of the U.S. average of 100. All figures are rounded.

Among retirement places, physicians' charges to Medicare patients are highest in Miami–Hialeah, Florida, and in the Tahoe Basin and the Other California region. In the rural parts of Arkansas, Kentucky, and Virginia, and on the South Carolina coast, they are lowest.

The Composite. Measuring local housing costs, taxes, and health care fees against a national average of 100 is all very interesting, you might say. What's the bottom line?

The bottom line is that these three items can account for half your living expenses—specifically, the Bureau of Labor's latest survey on spending among older households shows housing taking roughly 30 percent, taxes 10 percent, and health care another 10 percent. The remaining half is spent on consumer goods that together don't vary dramatically in cost between places—food, transportation, entertainment, personal insurance, clothing, and services.

Retirement Places Rated weights local costs for housing, taxes, and health care by their percent share in a typical budget, then adds 50 percentage points for consumer goods to produce a composite cost-of-living index. Against a national yardstick of 100, this composite ranges from a high of 121 in Maui, Hawaii, to 78 in Roswell, New Mexico, and in the twin Texas retirement places of McAllen–Edinburg–Mission and Brownsville–Harlingen. (Note that a place's composite cost-of-living index is derived from unrounded indexes for housing, taxes, and health care. The composite index is then rounded.)

Putting It All Together

LOWEST LIVING COSTS	Cost Index (U.S. Average = 100)
Brownsville–Harlingen, TX	78
McAllen–Edinburg–Mission, TX	78
Roswell, NM	78
Deming, NM	79
Canton–Lake Tawakoni, TX	80
Paris–Big Sandy, TN	80
Crossville, TN	81
Franklin County, TN	82
Athens–Cedar Creek Lake, TX	83
Branson–Cassville–Table Rock Lake, MO	83
Clayton–Clarkesville, GA	83
Grand Lake–Lake Tenkiller, OK	83
Las Cruces, NM	83
Murray–Kentucky Lake, KY	83

HIGHEST LIVING COSTS	Cost Index (U.S. Average = 100)
Maui, HI	121
Burlington, VT	115
San Diego, CA	114
Cape Cod, MA	113
Litchfield County, CT	113
Kauai, HI	112
Santa Rosa–Petaluma, CA	112
Ocean County, NJ	111
Salinas–Seaside–Monterey, CA	111
Cape May, NJ	110

PART-TIME JOBS

Here are three good reasons for including a part-time job in your retirement plans. First, employment earnings added to "mailbox income" help many an older household hang on to a comfortable lifestyle. Second, work itself offers psychic income in the form of human contact, challenge, activity that keeps your mind and body alert, and the feeling that you're still a producer on the job. Third, although Social Security benefits are cut if you earn more than $7,800 a year (if you're 70 or older, you can earn as much extra income as you like and still collect full benefits), they need not be if you limit the amount you earn by working only part-time.

"All of this is well and good," you say. "So why are four out of five people over 65 neither working nor looking for work?" Some don't need the money. Others are happy to relax and take it easy; still others don't work for reasons of health. The reason for most, however, is the discouragement that comes from having to search a long time to find a job.

Let's face it—age can be a handicap when convincing new employers that you can cut it. But employers are changing their attitudes, not entirely because the law protects anyone between 40 and 70 from being refused employment solely on the basis of age, but also because of demographics.

Right now, in certain thriving pockets of this country, many firms are having a hard time finding younger part-time workers. Their remedy: hire older adults. Consider that your age brings a big advantage that perhaps you hadn't thought of: younger workers want full-time jobs but are working part-time because that's all they can find. Employers know this and anticipate turnover as the local economy expands.

Not all employers offer part-time jobs, however. Forget manufacturing; even if you're a master machinist, an accomplished numerical control programmer, or have certification in a specialized area of production, plants operate on one or more eight-hour shifts, and there are too many other willing workers looking for the same opportunity. Forget construction, too. Unless you have a class-A license for operating a D-9 bulldozer or a master carpenter's ticket and want a full day's work in a short building season, construction jobs go to younger people.

What kinds of industries use part-timers? There are three that account for almost all of the short-schedule, temporary, or seasonal work in this country:

- Retail-trade establishments
- Finance, insurance, and real estate firms
- Service industries

What Are the Odds?

Consider your chances for tracking down a part-time job. Is the market overcrowded with short-schedule or seasonal job seekers, or are the odds more favorable in Phoenix than Colorado Springs or Albuquerque?

Competition for Part-time Jobs

MOST FAVORABLE	Ratio of College-Age Persons to Persons Over 55
Burnet–Marble Falls–Llano, TX	1 to 9
Sarasota, FL	3 to 26
Mountain Home–Bull Shoals, AR	5 to 42
Clear Lake, CA	5 to 39
St. Petersburg–Clearwater, FL	5 to 38
Bradenton, FL	10 to 71
Friday Harbor–San Juan Islands, WA	15 to 104
Eagle River, WI	12 to 83
Fredericksburg, TX	6 to 41
Kerrville, TX	6 to 41

LEAST FAVORABLE	Ratio of College-Age Persons to Persons Over 55
Blacksburg, VA	3 to 2
Iowa City, IA	5 to 4
Athens, GA	6 to 5
State College, PA	6 to 5
Chapel Hill, NC	9 to 8
Flagstaff, AZ	9 to 8
Bloomington–Brown County, IN	18 to 17
Ann Arbor, MI	1 to 1
Austin, TX	5 to 6
Hilton Head–Beaufort, SC	5 to 6

Source: Woods & Poole Economics, Inc., 1987 population forecasts.

The national average is two college-age persons for every five persons over 55.

In 1986, a Labor Department economist identified "voluntary" part-time workers as persons who want only part-time jobs rather than persons who take part-time jobs because there's nothing else available.

Who are these 11 million voluntary part-timers? Younger people and older adults account for a much higher proportion of them than any other age group for two practical reasons: (1) part-time schedules allow younger people to attend school while working and (2) they help older adults ease into retirement while supplementing their incomes.

Your competition for good available part-time work is likely to be younger people. To help you measure the level of competition, *Retirement Places Rated* compares the ratio of college-age persons 19 to 23 to persons over 55. Based on this comparison in each retirement place, the part-time job competition is

Favorable if the ratio of persons over 55 to college-age persons is *more* than 3.7 to 1.

Average if the ratio of persons over 55 to college-age persons is *between* 2.3 and 3.7 to 1.

Unfavorable if the ratio of persons over 55 to college-age persons is *less* than 2.3 to 1.

When you judge local job markets, one fact stands out: college towns, for all their lively attractions, aren't ideal grounds for retired people to hunt for part-time or seasonal work. Among retirement places in this book, the competition is particularly stiff in Athens

(University of Georgia), Blacksburg (Virginia Tech), Chapel Hill (University of North Carolina), Flagstaff (Northern Arizona University), Iowa City (University of Iowa), and State College (Penn State).

LOCAL INCOME AND JOB GROWTH: THE NEXT EIGHT YEARS

Having some idea of who and how numerous your competitors are for good part-time jobs isn't all you'll need to know if you plan to get back to work. It helps to know which retirement places will see rapidly expanding opportunities—and which ones will not.

Comparing living costs among these retirement places is certainly sensible, too. But be aware that the flip side of job growth usually means a rising cost of living. If local living costs rise faster than the national average (upon which your Social Security payments are boosted), you may be in trouble.

Job Growth Is a Good Sign . . .

Mark Twain wrote that if economists were to be joined end to end, they would never reach a conclusion. They do agree on one thing, though: the industries that will have the most job openings in the future are finance, insurance, and real estate; retail trade; and services. Precisely the industries, let us reiterate, where part-time employment is concentrated.

Job Growth Forecast, 1987–1995*

FASTEST	Growth Rate
Lake Havasu City–Kingman, AZ	65%
Kerrville, TX	51
Santa Fe, NM	51
Houghton Lake, MI	50
Ocala, FL	47
Twain Harte–Yosemite, CA	47
Maui, HI	45
Prescott, AZ	41
St. George–Zion, UT	41
West Palm Beach–Boca Raton–Delray Beach, FL	40

SLOWEST	Growth Rate
Deming, NM	−13%
Eagle River, WI	−8
Oscoda–Huron Shore, MI	−8
Franklin County, TN	−6
Monticello–Liberty, NY	−6
Athens, GA	−1
Columbia County, NY	0
Missoula, MT	0
Asheville, NC	2
Front Royal, VA	2
Oak Harbor–Whidbey Island, WA	2
Rhinelander, WI	2

Source: Woods & Poole Economics, Inc., employment projections.

* These forecasts are for total job growth, not just growth in the retail trades, finance and real estate, and service industries.

The projected national average for job growth is 11 percent. Among the 131 retirement places, it is 19 percent.

Income Growth Forecast, 1987–1995

FASTEST	Growth Rate
Clayton–Clarkesville, GA	31%
Eagle River, WI	28
Canton–Lake Tawakoni, TX	27
Gainesville–Lake Lanier, GA	27
St. George–Zion, UT	27
Franklin County, TN	26
Crossville, TN	25
Ocala, FL	25
Grand Lake–Lake Tenkiller, OK	23
Lakeland–Winter Haven, FL	23

SLOWEST	Growth Rate
Sarasota, FL	−4%
Fort Lauderdale–Hollywood–Pompano Beach, FL	−1
Friday Harbor–San Juan Islands, WA	−1
West Palm Beach–Boca Raton–Delray Beach, FL	−1
Naples, FL	0
Ann Arbor, MI	1
Kerrville, TX	2
Oak Harbor–Whidbey Island, WA	2
St. Petersburg–Clearwater, FL	2
Winchester, VA	2

Source: Woods & Poole Economics, Inc., personal income projections.

The national average for income growth is projected to be 11 percent; among the 131 retirement places, it is 12 percent.

But where among the 131 retirement places we've featured in *Retirement Places Rated* are you most likely to find a job? According to Woods & Poole Economics, Inc., the places with the fastest employment growth rates tend to be smaller places in the Desert Southwest and Metropolitan South Florida. And the slower-growing places? Surprisingly, they're not all found outside the Sun Belt.

. . . But Income Growth Isn't Always

If you had the choice, all other things being equal, where would you rather live? A place like Austin in Central Texas where incomes are high and income growth will be rapid? Or a place like Prescott, Arizona, in the Desert Southwest where people have lower incomes and more modest prospects for income growth?

Historically, many retired persons have moved from rich places where the benefits of big money are made empty by even bigger costs of living to poorer places where low costs of living more than make up for the liabilities of low incomes.

But heavens can become purgatories. One finding that came from a 1984 study of where retired persons moved was the large number who relocated to Florida in the late 1960s only to pack up and move to another state in the late 1970s. The major reason? Their fixed incomes couldn't keep up with the rapidly rising living costs in the Sunshine State.

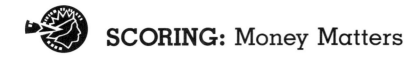

SCORING: Money Matters

If the money you and your spouse get from Social Security, a private pension, plus interest and dividends from investments you've made over the years comes to $20,000, will it stretch farther in the Desert Southwest than in the Ozarks and Ouachitas? Do costs of living really vary tremendously among the different places in these retirement regions, or can skillful budgeting keep your head above water anywhere you choose to live?

To help you compare each place's economic differences, *Retirement Places Rated* looks at three factors: (1) the average income for a two-person household, (2) cost-of-living indicators for taxes, health care, and housing, (3) the extent that average 1986 Social Security benefits for a retired couple ($8,376) can replace income adjusted by those cost-of-living indicators.

Each place starts with a base score of zero. Points are added or subtracted using these indicators:

1. *Average two-person household income adjusted for living costs.* The local average income is adjusted upward or downward by the local cost-of-living index. (See page 6 for an explanation of how costs for health care, housing, and state and local taxes are combined to determine a place's composite cost-of-living index.) For example, Maui's average household income—$27,886—is adjusted upward by 121 percent (since its cost-of-living index is 121) for an adjusted income of $33,742. Yuma's $20,402 household income is adjusted downward (multiplied by 85 percent, since its cost-of-living index is 85) to $17,342. (The composite cost-of-living index is derived from unrounded indexes for housing, taxes, and health care. The composite index is then rounded.)

2. *Social Security replacement rate.* The extent that annual Social Security benefits for a typical retired couple ($8,376) replaces the adjusted average household income in each place is determined. For example, typical Social Security benefits replace 24.09 percent of the adjusted income in San Diego and 57.72 percent in Franklin County, Tennessee. This local replacement rate is then multiplied by 100 to derive a score. San Diego's and Franklin County's scores, therefore, are 2,409 and 5,772, respectively.

SCORING EXAMPLES

One way to compare extremes in retirement money matters is to look at two places from sections of the country that represent economic opposites: McAllen–Edinburg–Mission on the bank of the Rio Grande in historically poor southernmost Texas, and the affluent Easton–Chesapeake Bay area on Maryland's Eastern Shore, a place attracting older exurbanites from Baltimore and Washington, DC.

McAllen–Edinburg–Mission, Texas (#1)

McAllen–Edinburg–Mission, a winter resort lined with palms, bougainvillea, poinsettias, and citrus trees, has the lowest income ($15,056) for a two-person household of 131 retirement places. This fact suggests poverty to some, but to others it means extremely low costs of living. Not for nothing did the number of retirement-age persons double here during the 1970s.

The Texas tax bite is notoriously forgiving. Since there are no levies on personal incomes nor any on interest and dividends, state and local taxes are just 34 percent of the U.S. average; physicians' fees are 93 percent; housing costs, exclusive of property taxes, 50 percent. All together, these items form a cost-of-living factor that is 78 percent of the national average. Adjusting local income downward (multiplying it by 78 percent), produces $11,744. Typical Social Security benefits will replace 71.32 percent of that adjusted income, giving this Texas retirement place a score of 7,132.

Easton–Chesapeake Bay, Maryland (#128)

Financially, people do quite well in Talbot County, Maryland, where Easton is the seat of local government. The place ranks near the top in personal income, not only in the Old Line State but in the nation. A retired couple here, however, may not do nearly so well as elsewhere. While the fees physicians bill Medicare are 94 percent of the U.S. average, basic home-ownership costs are 106 percent. Moreover, the impact of state sales and income taxes, plus residential property taxes, as in much of the country's northeastern quadrant, isn't lightly felt. These taxes amount to 129 percent of the national average. Annual Social Security benefits for a typical retired couple will replace only 21.75 percent of the $38,517 income (adjusted upward from $37,036 by living costs) that a two-person household gets by on in Talbot County. This produces a money matters score of 2,175.

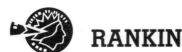

RANKINGS: Money Matters

Retirement Places Rated chooses three criteria to rank 131 places for money matters: (1) the average income for a two-person household, (2) cost-of-living indicators for taxes, health care, and housing, (3) the extent that average Social Security benefits for a retired couple ($8,376) can replace income adjusted for living costs.

Retirement Places from First to Last

Rank	Score
1. McAllen–Edinburg–Mission, TX	7,132
2. Brownsville–Harlingen, TX	6,357
3. Grand Lake–Lake Tenkiller, OK	6,003
4. Crossville, TN	5,930
5. Franklin County, TN	5,772
6. Deming, NM	5,768
7. Athens–Cedar Creek Lake, TX	5,463
8. Clayton–Clarkesville, GA	5,320
9. Southport, NC	5,165
10. Hamilton–Bitterroot Valley, MT	5,164
11. St. George–Zion, UT	5,067
12. Canton–Lake Tawakoni, TX	4,992
13. Houghton Lake, MI	4,946
14. Las Cruces, NM	4,915
15. Yuma, AZ	4,830
16. Lake Havasu City–Kingman, AZ	4,770
17. Murray–Kentucky Lake, KY	4,674
18. Oscoda–Huron Shore, MI	4,664
19. Eagle River, WI	4,634
20. Paris–Big Sandy, TN	4,575
21. Ocala, FL	4,558
22. Biloxi–Gulfport, MS	4,468
23. Flagstaff, AZ	4,425
24. Fayetteville, AR	4,404
25. Branson–Cassville–Table Rock Lake, MO	4,356
26. Roswell, NM	4,344
27. Blacksburg, VA	4,298
28. Front Royal, VA	4,278
29. Mountain Home–Bull Shoals, AR	4,194
30. Red Bluff–Sacramento Valley, CA	4,088
31. Lakeland–Winter Haven, FL	4,064
32. Bloomington–Brown County, IN	4,053
33. Fairhope–Gulf Shores, AL	4,015
34. Coeur d'Alene, ID	4,013
35. Panama City, FL	4,008
36. Myrtle Beach, SC	4,006
37. Kalispell, MT	3,962
38. Athens, GA	3,915
39. Twain Harte–Yosemite, CA	3,849
40. Asheville, NC	3,844
41. Prescott, AZ	3,841
42. San Antonio, TX	3,821
43. Camden–Penobscot Bay, ME	3,820
44. Hot Springs–Lake Ouachita, AR	3,789
45. Daytona Beach, FL	3,737
46. Brunswick–Golden Isles, GA	3,700
47. Fort Walton Beach, FL	3,690
48. Gainesville–Lake Lanier, GA	3,689
49. Charleston, SC	3,676
50. Rhinelander, WI	3,669
51. Bend, OR	3,659
52. Bellingham, WA	3,648
53. Chico–Paradise, CA	3,644
54. Springfield, MO	3,623
55. Bar Harbor–Frenchman Bay, ME	3,606
56. Medford–Ashland, OR	3,595
57. Missoula, MT	3,580
58. Hendersonville–Brevard, NC	3,559
59. Redding, CA	3,549
60. Port Angeles–Strait of Juan de Fuca, WA	3,546
61. Clear Lake, CA	3,536
62. Grand Junction, CO	3,532
63. Grass Valley–Truckee, CA	3,521
64. Ocean City–Assateague Island, MD	3,513
65. Newport–Lincoln City, OR	3,492
66. Oak Harbor–Whidbey Island, WA	3,456
67. Eugene–Springfield, OR	3,447
68. Fredericksburg, TX	3,414
69. State College, PA	3,411
70. Hilton Head–Beaufort, SC	3,394
71. Colorado Springs, CO	3,386
72. Olympia, WA	3,373
73. Burnet–Marble Falls–Llano, TX	3,358
74. Columbia County, NY	3,319
75. Winchester, VA	3,312
76. Petoskey–Straits of Mackinac, MI	3,304
77. Rehoboth Bay–Indian River Bay, DE	3,285
78. Bradenton, FL	3,261
79. Door County, WI	3,259
80. Melbourne–Titusville–Palm Bay, FL	3,227
81. Albuquerque, NM	3,207
82. Tucson, AZ	3,192
83. Orlando, FL	3,163
84. Fort Collins–Loveland, CO	3,122
85. Fort Myers–Cape Coral, FL	3,120
86. Traverse City–Grand Traverse Bay, MI	3,118
87. Laconia–Lake Winnipesaukee, NH	3,093
88. Amherst–Northampton, MA	3,083
89. Lexington, KY	3,071
90. Boise, ID	3,067
91. Kerrville, TX	3,061
92. Virginia Beach–Norfolk, VA	3,055
93. Monticello–Liberty, NY	3,024
94. Santa Fe, NM	3,016
95. Keene, NH	3,009
96. Kauai, HI	2,967
97. Phoenix, AZ	2,925
98. Charlottesville, VA	2,917
99. Austin, TX	2,915
100. Las Vegas, NV	2,912
101. Hanover, NH	2,893
102. Chapel Hill, NC	2,890
103. Bennington, VT	2,880
104. North Conway–White Mountains, NH	2,879
105. Lancaster, PA	2,843
106. San Luis Obispo, CA	2,789
107. St. Petersburg–Clearwater, FL	2,755
108. Iowa City, IA	2,726
109. New Paltz–Ulster County, NY	2,701
110. Miami–Hialeah, FL	2,650
111. Canandaigua, NY	2,599
112. Ocean County, NJ	2,586
113. Cape May, NJ	2,584
114. Carson City–Minden, NV	2,580
115. Friday Harbor–San Juan Islands, WA	2,531
116. Reno, NV	2,507
117. Maui, HI	2,482
118. San Diego, CA	2,409
119. Sarasota, FL	2,398
120. Burlington, VT	2,395
121. Portsmouth–Dover–Durham, NH	2,390
122. Salinas–Seaside–Monterey, CA	2,370
123. Madison, WI	2,369
124. Naples, FL	2,365
125. Santa Rosa–Petaluma, CA	2,296

Rank	Score		Rank	Score		Rank	Score
126. Ann Arbor, MI	2,222		129. Fort Lauderdale-Hollywood-			131. West Palm Beach-	
127. Litchfield County, CT	2,203		Pompano Beach, FL	2,167		Boca Raton-	
128. Easton-Chesapeake Bay,			130. Cape Cod, MA	2,165		Delray Beach, FL	2,139
MD	2,175						

Retirement Places Listed Alphabetically

Retirement Place	Rank	Retirement Place	Rank	Retirement Place	Rank
Albuquerque, NM	81	Flagstaff, AZ	23	Newport-Lincoln City, OR	65
Amherst-Northampton, MA	88	Fort Collins-Loveland, CO	84	North Conway-	
Ann Arbor, MI	126	Fort Lauderdale-Hollywood-		White Mountains, NH	104
Asheville, NC	40	Pompano Beach, FL	129	Oak Harbor-Whidbey	
Athens, GA	38	Fort Myers-Cape Coral, FL	85	Island, WA	66
		Fort Walton Beach, FL	47	Ocala, FL	21
Athens-Cedar Creek Lake, TX	7			Ocean City-	
Austin, TX	99	Franklin County, TN	5	Assateague Island, MD	64
Bar Harbor-		Fredericksburg, TX	68		
Frenchman Bay, ME	55	Friday Harbor-San Juan		Ocean County, NJ	112
Bellingham, WA	52	Islands, WA	115	Olympia, WA	72
Bend, OR	51	Front Royal, VA	28	Orlando, FL	83
		Gainesville-Lake Lanier, GA	48	Oscoda-Huron Shore, MI	18
Bennington, VT	103			Panama City, FL	35
Biloxi-Gulfport, MS	22	Grand Junction, CO	62		
Blacksburg, VA	27	Grand Lake-Lake Tenkiller, OK	3	Paris-Big Sandy, TN	20
Bloomington-		Grass Valley-Truckee, CA	63	Petoskey-Straits of Mackinac, MI	76
Brown County, IN	32	Hamilton-Bitterroot Valley, MT	10	Phoenix, AZ	97
Boise, ID	90	Hanover, NH	101	Port Angeles-Strait of	
				Juan de Fuca, WA	60
Bradenton, FL	78	Hendersonville-Brevard, NC	58	Portsmouth-Dover-Durham, NH	121
Branson-Cassville-		Hilton Head-Beaufort, SC	70		
Table Rock Lake, MO	25	Hot Springs-Lake Ouachita, AR	44	Prescott, AZ	41
Brownsville-Harlingen, TX	2	Houghton Lake, MI	13	Red Bluff-Sacramento Valley, CA	30
Brunswick-Golden Isles, GA	46	Iowa City, IA	108	Redding, CA	59
Burlington, VT	120			Rehoboth Bay-Indian River	
		Kalispell, MT	37	Bay, DE	77
Burnet-Marble Falls-Llano, TX	73	Kauai, HI	96	Reno, NV	116
Camden-Penobscot Bay, ME	43	Keene, NH	95		
Canandaigua, NY	111	Kerrville, TX	91	Rhinelander, WI	50
Canton-Lake Tawakoni, TX	12	Laconia-Lake Winnipesaukee, NH	87	Roswell, NM	26
Cape Cod, MA	130			St. George-Zion, UT	11
		Lake Havasu City-Kingman, AZ	16	St. Petersburg-Clearwater, FL	107
Cape May, NJ	113	Lakeland-Winter Haven, FL	31	Salinas-Seaside-	122
Carson City-Minden, NV	114	Lancaster, PA	105	Monterey, CA	
Chapel Hill, NC	102	Las Cruces, NM	14		
Charleston, SC	49	Las Vegas, NV	100	San Antonio, TX	42
Charlottesville, VA	98			San Diego, CA	118
		Lexington, KY	89	San Luis Obispo, CA	106
Chico-Paradise, CA	53	Litchfield County, CT	127	Santa Fe, NM	94
Clayton-Clarkesville, GA	8	Madison, WI	123	Santa Rosa-Petaluma, CA	125
Clear Lake, CA	61	Maui, HI	117		
Coeur d'Alene, ID	34	McAllen-Edinburg-Mission, TX	1	Sarasota, FL	119
Colorado Springs, CO	71			Southport, NC	9
		Medford-Ashland, OR	56	Springfield, MO	54
Columbia County, NY	74	Melbourne-Titusville-		State College, PA	69
Crossville, TN	4	Palm Bay, FL	80	Traverse City-Grand Traverse	
Daytona Beach, FL	45	Miami-Hialeah, FL	110	Bay, MI	86
Deming, NM	6	Missoula, MT	57		
Door County, WI	79	Monticello-Liberty, NY	93	Tucson, AZ	82
				Twain Harte-Yosemite, CA	39
Eagle River, WI	19	Mountain Home-Bull Shoals, AR	29	Virginia Beach-Norfolk, VA	92
Easton-Chesapeake Bay, MD	128	Murray-Kentucky Lake, KY	17	West Palm Beach-Boca Raton-	
Eugene-Springfield, OR	67	Myrtle Beach, SC	36	Delray Beach, FL	131
Fairhope-Gulf Shores, AL	33	Naples, FL	124	Winchester, VA	75
Fayetteville, AR	24	New Paltz-Ulster County, NY	109	Yuma, AZ	15

PLACE PROFILES: Money Matters

The following Place Profiles highlight certain economic features in the retirement places. These include the factors used to rank the places—estimated average income for a two-person household and indicators for the cost of housing, health care, and taxes against a national yardstick of 100.

The profiles also detail the number of new jobs forecast for 1987–1995 in finance and real estate, retail trade, and services (fields which employ the most part-time workers) as well as local income and job percent-growth forecasts during that period. A star preceding a place's name highlights it as one of the top 15 places for money matters.

The information comes from these sources: Commerce Clearing House, *State Tax Guide* (2 volumes), 1986; U.S. Department of Health and Human Services, Health Care Financing Administration, *Medicare Directory of Prevailing Charges*, 1984, and unpublished 1986 data; U.S. Department of Commerce, Bureau of the Census, *State Government Tax Collections*, 1986; U.S. Department of the Treasury, Internal Revenue Service, *Your Individual Income Tax*, 1986; and Woods & Poole Economics, Inc., Washington, DC, unpublished county income and employment forecasts, 1986.

Place	Household Income	Cost-of-Living Indexes (U.S. = 100)	New Jobs Forecast, 1987–1995	Growth Forecast, 1987–1995	Score	Rank
Albuquerque, NM	$29,022	Health care: 92 Housing: 84 State/local taxes: 54 Composite: 90	Finance and real estate: 1,540 Retail trade: 5,370 Services: 15,750 Part-time competition: Unfavorable	Income: 11% Jobs: 10%	3,207	81
Amherst–Northampton, MA	$26,900	Health care: 93 Housing: 98 State/local taxes: 128 Composite: 101	Finance and real estate: 60 Retail trade: −990 Services: 660 Part-time competition: Unfavorable	Income: 13% Jobs: 4%	3,083	88
Ann Arbor, MI	$34,576	Health care: 93 Housing: 103 State/local taxes: 190 Composite: 109	Finance and real estate: 690 Retail trade: −370 Services: 16,160 Part-time competition: Unfavorable	Income: 1% Jobs: 13%	2,222	126
Asheville, NC	$24,486	Health care: 91 Housing: 72 State/local taxes: 85 Composite: 89	Finance and real estate: −210 Retail trade: 670 Services: 920 Part-time competition: Unfavorable	Income: 18% Jobs: 2%	3,844	40
Athens, GA	$23,511	Health care: 85 Housing: 82 State/local taxes: 82 Composite: 91	Finance and real estate: 0 Retail trade: 670 Services: 640 Part-time competition: Unfavorable	Income: 15% Jobs: −1%	3,915	38
★ Athens–Cedar Creek Lake, TX	$18,471	Health care: 94 Housing: 63 State/local taxes: 44 Composite: 83	Finance and real estate: −20 Retail trade: 1,290 Services: 20 Part-time competition: Favorable	Income: 20% Jobs: 16%	5,463	7
Austin, TX	$30,569	Health care: 96 Housing: 92 State/local taxes: 68 Composite: 94	Finance and real estate: 6,050 Retail trade: 10,410 Services: 11,420 Part-time competition: Unfavorable	Income: 11% Jobs: 29%	2,915	99
Bar Harbor–Frenchman Bay, ME	$24,979	Health care: 87 Housing: 85 State/local taxes: 93 Composite: 93	Finance and real estate: −30 Retail trade: 180 Services: −60 Part-time competition: Average	Income: 10% Jobs: 8%	3,606	55
Bellingham, WA	$25,229	Health care: 106 Housing: 81 State/local taxes: 56 Composite: 91	Finance and real estate: −240 Retail trade: 1,750 Services: 1,730 Part-time competition: Unfavorable	Income: 8% Jobs: 10%	3,648	52
Bend, OR	$23,121	Health care: 97 Housing: 84 State/local taxes: 139 Composite: 99	Finance and real estate: −250 Retail trade: 1,340 Services: 2,160 Part-time competition: Average	Income: 6% Jobs: 22%	3,659	51

Place	Household Income	Cost-of-Living Indexes (U.S. = 100)	New Jobs Forecast, 1987–1995	Growth Forecast, 1987–1995	Score	Rank
Bennington, VT	$27,964	Health care: 101 Housing: 98 State/local taxes: 147 Composite: 104	Finance and real estate: 50 Retail trade: 160 Services: 10 Part-time competition: Average	Income: 13% Jobs: 6%	2,880	103
Biloxi–Gulfport, MS	$22,317	Health care: 82 Housing: 66 State/local taxes: 57 Composite: 84	Finance and real estate: − 160 Retail trade: 380 Services: 4,070 Part-time competition: Unfavorable	Income: 20% Jobs: 11%	4,468	22
Blacksburg, VA	$21,414	Health care: 80 Housing: 83 State/local taxes: 77 Composite: 91	Finance and real estate: 80 Retail trade: 970 Services: 650 Part-time competition: Unfavorable	Income: 11% Jobs: 30%	4,298	27
Bloomington– Brown County, IN	$23,220	Health care: 89 Housing: 74 State/local taxes: 76 Composite: 89	Finance and real estate: 330 Retail trade: 1,870 Services: 2,040 Part-time competition: Unfavorable	Income: 15% Jobs: 25%	4,053	32
Boise, ID	$29,370	Health care: 94 Housing: 80 State/local taxes: 91 Composite: 93	Finance and real estate: 790 Retail trade: 3,100 Services: 4,120 Part-time competition: Unfavorable	Income: 15% Jobs: 17%	3,067	90
Bradenton, FL	$27,922	Health care: 100 Housing: 90 State/local taxes: 44 Composite: 92	Finance and real estate: 1,120 Retail trade: 1,120 Services: 1,030 Part-time competition: Favorable	Income: 5% Jobs: 14%	3,261	78
Branson–Cassville–Table Rock Lake, MO	$23,168	Health care: 89 Housing: 62 State/local taxes: 60 Composite: 83	Finance and real estate: 430 Retail trade: 740 Services: 730 Part-time competition: Favorable	Income: 14% Jobs: 17%	4,356	25
★ Brownsville– Harlingen, TX	$16,893	Health care: 91 Housing: 50 State/local taxes: 35 Composite: 78	Finance and real estate: 350 Retail trade: 4,310 Services: 1,880 Part-time competition: Average	Income: 22% Jobs: 26%	6,357	2
Brunswick– Golden Isles, GA	$25,727	Health care: 85 Housing: 71 State/local taxes: 79 Composite: 88	Finance and real estate: − 60 Retail trade: 560 Services: 1,230 Part-time competition: Average	Income: 18% Jobs: 9%	3,700	46
Burlington, VT	$30,413	Health care: 101 Housing: 124 State/local taxes: 181 Composite: 115	Finance and real estate: 30 Retail trade: 1,410 Services: 5,690 Part-time competition: Unfavorable	Income: 11% Jobs: 22%	2,395	120
Burnet–Marble Falls– Llano, TX	$29,349	Health care: 86 Housing: 71 State/local taxes: 51 Composite: 85	Finance and real estate: 160 Retail trade: 620 Services: 320 Part-time competition: Favorable	Income: 8% Jobs: 32%	3,358	73
Camden– Penobscot Bay, ME	$23,578	Health care: 86 Housing: 85 State/local taxes: 91 Composite: 93	Finance and real estate: 50 Retail trade: 770 Services: 50 Part-time competition: Favorable	Income: 8% Jobs: 7%	3,820	43
Canandaigua, NY	$29,837	Health care: 113 Housing: 93 State/local taxes: 191 Composite: 108	Finance and real estate: 30 Retail trade: 430 Services: 140 Part-time competition: Average	Income: 15% Jobs: 15%	2,599	111

Place	Household Income	Cost-of-Living Indexes (U.S. = 100)	New Jobs Forecast, 1987–1995	Growth Forecast, 1987–1995	Score	Rank
★ Canton–Lake Tawakoni, TX	$20,973	Health care: 94 Housing: 55 State/local taxes: 39 Composite: 80	Finance and real estate: 100 Retail trade: −60 Services: 660 Part-time competition: Favorable	Income: 27% Jobs: 14%	4,992	12
Cape Cod, MA	$34,244	Health care: 84 Housing: 125 State/local taxes: 167 Composite: 113	Finance and real estate: 250 Retail trade: 1,530 Services: 3,740 Part-time competition: Favorable	Income: 6% Jobs: 16%	2,165	130
Cape May, NJ	$29,464	Health care: 100 Housing: 110 State/local taxes: 165 Composite: 110	Finance and real estate: −180 Retail trade: 1,310 Services: −50 Part-time competition: Unfavorable	Income: 6% Jobs: 4%	2,584	113
Carson City–Minden, NV	$31,830	Health care: 123 Housing: 115 State/local taxes: 48 Composite: 102	Finance and real estate: 570 Retail trade: 1,260 Services: 5,250 Part-time competition: Average	Income: 8% Jobs: 29%	2,580	114
Chapel Hill, NC	$28,696	Health care: 91 Housing: 102 State/local taxes: 109 Composite: 101	Finance and real estate: 320 Retail trade: 880 Services: 1,740 Part-time competition: Unfavorable	Income: 11% Jobs: 21%	2,890	102
Charleston, SC	$25,602	Health care: 77 Housing: 79 State/local taxes: 79 Composite: 89	Finance and real estate: 1,190 Retail trade: 170 Services: 4,540 Part-time competition: Unfavorable	Income: 13% Jobs: 8%	3,676	49
Charlottesville, VA	$29,303	Health care: 88 Housing: 99 State/local taxes: 98 Composite: 98	Finance and real estate: 1,210 Retail trade: 800 Services: 1,740 Part-time competition: Unfavorable	Income: 12% Jobs: 20%	2,917	98
Chico–Paradise, CA	$23,698	Health care: 120 Housing: 86 State/local taxes: 91 Composite: 97	Finance and real estate: 710 Retail trade: −110 Services: 4,230 Part-time competition: Average	Income: 11% Jobs: 15%	3,644	53
★ Clayton–Clarkesville, GA	$18,969	Health care: 83 Housing: 61 State/local taxes: 63 Composite: 83	Finance and real estate: 290 Retail trade: 560 Services: 70 Part-time competition: Average	Income: 31% Jobs: 11%	5,320	8
Clear Lake, CA	$23,926	Health care: 125 Housing: 92 State/local taxes: 91 Composite: 99	Finance and real estate: 60 Retail trade: 510 Services: 170 Part-time competition: Favorable	Income: 17% Jobs: 28%	3,536	61
Coeur d'Alene, ID	$23,454	Health care: 89 Housing: 75 State/local taxes: 79 Composite: 89	Finance and real estate: 100 Retail trade: 220 Services: 1,230 Part-time competition: Average	Income: 11% Jobs: 19%	4,013	34
Colorado Springs, CO	$27,180	Health care: 89 Housing: 82 State/local taxes: 73 Composite: 91	Finance and real estate: 1,050 Retail trade: 3,920 Services: 3,760 Part-time competition: Unfavorable	Income: 17% Jobs: 16%	3,386	71
Columbia County, NY	$24,268	Health care: 92 Housing: 90 State/local taxes: 176 Composite: 104	Finance and real estate: −20 Retail trade: 80 Services: −590 Part-time competition: Unfavorable	Income: 17% Jobs: 0%	3,319	74

Place	Household Income	Cost-of-Living Indexes (U.S. = 100)	New Jobs Forecast, 1987–1995	Growth Forecast, 1987–1995	Score	Rank
★ Crossville, TN	$17,438	Health care: 91 Housing: 59 State/local taxes: 42 Composite: 81	Finance and real estate: 920 Retail trade: −90 Services: 190 Part-Time competition: Average	Income: 25% Jobs: 12%	5,930	4
Daytona Beach, FL	$25,467	Health care: 100 Housing: 81 State/local taxes: 40 Composite: 88	Finance and real estate: −960 Retail trade: 1,890 Services: −910 Part-time competition: Favorable	Income: 11% Jobs: 7%	3,737	45
★ Deming, NM	$18,383	Health care: 92 Housing: 54 State/local taxes: 35 Composite: 79	Finance and real estate: −40 Retail trade: −290 Services: −90 Part-time competition: Unfavorable	Income: 11% Jobs: −13%	5,768	6
Door County, WI	$26,770	Health care: 91 Housing: 80 State/local taxes: 132 Composite: 96	Finance and real estate: 200 Retail trade: 1,830 Services: 1,450 Part-time competition: Average	Income: 10% Jobs: 28%	3,259	79
Eagle River, WI	$19,027	Health care: 96 Housing: 80 State/local taxes: 115 Composite: 95	Finance and real estate: 10 Retail trade: −150 Services: −400 Part-time competition: Favorable	Income: 28% Jobs: −8%	4,634	19
Easton– Chesapeake Bay, MD	$37,036	Health care: 94 Housing: 106 State/local taxes: 129 Composite: 104	Finance and real estate: −80 Retail trade: 580 Services: 2,950 Part-time competition: Favorable	Income: 9% Jobs: 26%	2,175	128
Eugene–Springfield, OR	$24,300	Health care: 99 Housing: 85 State/local taxes: 146 Composite: 100	Finance and real estate: −380 Retail trade: 2,580 Services: 1,740 Part-time competition: Unfavorable	Income: 9% Jobs: 9%	3,447	67
Fairhope– Gulf Shores, AL	$23,978	Health care: 88 Housing: 78 State/local taxes: 50 Composite: 87	Finance and real estate: 880 Retail trade: 2,820 Services: 810 Part-time competition: Average	Income: 20% Jobs: 23%	4,015	33
Fayetteville, AR	$21,860	Health care: 83 Housing: 70 State/local taxes: 78 Composite: 87	Finance and real estate: 150 Retail trade: −520 Services: 730 Part-time competition: Unfavorable	Income: 15% Jobs: 8%	4,404	24
Flagstaff, AZ	$21,030	Health care: 97 Housing: 81 State/local taxes: 57 Composite: 90	Finance and real estate: 210 Retail trade: 1,420 Services: 460 Part-time competition: Unfavorable	Income: 18% Jobs: 24%	4,425	23
Fort Collins– Loveland, CO	$27,948	Health care: 89 Housing: 96 State/local taxes: 80 Composite: 96	Finance and real estate: −90 Retail trade: 4,000 Services: 3,750 Part-time competition: Unfavorable	Income: 13% Jobs: 28%	3,122	84
Fort Lauderdale– Hollywood– Pompano Beach, FL	$37,534	Health care: 119 Housing: 119 State/local taxes: 59 Composite: 103	Finance and real estate: 12,570 Retail trade: 5,410 Services: 35,110 Part-time competition: Favorable	Income: −1% Jobs: 22%	2,167	129
Fort Myers– Cape Coral, FL	$27,964	Health care: 100 Housing: 103 State/local taxes: 50 Composite: 96	Finance and real estate: 5,060 Retail trade: 8,190 Services: 9,400 Part-time competition: Favorable	Income: 9% Jobs: 33%	3,120	85

Place	Household Income	Cost-of-Living Indexes (U.S. = 100)	New Jobs Forecast, 1987–1995	Growth Forecast, 1987–1995	Score	Rank
Fort Walton Beach, FL	$25,218	Health care: 100 Housing: 84 State/local taxes: 43 Composite: 90	Finance and real estate: 480 Retail trade: 1,580 Services: 4,970 Part-time competition: Unfavorable	Income: 7% Jobs: 24%	3,690	47
★ Franklin County, TN	$17,698	Health care: 91 Housing: 61 State/local taxes: 42 Composite: 82	Finance and real estate: 50 Retail trade: −10 Services: −190 Part-time competition: Average	Income: 26% Jobs: −6%	5,772	5
Fredericksburg, TX	$28,202	Health care: 86 Housing: 77 State/local taxes: 57 Composite: 87	Finance and real estate: 60 Retail trade: 370 Services: 140 Part-time competition: Favorable	Income: 6% Jobs: 18%	3,414	68
Friday Harbor–San Juan Islands, WA	$31,815	Health care: 106 Housing: 120 State/local taxes: 79 Composite: 104	Finance and real estate: 30 Retail trade: 370 Services: 130 Part-time competition: Favorable	Income: −1% Jobs: 37%	2,531	115
Front Royal, VA	$22,000	Health care: 80 Housing: 78 State/local taxes: 76 Composite: 89	Finance and real estate: 50 Retail trade: −250 Services: 240 Part-time competition: Average	Income: 22% Jobs: 2%	4,278	28
Gainesville–Lake Lanier, GA	$25,799	Health care: 85 Housing: 73 State/local taxes: 80 Composite: 88	Finance and real estate: 460 Retail trade: 140 Services: −470 Part-time competition: Average	Income: 27% Jobs: 3%	3,689	48
Grand Junction, CO	$25,779	Health care: 89 Housing: 87 State/local taxes: 72 Composite: 92	Finance and real estate: 700 Retail trade: 2,120 Services: 1,110 Part-time competition: Unfavorable	Income: 14% Jobs: 16%	3,532	62
★ Grand Lake–Lake Tenkiller, OK	$16,810	Health care: 88 Housing: 63 State/local taxes: 51 Composite: 83	Finance and real estate: 0 Retail trade: 440 Services: −670 Part-time competition: Average	Income: 23% Jobs: 9%	6,003	3
Grass Valley–Truckee, CA	$22,026	Health care: 117 Housing: 119 State/local taxes: 102 Composite: 108	Finance and real estate: 410 Retail trade: 920 Services: 830 Part-time competition: Favorable	Income: 10% Jobs: 35%	3,521	63
★ Hamilton–Bitterroot Valley, MT	$18,642	Health care: 98 Housing: 70 State/local taxes: 57 Composite: 87	Finance and real estate: 10 Retail trade: 90 Services: 40 Part-time competition: Favorable	Income: 9% Jobs: 10%	5,164	10
Hanover, NH	$29,843	Health care: 93 Housing: 96 State/local taxes: 88 Composite: 97	Finance and real estate: 350 Retail trade: 140 Services: 2,430 Part-time competition: Unfavorable	Income: 9% Jobs: 9%	2,893	101
Hendersonville–Brevard, NC	$25,582	Health care: 83 Housing: 81 State/local taxes: 92 Composite: 92	Finance and real estate: 30 Retail trade: 680 Services: −30 Part-time competition: Favorable	Income: 5% Jobs: 13%	3,559	58
Hilton Head–Beaufort, SC	$25,981	Health care: 77 Housing: 97 State/local taxes: 85 Composite: 95	Finance and real estate: −50 Retail trade: 3,520 Services: 3,370 Part-time competition: Unfavorable	Income: 22% Jobs: 9%	3,394	70

Place	Household Income	Cost-of-Living Indexes (U.S. = 100)	New Jobs Forecast, 1987–1995	Growth Forecast, 1987–1995	Score	Rank
Hot Springs–Lake Ouachita, AR	$26,007	Health care: 83 Housing: 63 State/local taxes: 78 Composite: 85	Finance and real estate: 470 Retail trade: 760 Services: 2,730 Part-time competition: Favorable	Income: 9% Jobs: 12%	3,789	44
★ Houghton Lake, MI	$19,691	Health care: 93 Housing: 56 State/local taxes: 98 Composite: 86	Finance and real estate: 180 Retail trade: 760 Services: 880 Part-time competition: Favorable	Income: 6% Jobs: 50%	4,946	13
Iowa City, IA	$30,128	Health care: 89 Housing: 101 State/local taxes: 125 Composite: 102	Finance and real estate: 150 Retail trade: 1,380 Services: −1,750 Part-time competition: Unfavorable	Income: 7% Jobs: 10%	2,726	108
Kalispell, MT	$24,300	Health care: 98 Housing: 70 State/local taxes: 63 Composite: 87	Finance and real estate: −40 Retail trade: 230 Services: −210 Part-time competition: Average	Income: 3% Jobs: 4%	3,962	37
Kauai, HI	$25,208	Health care: 115 Housing: 137 State/local taxes: 90 Composite: 112	Finance and real estate: −70 Retail trade: 920 Services: 660 Part-time competition: Average	Income: 17% Jobs: 18%	2,967	96
Keene, NH	$28,696	Health care: 93 Housing: 97 State/local taxes: 88 Composite: 97	Finance and real estate: −390 Retail trade: 550 Services: 1,160 Part-time competition: Average	Income: 13% Jobs: 13%	3,009	95
Kerrville, TX	$31,093	Health care: 86 Housing: 78 State/local taxes: 58 Composite: 88	Finance and real estate: 200 Retail trade: 2,400 Services: 2,160 Part-time competition: Favorable	Income: 2% Jobs: 51%	3,061	91
Laconia–Lake Winnipesaukee, NH	$27,351	Health care: 93 Housing: 102 State/local taxes: 94 Composite: 99	Finance and real estate: 120 Retail trade: −250 Services: 1,920 Part-time competition: Average	Income: 18% Jobs: 8%	3,093	87
Lake Havasu City–Kingman, AZ	$19,509	Health care: 102 Housing: 81 State/local taxes: 51 Composite: 90	Finance and real estate: 1,390 Retail trade: 4,840 Services: 720 Part-time competition: Favorable	Income: 20% Jobs: 65%	4,770	16
Lakeland–Winter Haven, FL	$23,967	Health care: 100 Housing: 73 State/local taxes: 37 Composite: 86	Finance and real estate: 660 Retail trade: 3,180 Services: 4,040 Part-time competition: Average	Income: 23% Jobs: 9%	4,064	31
Lancaster, PA	$28,332	Health care: 96 Housing: 109 State/local taxes: 113 Composite: 104	Finance and real estate: 110 Retail trade: 2,200 Services: 4,700 Part-time competition: Average	Income: 16% Jobs: 9%	2,843	105
★ Las Cruces, NM	$20,532	Health care: 92 Housing: 65 State/local taxes: 41 Composite: 83	Finance and real estate: −260 Retail trade: −750 Services: −1,010 Part-time competition: Unfavorable	Income: 5% Jobs: 3%	4,915	14
Las Vegas, NV	$29,962	Health care: 123 Housing: 97 State/local taxes: 42 Composite: 96	Finance and real estate: 3,880 Retail trade: 9,130 Services: 18,450 Part-time competition: Unfavorable	Income: 11% Jobs: 18%	2,912	100

Place	Household Income	Cost-of-Living Indexes (U.S. = 100)	New Jobs Forecast, 1987–1995	Growth Forecast, 1987–1995	Score	Rank
Lexington, KY	$29,329	Health care: 76 Housing: 89 State/local taxes: 83 Composite: 93	Finance and real estate: −80 Retail trade: 2,330 Services: 10,420 Part-time competition: Unfavorable	Income: 9% Jobs: 14%	3,071	89
Litchfield County, CT	$33,647	Health care: 92 Housing: 137 State/local taxes: 131 Composite: 113	Finance and real estate: 10 Retail trade: 1,780 Services: 2,120 Part-time competition: Favorable	Income: 14% Jobs: 11%	2,203	127
Madison, WI	$33,045	Health care: 91 Housing: 102 State/local taxes: 168 Composite: 107	Finance and real estate: 580 Retail trade: 1,720 Services: 3,050 Part-time competition: Unfavorable	Income: 8% Jobs: 15%	2,369	123
Maui, HI	$27,886	Health care: 115 Housing: 164 State/local taxes: 103 Composite: 121	Finance and real estate: 340 Retail trade: 3,760 Services: 11,680 Part-time competition: Average	Income: 9% Jobs: 45%	2,482	117
★ **McAllen–Edinburg– Mission, TX**	$15,056	Health care: 93 Housing: 50 State/local taxes: 34 Composite: 78	Finance and real estate: 280 Retail trade: 5,620 Services: 1,740 Part-time competition: Unfavorable	Income: 21% Jobs: 19%	7,132	1
Medford–Ashland, OR	$23,775	Health care: 88 Housing: 85 State/local taxes: 141 Composite: 98	Finance and real estate: 750 Retail trade: 2,610 Services: 2,650 Part-time competition: Average	Income: 9% Jobs: 20%	3,595	56
Melbourne–Titusville– Palm Bay, FL	$27,907	Health care: 100 Housing: 96 State/local taxes: 47 Composite: 93	Finance and real estate: −110 Retail trade: 1,030 Services: 1,360 Part-time competition: Average	Income: 11% Jobs: 8%	3,227	80
Miami–Hialeah, FL	$31,291	Health care: 130 Housing: 109 State/local taxes: 54 Composite: 101	Finance and real estate: 25,100 Retail trade: 2,360 Services: 38,610 Part-time competition: Average	Income: 8% Jobs: 13%	2,650	110
Missoula, MT	$25,161	Health care: 98 Housing: 87 State/local taxes: 74 Composite: 93	Finance and real estate: −90 Retail trade: 290 Services: −470 Part-time competition: Unfavorable	Income: 4% Jobs: 0%	3,580	57
Monticello–Liberty, NY	$26,635	Health care: 92 Housing: 88 State/local taxes: 178 Composite: 104	Finance and real estate: −120 Retail trade: −840 Services: −180 Part-time competition: Unfavorable	Income: 12% Jobs: −6%	3,024	93
Mountain Home– Bull Shoals, AR	$22,955	Health care: 83 Housing: 70 State/local taxes: 78 Composite: 87	Finance and real estate: 0 Retail trade: 150 Services: 1,790 Part-time competition: Favorable	Income: 4% Jobs: 28%	4,194	29
Murray– Kentucky Lake, KY	$21,590	Health care: 76 Housing: 65 State/local taxes: 62 Composite: 83	Finance and real estate: 0 Retail trade: 60 Services: 590 Part-time competition: Average	Income: 12% Jobs: 11%	4,674	17
Myrtle Beach, SC	$23,230	Health care: 77 Housing: 83 State/local taxes: 76 Composite: 90	Finance and real estate: 1,800 Retail trade: 4,480 Services: 1,170 Part-time competition: Unfavorable	Income: 20% Jobs: 14%	4,006	36

Place	Household Income	Cost-of-Living Indexes (U.S. = 100)	New Jobs Forecast, 1987–1995	Growth Forecast, 1987–1995	Score	Rank
Naples, FL	$32,790	Health care: 119 Housing: 132 State/local taxes: 63 Composite: 108	Finance and real estate: 1,040 Retail trade: 1,170 Services: 3,340 Part-time competition: Favorable	Income: 0% Jobs: 26%	2,365	124
New Paltz–Ulster County, NY	$29,531	Health care: 92 Housing: 92 State/local taxes: 186 Composite: 105	Finance and real estate: −470 Retail trade: −820 Services: 1,580 Part-time competition: Average	Income: 18% Jobs: 17%	2,701	109
Newport–Lincoln City, OR	$24,730	Health care: 97 Housing: 79 State/local taxes: 137 Composite: 97	Finance and real estate: 30 Retail trade: 460 Services: 1,200 Part-time competition: Favorable	Income: 12% Jobs: 14%	3,492	65
North Conway–White Mountains, NH	$28,805	Health care: 93 Housing: 105 State/local taxes: 97 Composite: 101	Finance and real estate: 30 Retail trade: 1,110 Services: 1,490 Part-time competition: Favorable	Income: 9% Jobs: 24%	2,879	104
Oak Harbor–Whidbey Island, WA	$25,514	Health care: 106 Housing: 94 State/local taxes: 62 Composite: 95	Finance and real estate: −60 Retail trade: 160 Services: 150 Part-time competition: Unfavorable	Income: 2% Jobs: 2%	3,456	66
Ocala, FL	$21,367	Health care: 100 Housing: 74 State/local taxes: 36 Composite: 86	Finance and real estate: 1,940 Retail trade: 5,370 Services: 2,920 Part-time competition: Favorable	Income: 25% Jobs: 47%	4,558	21
Ocean City–Assateague Island, MD	$25,914	Health care: 94 Housing: 77 State/local taxes: 90 Composite: 92	Finance and real estate: 350 Retail trade: 2,500 Services: 900 Part-time competition: Average	Income: 15% Jobs: 16%	3,513	64
Ocean County, NJ	$29,178	Health care: 101 Housing: 112 State/local taxes: 168 Composite: 111	Finance and real estate: 440 Retail trade: 1,580 Services: 1,090 Part-time competition: Favorable	Income: 3% Jobs: 9%	2,586	112
Olympia, WA	$26,988	Health care: 106 Housing: 84 State/local taxes: 58 Composite: 92	Finance and real estate: 160 Retail trade: 2,550 Services: 3,820 Part-time competition: Average	Income: 13% Jobs: 28%	3,373	72
Orlando, FL	$29,100	Health care: 100 Housing: 87 State/local taxes: 45 Composite: 91	Finance and real estate: −660 Retail trade: 23,910 Services: 40,960 Part-time competition: Average	Income: 11% Jobs: 26%	3,163	83
Oscoda–Huron Shore, MI	$20,641	Health care: 93 Housing: 59 State/local taxes: 104 Composite: 87	Finance and real estate: −70 Retail trade: −430 Services: −240 Part-time competition: Average	Income: 13% Jobs: −8%	4,664	18
Panama City, FL	$24,881	Health care: 100 Housing: 69 State/local taxes: 36 Composite: 84	Finance and real estate 120 Retail trade: 1,260 Services: 1,230 Part-time competition: Unfavorable	Income: 11% Jobs: 15%	4,008	35
Paris–Big Sandy, TN	$22,883	Health care: 91 Housing: 56 State/local taxes: 42 Composite: 80	Finance and real estate: 220 Retail trade: 370 Services: 600 Part-time competition: Unfavorable	Income: 21% Jobs: 3%	4,575	20

Place	Household Income	Cost-of-Living Indexes (U.S. = 100)	New Jobs Forecast, 1987–1995	Growth Forecast, 1987–1995	Score	Rank
Petoskey–Straits of Mackinac, MI	$26,967	Health care: 93 Housing: 72 State/local taxes: 134 Composite: 94	Finance and real estate: 70 Retail trade: −260 Services: 1,060 Part-time competition: Average	Income: 5% Jobs: 15%	3,304	76
Phoenix, AZ	$30,460	Health care: 107 Housing: 88 State/local taxes: 71 Composite: 94	Finance and real estate: 16,240 Retail trade: 28,150 Services: 33,440 Part-time competition: Average	Income: 10% Jobs: 23%	2,925	97
Port Angeles–Strait of Juan de Fuca, WA	$25,960	Health care: 106 Housing: 82 State/local taxes: 57 Composite: 91	Finance and real estate: 0 Retail trade: −40 Services: −30 Part-time competition: Average	Income: 6% Jobs: 11%	3,546	60
Portsmouth–Dover–Durham, NH	$34,020	Health care: 93 Housing: 112 State/local taxes: 104 Composite: 103	Finance and real estate: 3,570 Retail trade: 1,700 Services: 8,040 Part-time competition: Unfavorable	Income: 20% Jobs: 35%	2,390	121
Prescott, AZ	$24,227	Health care: 104 Housing: 78 State/local taxes: 59 Composite: 90	Finance and real estate: −160 Retail trade: 2,500 Services: 1,690 Part-time competition: Favorable	Income: 8% Jobs: 41%	3,841	41
Red Bluff–Sacramento Valley, CA	$22,270	Health care: 120 Housing: 72 State/local taxes: 82 Composite: 92	Finance and real estate: 240 Retail trade: 550 Services: 120 Part-time competition: Favorable	Income: 11% Jobs: 21%	4,088	30
Redding, CA	$24,331	Health care: 120 Housing: 85 State/local taxes: 94 Composite: 97	Finance and real estate: 140 Retail trade: 1,490 Services: 2,330 Part-time competition: Average	Income: 7% Jobs: 21%	3,549	59
Rehoboth Bay–Indian River Bay, DE	$27,715	Health care: 101 Housing: 76 State/local taxes: 88 Composite: 92	Finance and real estate: 510 Retail trade: 3,410 Services: 3,120 Part-time competition: Favorable	Income: 11% Jobs: 21%	3,285	77
Reno, NV	$35,162	Health care: 123 Housing: 95 State/local taxes: 43 Composite: 95	Finance and real estate: 1,260 Retail trade: 4,140 Services: 13,280 Part-time competition: Unfavorable	Income: 9% Jobs: 25%	2,507	116
Rhinelander, WI	$24,284	Health care: 96 Housing: 75 State/local taxes: 121 Composite: 94	Finance and real estate: 80 Retail trade: −160 Services: 480 Part-time competition: Unfavorable	Income: 13% Jobs: 2%	3,669	50
Roswell, NM	$24,720	Health care: 92 Housing: 50 State/local taxes: 38 Composite: 78	Finance and real estate: 180 Retail trade: 250 Services: 910 Part-time competition: Average	Income: 5% Jobs: 15%	4,344	26
★ St. George–Zion, UT	$18,165	Health care: 89 Housing: 82 State/local taxes: 76 Composite: 91	Finance and real estate: 50 Retail trade: 570 Services: 2,000 Part-time competition: Average	Income: 27% Jobs: 41%	5,067	11
St. Petersburg–Clearwater, FL	$33,777	Health care: 100 Housing: 85 State/local taxes: 45 Composite: 90	Finance and real estate: 8,100 Retail trade: 24,210 Services: 180 Part-time competition: Favorable	Income: 2% Jobs: 24%	2,755	107

Place	Household Income	Cost-of-Living Indexes (U.S. = 100)	New Jobs Forecast, 1987–1995	Growth Forecast, 1987–1995	Score	Rank
Salinas–Seaside–Monterey, CA	$31,846	Health care: 121 Housing: 121 State/local taxes: 125 Composite: 111	Finance and real estate: 80 Retail trade: 1,670 Services: 4,230 Part-time competition: Unfavorable	Income: 9% Jobs: 10%	2,370	122
San Antonio, TX	$26,095	Health care: 103 Housing: 65 State/local taxes: 47 Composite: 84	Finance and real estate: 7,540 Retail trade: 22,030 Services: 16,240 Part-time competition: Unfavorable	Income: 12% Jobs: 20%	3,821	42
San Diego, CA	$30,496	Health care: 128 Housing: 129 State/local taxes: 126 Composite: 114	Finance and real estate: 16,940 Retail trade: 34,420 Services: 67,020 Part-time competition: Unfavorable	Income: 9% Jobs: 20%	2,409	118
San Luis Obispo, CA	$28,332	Health care: 119 Housing: 109 State/local taxes: 113 Composite: 106	Finance and real estate: 1,240 Retail trade: 2,530 Services: 3,290 Part-time competition: Unfavorable	Income: 7% Jobs: 28%	2,789	106
Santa Fe, NM	$29,547	Health care: 92 Housing: 96 State/local taxes: 58 Composite: 94	Finance and real estate: 710 Retail trade: 5,310 Services: 5,800 Part-time competition: Average	Income: 6% Jobs: 51%	3,016	94
Santa Rosa–Petaluma, CA	$32,567	Health care: 124 Housing: 123 State/local taxes: 128 Composite: 112	Finance and real estate: 1,880 Retail trade: 6,080 Services: 6,790 Part-time competition: Average	Income: 6% Jobs: 29%	2,296	125
Sarasota, FL	$36,322	Health care: 100 Housing: 103 State/local taxes: 53 Composite: 96	Finance and real estate: 4,330 Retail trade: 5,750 Services: 6,400 Part-time competition: Favorable	Income: −4% Jobs: 27%	2,398	119
★ Southport, NC	$19,078	Health care: 83 Housing: 65 State/local taxes: 71 Composite: 85	Finance and real estate: −50 Retail trade: 370 Services: −10 Part-time competition: Average	Income: 21% Jobs: 20%	5,165	9
Springfield, MO	$27,196	Health care: 91 Housing: 64 State/local taxes: 67 Composite: 85	Finance and real estate: 640 Retail trade: 250 Services: 2,710 Part-time competition: Unfavorable	Income: 8% Jobs: 9%	3,623	54
State College, PA	$23,843	Health care: 105 Housing: 106 State/local taxes: 105 Composite: 103	Finance and real estate: 340 Retail trade: 1,280 Services: −690 Part-time competition: Unfavorable	Income: 8% Jobs: 16%	3,411	69
Traverse City–Grand Traverse Bay, MI	$27,414	Health care: 93 Housing: 80 State/local taxes: 144 Composite: 98	Finance and real estate: −20 Retail trade: −550 Services: 620 Part-time competition: Average	Income: 12% Jobs: 8%	3,118	86
Tucson, AZ	$28,519	Health care: 107 Housing: 84 State/local taxes: 67 Composite: 92	Finance and real estate: 2,130 Retail trade: 12,960 Services: 19,250 Part-time competition: Average	Income: 9% Jobs: 25%	3,192	82
Twain Harte–Yosemite, CA	$21,544	Health care: 121 Housing: 97 State/local taxes: 93 Composite: 101	Finance and real estate: 540 Retail trade: 2,340 Services: 2,100 Part-time competition: Favorable	Income: 12% Jobs: 47%	3,849	39

Place	Household Income	Cost-of-Living Indexes (U.S. = 100)	New Jobs Forecast, 1987–1995	Growth Forecast, 1987–1995	Score	Rank
Virginia Beach– Norfolk, VA	$28,265	Health care: 102 Housing: 92 State/local taxes: 93 Composite: 97	Finance and real estate: 3,350 Retail trade: −630 Services: 4,490 Part-time competition: Unfavorable	Income: 14% Jobs: 6%	3,055	92
West Palm Beach– Boca Raton– Delray Beach, FL	$38,764	Health care: 119 Housing: 110 State/local taxes: 56 Composite: 101	Finance and real estate: 12,700 Retail trade: 24,120 Services: 56,050 Part-time competition: Favorable	Income: −1% Jobs: 40%	2,139	131
Winchester, VA	$27,190	Health care: 80 Housing: 86 State/local taxes: 88 Composite: 93	Finance and real estate: −90 Retail trade: 1,310 Services: 1,430 Part-time competition: Average	Income: 2% Jobs: 14%	3,312	75
★ Yuma, AZ	$20,402	Health care: 99 Housing: 66 State/local taxes: 49 Composite: 85	Finance and real estate: 320 Retail trade: 730 Services: 350 Part-time competition: Unfavorable	Income: 20% Jobs: 9%	4,830	15

 ET CETERA: Money Matters

YOUR RETIREMENT STATE TAX GUIDE

Question: Where in America can you find rock-bottom property taxes, no personal income tax on any of your retirement income, no sales tax on the basics you'll need like food and medicine, no inheritance taxes for your heirs to pay, and a minimum of nickel-and-dime fees for licensing a car or for taking out a fishing license?

Answer: Dream on. To fit the requirements for an ideal retirement tax haven, this place would have to have the low property taxes of Louisiana, Alaska's forgiveness of taxes on personal income, and the absence of retail sales taxes as in Oregon. Unfortunately, you just can't find all these wonderful tax breaks together in any one state.

When you retire, federal taxes on private pensions and any income you may have from investments will take the same bite whether you live in Kauai, Keene, or Kerrville, but state taxes differ dramatically around the country. Sales taxes, excise taxes, license taxes, income taxes, property taxes, inheritance taxes, and gift taxes are just some of the forms state taxes can take. Depending on where you want to live, you may encounter all of them or only a few.

Property Taxes. Taxes on land and the buildings on it—whether they are homes, farms, industrial plants, or commercial buildings—are the biggest sources of cash for local governments. Property taxes are imposed not by states but by more than 20,000 cities,

townships, counties, school districts, sanitary districts, hospital districts, and other special districts in the nation. All the states do is specify the maximum rate on the market value of the property, or a percentage of it, as the legal standard for local assessors to follow. The local assessor determines the value to be taxed. If you think the valuation is too high, you have a limited right of appeal.

You can't escape property taxes in any state except Alaska (there you must be over 65 to take advantage of that break), but you can find dramatically low rates in certain parts of the country. Nationally, the average bills on homes amount to 1.23 percent of their market value, while the average bills in Alabama, Hawaii, Louisiana, and West Virginia are based on less than half that rate. In addition, nine states allow specific exemptions, without any income qualification, on property valuation for older homeowners.

Sales Taxes. Sometimes called "retail taxes" or consumption taxes, sales taxes are collected on the purchase of goods at the store level. After property taxes, sales taxes account for the largest source of revenue for state and local governments. Unlike property taxes, however, they will not be deductible from your federal tax return after 1991.

Nationally, sales taxes average 6.6 percent of retail sales. If you're living in Connecticut, you're paying the nation's highest state rate, 7.5 percent. But the highest rate paid by anyone in the country is the 8.5 percent levied on purchase of retail goods in New York City, a

---

Taxing the Necessities

You'll pay sales tax on groceries in . . .

Alabama	Missouri	Tennessee
Arkansas	New Mexico	Utah
Georgia	North Carolina	Virginia
Hawaii	Oklahoma	Wyoming
Idaho	South Carolina	
Kansas	South Dakota	
Mississippi		

And sales tax on medicine in . . .

New Mexico

But NO sales tax on clothing in . . .

Connecticut	New Jersey
Massachusetts	Pennsylvania
Minnesota	Rhode Island

And NO sales tax, period, in . . .

Alaska	New Hampshire
Delaware	Oregon
Montana	

Source: Commerce Clearing House, *State Tax Guide,* 1987.

Taxes are paid by all taxpayers, not just those of retirement age.

---

rate created in 1975 to help the Big Apple pay its debts.

Five states—Alaska, Delaware, Montana, New Hampshire, and Oregon—collect no sales taxes at all. To a retired couple, this could mean $300 to $600 a year in avoided costs. But you can avoid much of that cost in states where such basics as food, medicine, and clothing are exempt from sales taxes.

Personal Income Taxes. When federal income taxes were enacted in 1914, two states—Mississippi and Wisconsin—were already collecting income taxes on their own. It was only during the 1920s and 1930s that the majority of states began to raise cash by tapping personal incomes. Today, 40 states impose the tax; 2 (New Hampshire and Tennessee) apply it only to income from interest and dividends; 1 (Connecticut) applies it only to income from capital gains and dividends; and 7 (Alaska, Florida, Nevada, South Dakota, Texas, Washington, and Wyoming) don't tax incomes at all.

License Taxes. These usually are enacted as flat fees for regulating certain kinds of privileges. For example, you'll pay a license tax on the family car for the right to use it on public highways; you'll buy a fishing license for the privilege of trolling for bass at the lake maintained by the state. Together, these license taxes and fees make up a small part of a state's revenues.

Excise Taxes. In most states, when you return from buying a tankful of gas for the family car, a bottle of gin, and a pack of cigarettes, you've also just paid excise taxes.

Excise taxes are related to sales taxes but are different in that they are levied only on specific items. Gasoline at the pump, for example, is taxed in every state at a higher rate than the local sales tax rate (excise taxes on gasoline are heaviest in Hawaii, lightest in Texas). Tobacco and alcohol, too, are big targets for excise taxes, usually at rates that suggest social disap-

proval. In fact, taxes on cigarettes and liquor are popularly called "sin taxes."

STATE TAX PROFILES

The difference between Montana and New York is more than one between Big Sky Country and the grimy and glittery megalopolitan Northeast. In the five most common taxes that come out of the pockets of residents—personal income, retail sales, residential property, gasoline excise, and auto registration—New Yorkers shoulder more in tax dollars per capita than do citizens in any other state, and their burden is more than three times that of Montana citizens, whose tax burden is the least in the Union.

To help you compare state taxes, *Retirement Places Rated* totals the taxes from personal income, retail sales, residential property, gasoline excise, and auto registration fees that each state collects per capita. Measured against the U.S. average per capita collections from these sources, each state's taxes can be expressed as a percentage. New York's taxes, for example, are 157 percent of the U.S. average; Montana's are 48 percent.

ALABAMA
Per Capita Tax Burden: 60 percent of U.S. average
After Mississippi, Alabama is the poorest state in the

RELOCATION RESOURCES

For many, money matters are a major consideration when choosing where to retire. The following resources provide information on money.

General living costs. Every three months, the American Chamber of Commerce Researchers Association (ACCRA) surveys the costs of housing, food, services, transportation, and health care in 250 locations around the United States. While the ACCRA survey is modeled on what a young family of four buys and hence isn't meant for retirement purposes, it is still enormously useful for making comparisons.

You can order a four-quarter subscription for $75 or the latest quarter's survey for $40 from:

ACCRA
1 Riverfront Plaza
Louisville, KY 40202

Better yet, save your money. If you're thinking of only one or two destinations, call your local chamber of commerce. If it belongs to ACCRA, it can readily give you cost comparisons over the telephone.

Doctors' fees. The maximum dollar amounts that physicians can legally bill their Medicare patients vary tremendously, depending on geography. Indeed, it is possible for two specialists, each practicing in adjacent counties, to charge dramatically different amounts for the same service.

Look up the U.S. Department of Health and Human Services *Medicare Directory of Prevailing Charges* in your library. It breaks the entire United States into 230 geographic areas and details the fees for 29 common medical services performed by general practitioners and 100 physician services performed by specialists in each area.

One caveat: the fees in the directory that doctors can charge you were frozen in 1984. This freeze, which was to have lasted 15 months, has been extended three times, and is, as of this writing, scheduled to thaw in 1987.

country in taxable resources. The state's per capita take from personal income, sales, and property taxes ranks 46th among the 50 states. Like many other Sun Belt states, the Cotton State makes up much of this deficiency with heavy sin taxes on alcohol and tobacco.

Retirement Tax Breaks: Alabama excludes income from public pensions and fully exempts Social Security benefits.

ALASKA
Per Capita Tax Burden: 56 percent of U.S. average
This state holds so many fiscal records that it's in a class by itself. In recent years, it was the richest state in taxable wealth and annually sent checks from its billion dollar permanent fund to each of its citizens. Most of the revenue still comes not from residents' pockets but from North Slope oil and gas drillers. Alaska is the only state ever to have repealed its income tax (1979).

Retirement Tax Breaks: Persons over 65 are exempt from any residential property tax, regardless of gross income.

Other Pluses: There is no income tax or state sales tax. Cities and boroughs, however, may impose local sales tax rates of 1 percent to 5 percent.

Minuses: The state's oil and gas royalties have plunged; Governor Cowper is urging repeal of the property tax exemption and the return of the state personal income tax.

ARIZONA
Per Capita Tax Burden: 89 percent of U.S. average
Without question, the Grand Canyon State overuses its sales tax. It was the second state in the nation to adopt a sales tax (Mississippi was first), doing so in 1933, and currently its collections per capita from that source rank 11th in the country. In contrast, property taxes and personal income taxes rank 32nd and 33rd, respectively, among all 50 states in per capita dollars levied.

Retirement Tax Breaks: Arizona excludes up to $2,500 in Federal Civil Service benefits, doesn't tax Social Security or Railroad Retirement benefits, and allows additional personal exemptions.

Other Pluses: All taxpayers have a hefty ($1,996 if single, $3,992 if married) personal exemption. Food and prescription drugs are exempt from the state's 5 percent sales tax, and Governor Mecham wants sales taxes reduced to 4 percent.

ARKANSAS
Per Capita Tax Burden: 64 percent of U.S. average
Perhaps there is another meaning to Arkansas' nickname, Land of Opportunity. The per capita burden here is one of the lightest in the country. Can there be a connection between this and the rapid growth of certain retirement spots within the state? Among the 45 states that tax retail sales, Arkansas ranks 36th in per capita collections; among the 40 states with a broad-based tax on personal incomes, the state ranks 32nd.

Retirement Tax Breaks: The Arkansas tax code has

provisions for excluding income from private and public pensions, fully exempts Social Security benefits, and allows additional personal tax credits.

Minuses: The combined 5 percent state and local sales tax doesn't exempt groceries and clothing.

CALIFORNIA
Per Capita Tax Burden: 121 percent of U.S. average
California's per capita taxable wealth ranks 7th in the country. After the state's voters approved Proposition 13 in late 1978, California's residential property taxes plunged. The state now ranks 20th in per capita property tax collections. Offsetting that are the 7th highest sales tax collections and the 10th highest income tax collections.

Retirement Tax Breaks: California tax code has provisions for excluding income from public pensions and fully exempts Social Security benefits. The state also has a property tax deferral program for older homeowners.

Pluses: Californians recently approved the Taxpayers' Voting Rights Initiative, requiring voter approval of local property tax increases.

COLORADO
Per Capita Tax Burden: 108 percent of U.S. average
Since the 1960s, the Silver State's economy has rapidly shifted from agriculture and mining to high-technology manufacturing and services. This state was the first to impose an excise tax on gasoline (1919). Per capita retail sales taxes and personal income taxes rank 17th and 24th, respectively, in the country; taxpayers recently rejected an initiative requiring voter approval of new tax increases.

Retirement Tax Breaks: Colorado tax code has provisions for excluding income from private and public pensions and allows additional personal exemptions. The state also has a property tax deferral program for older homeowners.

Minuses: Even though food and medicines are exempt from the sales tax, the combined state and local rate of 7 percent is one of the nation's highest.

CONNECTICUT
Per Capita Tax Burden: 118 percent of U.S. average
Connecticut is well-off in the amount of taxable wealth within its borders, and the state's effort to mine that wealth, in the form of tax revenues, ranks 10th in the country. There is no tax on earned income, but dividends and capital gains are taxed. Two overused taxes here are the property tax and the sales tax.

Retirement Tax Breaks: Persons over 65 who sell their homes at a profit are exempt from the 7 percent capital gains tax (the house must have been their principal residence for five of the last eight years).

Other Pluses: The state has reduced its dividends tax rate and may cut sales taxes to 6.5 percent.

Minuses: Connecticut has high property taxes (1st in per capita collections) and the highest statewide sales tax rate (7.5 percent), though with exemptions on groceries, medicine, and clothing under $75.

DELAWARE
Per Capita Tax Burden: 91 percent of U.S. average

Although you won't pay any sales taxes here, and property taxes are the lowest in the northeastern quarter of the United States, the state compensates for these breaks by having the second-highest per capita personal income tax collections in the country.

Retirement Tax Breaks: Delaware tax code has provisions for excluding income from private and public pensions, fully exempts Social Security benefits, and allows additional personal exemptions.

Other Pluses: There is no sales tax.

Minuses: In spite of cuts approved for 1987 and beyond, taxes on personal incomes will remain among the highest in the country.

FLORIDA
Per Capita Tax Burden: 80 percent of U.S. average

Since the 1950s, this has been *the* retirement state, and its tax effort shows it. Ranking 18th in per capita taxable wealth, the Sunshine State limps in at 37th in actual tax dollars. But Floridians realize that quality services aren't free; recently, they defeated a measure to further increase the homestead exemption.

Retirement Tax Breaks: Florida has a local option property tax deferral program for older homeowners.

Other Pluses: Florida has no tax on personal income, and the state has a low property tax rate with a $25,000 homestead exemption from school district levies for permanent residents.

GEORGIA
Per Capita Tax Burden: 89 percent of U.S. average

Outside of metropolitan Atlanta, Georgia isn't a wealthy state, but it does take pains to tap all sources for revenue. Two overused taxes are retail sales and personal income.

Retirement Tax Breaks: Georgia tax code has provisions for excluding income from private and public pensions, fully exempts Social Security benefits, and allows additional personal exemptions. The state also has a property tax deferral program for older homeowners.

Other Pluses: Governor Harris has recommended no tax increases. The state has surplus funds and may gradually cut income taxes over the next four years.

Minuses: Georgia's sales taxes per capita rank 22nd nationally, with no exemptions for food or clothing.

HAWAII
Per Capita Tax Burden: 144 percent of U.S. average

In 1901, well before any state on the mainland, the Hawaiian Islands began taxing personal income. This tax continues to be the Aloha State's most overused levy. The sales tax is also high by mainland standards.

Retirement Tax Breaks: Hawaii tax code has provisions for excluding income from private and public pensions, fully exempts Social Security benefits, and allows additional personal exemptions. The state also has a special homestead exemption, without income qualification, for older homeowners.

IDAHO
Per Capita Tax Burden: 73 percent of U.S. average

The Gem State's per capita tax collections from all possible sources are the lowest in the Pacific Northwest. There's very little that is exceptional about Idaho's taxes (except perhaps to residents of New York or Massachusetts): the state occupies the low to middle ground in its per capita revenues from sales (44th), personal income (19th), and property (33rd).

Retirement Tax Breaks: Idaho tax code has provisions for excluding income from public pensions, fully exempts Social Security benefits, and allows additional personal exemptions. The state has a special property tax reduction program for older homeowners.

Minuses: There is an inheritance tax; groceries and clothing are not exempt from the 4 percent sales tax.

ILLINOIS
Per Capita Tax Burden: 98 percent of U.S. average

Illinois takes 2.5 percent of your federal adjusted gross income as its tax on personal income. Also, two overused taxes are levies on retail sales and residential property.

Retirement Tax Breaks: For retired persons, the state has a broad range of tax breaks. Illinois excludes income from public pensions, fully exempts Social Security benefits, and allows additional personal exemptions. The state has a property tax deferral program, a special homestead exemption for older homeowners, and has repealed the inheritance tax.

Minuses: Illinois sales tax collections are the country's 17th highest per capita in spite of the reduced rate on groceries and medicine. Property taxes are 15th.

INDIANA
Per Capita Tax Burden: 84 percent of U.S. average

This state fits most people's idea of Middle America, and in fact Indiana's per capita collections of income taxes and property taxes tend to place it in the middle rank among the 50 states.

Retirement Tax Breaks: Indiana tax code has provisions for excluding income from public pensions, fully exempts Social Security benefits, and allows additional personal exemptions.

Other Pluses: Income tax collections are modest (34th per capita nationally); food and medicine are exempt from the state's 5 percent tax.

Minuses: There are no significant property tax breaks without income qualifiers for older homeowners; an inheritance tax is coupled with an estate tax.

IOWA
Per Capita Tax Burden: 90 percent of U.S. average

The Hawkeye State was the first (1921) to spot tobacco as a weed worthy of a tax. Like neighboring Minnesota, Iowa overuses the personal income tax and underuses the retail sales tax. Property taxes rank 24th in the nation in per capita dollars collected.

Retirement Tax Breaks: Iowa tax code has provisions for excluding income from public pensions and allows additional personal tax credits. The state also has a local option property tax deferral program for older homeowners.

Other Pluses: There is a low (4 percent) statewide sales tax with exemptions for food and prescription medicine.

KANSAS
Per Capita Tax Burden: 85 percent of U.S. average
Kansas is richer in taxable wealth than 30 other states, and it takes appropriate steps to collect the revenue, particularly from homeowners.

Retirement Tax Breaks: Kansas excludes income from public pensions and allows additional personal exemptions.

Other Pluses: Sales taxes are low (3 percent), and they are further reduced by exemptions on medicine and disability appliances.

Minuses: There are no significant property tax breaks for older homeowners.

KENTUCKY
Per Capita Tax Burden: 72 percent of U.S. average
One might say the Bluegrass State doesn't tax beyond its means. Taxable wealth here ranks 46th in the country, and so do tax revenues. Property is taxed at bargain rates, but low property tax rates are offset by high rates on personal income. The state ranks 18th in revenue from personal income taxes.

State Tax Treatment of Retirement Income

State	Pension Income Exclusions		Social Security Benefits Fully Exempted	Additional Personal Exemptions	Additional Credit
	Public	Private			
Alabama	•		•		
Arizona	•		•	•	
Arkansas	•	•	•		•
California	•		•		
Colorado	•	•		•	
Delaware	•	•	•	•	
Georgia	•	•	•	•	
Hawaii	•		•	•	
Idaho	•		•	•	
Illinois	•		•	•	
Indiana	•				
Iowa	•				•
Kansas	•			•	
Kentucky	•		•		•
Louisiana	•	•		•	
Maine			•	•	
Maryland	•	•	•	•	
Massachusetts	•		•	•	
Michigan	•	•	•	•	
Minnesota	•	•	•		•
Mississippi	•	•		•	
Missouri	•				
Montana	•	•		•	
Nebraska					
New Jersey	•	•	•	•	
New Mexico	•	•	•	•	
New York	•	•	•	•	
North Carolina	•		•	•	
North Dakota	•			•	
Ohio			•		
Oklahoma	•		•		
Oregon	•		•		
Pennsylvania	•	•		•	
Rhode Island				•	
South Carolina	•	•	•	•	
Utah	•	•			
Vermont				•	
Virginia	•		•	•	
West Virginia	•		•		
Wisconsin	•				•

Source: National Conference of State Legislators, *State Tax Policy & Senior Citizens,* 1985.

Alaska, Florida, Nevada, South Dakota, Texas, Washington, and Wyoming do not tax personal income from any source. Nebraska, Rhode Island, and Vermont calculate personal income taxes as a percentage of federal income tax; therefore, provisions in the federal tax code are implicitly recognized.

Retirement Tax Breaks: Kentucky tax code has provisions for excluding income from public pensions, fully exempts Social Security benefits, and allows additional personal tax credits. The state also has a special $6,500 homestead exemption for older homeowners.

Minuses: There are high personal income taxes.

LOUISIANA
Per Capita Tax Burden: 66 percent of U.S. average
In good times, the Pelican State had an enviable amount of taxable wealth from oil and natural gas production. This wealth took some of the tax pressure off average citizens, but not any longer. Because of a severe budget crunch, the state is aggressively looking for ways to raise cash. Currently, the only overused tax is the sales tax; indeed, Louisiana ranks sixth in the nation in per capita revenues from this source.

Retirement Tax Breaks: Louisiana tax code has provisions for excluding income from private and public pensions, fully exempts Social Security benefits, and allows additional personal exemptions.

Other Pluses: Louisiana has the lowest effective property tax rate of any state in America.

Minuses: High combined state and parish sales tax rate (up to 8 percent) is relieved somewhat by exemptions on groceries and medicine.

MAINE
Per Capita Tax Burden: 101 percent of U.S. average
Maine, it is said, gets the most revenue from the least resources. After Rhode Island, the Pine Tree State is the poorest of all the states in the country's northeastern quarter and ranks 32nd in the nation in per capita taxable wealth. Because of this, the state taps all possible resources for cash.

Retirement Tax Breaks: Maine fully exempts Social Security benefits and allows additional personal exemptions.

Minuses: There is no significant property tax relief for retired homeowners, and there are high estate taxes.

MARYLAND
Per Capita Tax Burden: 124 percent of U.S. average
After New York and Delaware, the Old Line State collects the most dollars per capita from personal income taxes each year. On the other hand, the state ranks in the middle in revenue from sales and property taxes.

Retirement Tax Breaks: Maryland tax code has provisions for excluding income from private and public pensions, fully exempts Social Security benefits, and allows additional personal exemptions.

Minuses: There are no significant property tax breaks for older homeowners.

MASSACHUSETTS
Per Capita Tax Burden: 133 percent of U.S. average
"Taxachusetts," a name pinned on the Bay State during the 1970s, still applies. In spite of the 1980 approval by voters of Proposition 2½ (an initiative to reduce property taxes), the state's take on property taxes ranks sixth in the country. One other overused levy here is the personal income tax.

Retirement Tax Breaks: Massachusetts excludes income from public pensions, fully exempts Social Security benefits, and allows additional personal exemptions. The state also has a local option property tax deferral program for older homeowners.

Other Pluses: The state has a $1 billion surplus. Voters recently approved initiatives to reduce personal income taxes and to limit state revenue growth; sales tax (5 percent) exempts food, clothing, and medicine.

Minuses: There are no significant property tax concessions for older homeowners.

MICHIGAN
Per Capita Tax Burden: 124 percent of U.S. average
Michigan's taxable wealth ranks a modest 31st in the country, but its revenues from taxing residential property and personal incomes rank 4th and 9th, respectively, in per capita dollars.

Retirement Tax Breaks: Michigan tax code has provisions for excluding income from private and public pensions, fully exempts Social Security benefits, and allows additional personal exemptions. The state also has a property tax deferral program for older homeowners.

Other Pluses: Food and medicine are exempt from the state's 4 percent sales tax.

Minuses: Despite modest concessions for people over 65, income and property taxes here are high compared with those of other states.

MINNESOTA
Per Capita Tax Burden: 128 percent of U.S. average
Not only is Minnesota's tax on personal income the highest in the Midwest, but it is also one of the highest in the entire country; the state ranks fourth in per capita dollars collected. Property taxes are also overused in the Gopher State.

Retirement Tax Breaks: Minnesota tax code has provisions for excluding income from private and public pensions, fully exempts Social Security benefits, and allows additional personal tax credits.

Other Pluses: Food, clothing, and medicine are exempt from the 6 percent sales tax.

MISSISSIPPI
Per Capita Tax Burden: 57 percent of U.S. average
In 1900, this state was the poorest in the country; in 1932, it became the first state to adopt a tax on retail sales. Today Mississippi is still the poorest of the 50 states in taxable wealth. Its 55-year-old sales tax, therefore, is its biggest single source of revenue.

Retirement Tax Breaks: Mississippi tax code has provisions for excluding income from private and public pensions, fully exempts Social Security benefits, and allows additional personal exemptions.

MISSOURI
Per Capita Tax Burden: 83 percent of U.S. average
When it comes to per capita taxable wealth, Missouri ranks 34th in the country. The state takes a moderate

approach to tapping revenue from residents; none of its taxes are exceptionally high or low.

Retirement Tax Breaks: Missouri excludes income from public pensions.

Other Pluses: Missouri has low property taxes, ranking 35th nationally in per capita receipts.

MONTANA
Per Capita Tax Burden: 48 percent of U.S. average

In flusher times, Montana enjoyed a stream of revenue from coal and lumber producers that sheltered residents from higher income and property taxes. Today, the state has a budget deficit. Voters recently defeated an initiative that would have eliminated property taxes completely, but it is likely the state will have a 3 percent sales tax in 1989.

Retirement Tax Breaks: Montana tax code has provisions for excluding income from private and public pensions, partially exempts Social Security benefits, and allows additional personal exemptions.

Other Pluses: The state has no sales tax.

Minuses: The agriculture, lumber, and mining sectors of the economy are depressed. Voters may decide on the imposition of a 3 percent sales tax in 1988.

NEBRASKA
Per Capita Tax Burden: 89 percent of U.S. average

The Cornhusker State, like so many other states in America's Heartland, doesn't tax its citizens beyond their capacity to pay. Per capita taxable wealth here ranks 20th in the country, and taxes from all sources rank 21st.

Retirement Tax Breaks: There are none. Nebraska claims a flat 19 percent of taxpayer's federal income tax liability.

Minuses: The farm economy is in a slump. Nebraska will boost personal income tax rates in the face of revenue losses from federal tax reform. Sales taxes have already been boosted, effective January 1987.

NEVADA
Per Capita Tax Burden: 77 percent of U.S. average

Gambling is Nevada's biggest man-made tax resource. If it weren't for the tables and slots in Reno and Las Vegas, the local citizenry would be shelling out money in the form of income taxes and dramatically higher property taxes.

Retirement Tax Breaks: Nevada has no inheritance taxes.

Other Pluses: There is no tax on personal income.

Minuses: In spite of exemptions on food and medicine, Nevada's high sales tax (6 percent in Reno, 5.75 percent elsewhere) results in the fourth highest per capita receipts in the nation. Beginning in 1987, an estate tax will be imposed.

NEW HAMPSHIRE
Per Capita Tax Burden: 65 percent of U.S. average

Southern New Hampshire has been filling up with Boston commuters for a good reason. Compared with Massachusetts (and all other states in the Northeast), the Granite State is a tax haven. There are no sales

taxes here, nor are there taxes on earned income (dividend and interest income, however, is taxed at 5 percent). On the other hand, property and excise taxes are high, a pattern typical throughout New England.

Retirement Tax Breaks: New Hampshire has a local option property tax deferral program for older homeowners.

Other Pluses: There is no sales tax or tax on earned income.

Minuses: Property taxes per capita rank third highest in the country with no significant exemptions for older homeowners.

NEW JERSEY
Per Capita Tax Burden: 117 percent of U.S. average

This state was the last to adopt the income tax, doing so in 1976 to tap the earnings of New York City and Philadelphia commuters.

Retirement Tax Breaks: New Jersey tax code has provisions for excluding income from private pensions and public pensions, fully exempts Social Security benefits, and allows additional personal exemptions. The state also allows a special property tax credit to older homeowners.

Other Pluses: Food, clothing, and medicines are exempt from the state's 6 percent sales tax.

Minuses: The Garden State's per capita property tax collections are second highest in the United States.

NEW MEXICO
Per Capita Tax Burden: 66 percent of U.S. average

The Land of Enchantment has attracted many older adults for three decades, and one of the reasons is its relatively small effort to tax property and income. Nationally, the state ranks 13th in taxable wealth per capita but only 33rd in the pains it takes to tap that wealth for revenue.

Retirement Tax Breaks: New Mexico tax code has provisions for excluding income from private and public pensions, fully exempts Social Security benefits, and allows additional personal exemptions.

Other Pluses: The lowest property taxes in the Desert Southwest are found here.

Minuses: The state has high combined state and local sales taxes (fifth in the nation in per capita collections) with no exemptions.

NEW YORK
Per Capita Tax Burden: 157 percent of U.S. average

The Empire State collects more direct taxes from its residents than any other state. (Alaska collects more per capita revenue, but most of it comes from oil and gas drillers.) There are three glaringly overused taxes here: personal income (highest in the country in per capita dollars collected), sales (eighth highest), and property (ninth highest).

Retirement Tax Breaks: New York tax code has provisions for excluding income from private and public pensions, fully exempts Social Security benefits, and allows additional personal exemptions.

Minuses: Combined state and local sales tax averages 7 percent but is softened somewhat by exemptions on food and medicine. No significant tax breaks for retired persons on earned income, interest and dividends, business profits, or residential property.

NORTH CAROLINA
Per Capita Tax Burden: 78 percent of U.S. average
Like South Carolina, the Tar Heel State has no abundance of taxable resources and therefore doesn't make a strenuous effort to extract money from taxpayers. Two overused taxes, however, are income (15th highest per capita in the country) and excise (in 1969, North Carolina became the last state in the country to tax cigarettes).

Retirement Tax Breaks: North Carolina tax code has provisions for excluding income from public pensions, fully exempts Social Security benefits, and allows additional personal exemptions.

NORTH DAKOTA
Per Capita Tax Burden: 58 percent of U.S. average
The popular conception of the Flickertail State is that it is out of the mainstream, and that the state and its windblown prairie deserve each other. Actually, this agrarian state ranks 12th in taxable wealth per capita, ahead of such industrial states as Michigan and Pennsylvania. Unlike those two states, however, North Dakota still keeps to the agrarian tradition and doesn't exhaust its taxable wealth for revenue.

Retirement Tax Breaks: North Dakota tax code has provisions for excluding income from public pensions and allows additional personal exemptions.

Minuses: North Dakota has increased personal income taxes effective for tax years after 1986.

OHIO
Per Capita Tax Burden: 92 percent of U.S. average
The Buckeye State ranks 20th among the states in the per capita amount of revenue it extracts from citizens. It overuses personal income taxes, property taxes, and retail sales taxes.

Retirement Tax Breaks: Ohio fully exempts Social Security benefits and allows additional personal exemptions.

OKLAHOMA
Per Capita Tax Burden: 74 percent of U.S. average
The Sooner State is surviving the slump in the oil patch with difficulty. All of its taxes except retail sales are underused. This may change as the state struggles to overcome a severe budget crunch.

Retirement Tax Breaks: Oklahoma tax code has provisions for excluding income from public pensions and fully exempts Social Security benefits.

Other Pluses: The state's effective property tax rate is one of the country's lowest.

Minuses: Food and over-the-counter medicines aren't exempt from a combined state and local sales tax that, in some cities, tops 7 percent.

OREGON
Per Capita Tax Burden: 102 percent of U.S. average
Oregon's property taxes are the highest of all states west of the Rocky Mountains; its income tax collections rank fifth per capita in the country, highest of any state west of Mississippi.

Retirement Tax Breaks: Oregon tax code has provisions for excluding income from public pensions, fully exempts Social Security benefits, and allows additional personal exemptions. The state also has a property tax deferral program for older homeowners.

Other Pluses: Oregon has no sales tax. Voters recently rejected an amendment to the state constitution imposing a new 5 percent sales tax starting in 1988.

PENNSYLVANIA
Per Capita Tax Burden: 93 percent of U.S. average
For a relatively poor state (35th in potential tax revenues), the Keystone State resembles others in the northeastern portion of the country in leaving no possible tax untried.

Retirement Tax Breaks: Pennsylvania tax code has provisions for excluding income from private and public pensions, and fully exempts Social Security benefits.

Minuses: Two greatly overused levies here are personal income taxes and inheritance taxes. Pennsylvania has a heavy (6 percent) sales tax, somewhat lightened by exemptions for food, clothing, and medicine.

RHODE ISLAND
Per Capita Tax Burden: 119 percent of U.S. average
Like Maine, Rhode Island gets the most with the least. The state ranks only 42nd in taxable wealth but 12th in the per capita amount of revenue it extracts from all sources. Of these sources, the biggest are residential property and personal income.

Retirement Tax Breaks: Rhode Island claims a flat 22.21 percent of taxpayer's federal tax liability but allows additional personal exemptions.

Minuses: Rhode Island has high estate taxes and extremely high property taxes with no significant breaks for older homeowners.

SOUTH CAROLINA
Per Capita Tax Burden: 73 percent of U.S. average
For all of South Carolina's industrial growth, particularly in textiles and high technology, the state ranks 48th in taxable wealth (higher than only Mississippi and Alabama).

Retirement Tax Breaks: South Carolina tax code has provisions for excluding income from private and public pensions, fully exempts Social Security benefits, and allows additional personal exemptions. The state also has a special homestead exemption, without income qualification, for older homeowners.

Minuses: Two taxes that the Palmetto State overuses are income taxes (20th in per capita collections) and sales taxes (34th) with only residential fuel and medicine exempt.

SOUTH DAKOTA
Per Capita Tax Burden: 64 percent of U.S. average
All else being equal, demographers say, South Dakota will continue to lose population. This state is a contrast

to neighboring North Dakota. It is poorer in taxable wealth but doesn't make up for this deficiency by imposing an income tax.

Retirement Tax Breaks: There are none.

Other Pluses: There is no tax on personal income.

Minuses: South Dakota has high sales taxes (18th nationally in per capita collections) with only one significant exemption: medicine.

TENNESSEE
Per Capita Tax Burden: 64 percent of U.S. average
The Volunteer State adopted the sales tax somewhat late (1947); today retail sales taxes and special taxes on liquor, tobacco, and gasoline are the state's major sources for revenue. Like other states in the country's southern quarter, Tennessee isn't tax-rich by any standard, nor does it take pains to tap citizens beyond their capacity to pay.

Retirement Tax Breaks: Tennessee has a local option property tax deferral program for older homeowners.

Other Pluses: There is no tax on earned income.

Minuses: The combined state and local sales tax rate can be as much as 7.75 percent; income from dividends and interest is taxed at 6 percent.

TEXAS
Per Capita Tax Burden: 68 percent of U.S. average
Prior to the collapse of the oil patch, Texas once was so wealthy in taxable resources that, if it had levied average U.S. taxes on oil, gas, personal income, property, and retail sales, it could have collected another $6 billion a year in revenue. As it stands, the Lone Star State ranks only 39th in its effort to tap citizens for revenue; indeed, there is really no tax that can be regarded as overused here.

Retirement Tax Breaks: Texas has a property tax deferral program and a special homestead exemption for older homeowners.

Other Pluses: Texas has no tax on personal income.

UTAH
Per Capita Tax Burden: 89 percent of U.S. average
Utah ranks 44th in taxable resources but manages to extract enough tax dollars to push it into the middle rank in tax collections. Its most overused levy is the sales tax.

Retirement Tax Breaks: Utah tax code has provisions for excluding income from private and public pensions. The state also has a property tax deferral program for older homeowners.

Minuses: High (5 percent) sales taxes are relieved only by an exemption on medicine. The state will likely boost its personal income tax because of a budget crunch.

VERMONT
Per Capita Tax Burden: 93 percent of U.S. average
The Green Mountain State was the last state in the Union to adopt a sales tax (1969). Most of its revenue comes from property taxes that it taps from the owners of vacation homes and Vermonters with equal energy. In fact, property tax collections are the eighth highest

per capita in the country. Another tax Vermont overuses is the personal income tax.

Retirement Tax Breaks: Vermont claims a flat 25.85 percent of taxpayer's federal tax liability for 1987 but allows additional personal exemptions.

Other Pluses: Vermont has a low 4 percent statewide sales tax that exempts food and prescription medicines.

VIRGINIA
Per Capita Tax Burden: 94 percent of U.S. average
The Old Dominion State has been rising in taxable wealth since World War II. Its most overused tax is the one on personal income. Another overused tax is the "sin" excise tax on tobacco, liquor, and gasoline.

Retirement Tax Breaks: Virginia tax code has provisions for excluding income from public pensions, fully exempts Social Security benefits, and allows additional personal exemptions. The state also has a local option property tax deferral program.

Minuses: While the combined state and local 4 percent sales tax is a modest one, groceries aren't exempt.

WASHINGTON
Per Capita Tax Burden: 117 percent of U.S. average
Washington ranks first in the country in per capita collections from the retail sales tax, but this levy that residents encounter daily is partially offset on April 15 by the absence of a tax on personal incomes.

Retirement Tax Breaks: Washington has a property tax deferral program for older homeowners.

Other Pluses: There is no tax on personal income. Washington voters recently defeated a measure to boost sales taxes.

Minuses: Though groceries and prescription medicines are exempt, cities and counties add .5 percent to 1.6 percent to the state's already high 6.5 percent sales tax.

WEST VIRGINIA
Per Capita Tax Burden: 76 percent of U.S. average
West Virginia isn't quite as poor as its 1960s Appalachian image. The state ranks 38th in taxable wealth. The overused sales tax is offset by low taxes on personal income and residential property.

Retirement Tax Breaks: West Virginia tax code has provisions for excluding income from public pensions and fully exempts Social Security benefits. The state also has a $20,000 homestead exemption for older homeowners.

Other Pluses: West Virginia's effective property tax rate is the fourth lowest in the country, after Louisiana's, Wyoming's, and Hawaii's. West Virginia voters recently defeated a measure to boost sales taxes from 5 percent to 6 percent. In spite of the state's budget deficit, Governor Moore is urging that taxes on personal incomes be reduced.

WISCONSIN
Per Capita Tax Burden: 132 percent of U.S. average
Like neighboring Minnesota, the Badger State has a tax

package with an onerous reputation. Wisconsin's taxable wealth ranks 37th in the country, but its tax collections rank 4th. The state taps every possible source for revenue, and it overuses three taxes: personal income, inheritance and estate, and residential property.

Retirement Tax Breaks: Wisconsin tax code has provisions for excluding income from public pensions, partially exempts Social Security benefits, and allows additional personal tax credits.

Other Pluses: Governor-elect Thompson has pledged a 5 percent reduction in personal income taxes and a reduction in the state's inheritance tax.

WYOMING
Per Capita Tax Burden: 76 percent of U.S. average
Until the slump in the oil and natural gas business, this state was the second richest in potential tax wealth per capita. Three features of Wyoming's fiscal scene are its absence of a state income tax, its extremely low property taxes, and the highest taxes for using the automobile (license, registration, and gasoline) in the country.

Retirement Tax Breaks: There are none.

Other Pluses: Wyoming has no tax on personal income, no inheritance tax, a low (3 percent) sales tax exempting medicine and disability appliances, and one of country's lowest effective property tax rates.

Minuses: Sales taxes and property taxes may rise to offset lagging royalties from natural resources.

MUNICIPAL BONDS AREN'T TAX EXEMPT EVERYWHERE

Even though income from state and local government obligations, collectively called "municipal bonds," is exempt from federal income tax, it isn't necessarily exempt from state personal income taxes. Thirty-eight

---

State Tax Burdens

Tax burdens in each state are typically determined by dividing total tax collections by the state's population. Doing it this way makes Alaska's $4,585 per capita tax burden seem the heaviest in the nation.

Almost all of Alaska's revenues, however, come from royalty fees on natural resources. If you consider the revenue that states routinely collect from the pockets of residents—personal income taxes, residential property taxes, retail sales taxes, gasoline taxes, and automobile registration taxes—Alaska actually has the second lowest per capita tax burden of the 50 states.

Comparing Tax Burdens: The States Ranked from Lowest to Highest

State	Per Capita Tax Burden	State	Per Capita Tax Burden
1. Montana	$ 390	26. Utah	$ 718
2. Alaska	454	26. Georgia	718
3. Mississippi	462	28. Arizona	719
4. North Dakota	463	29. Iowa	725
5. Alabama	487	30. Delaware	736
6. Arkansas	513	31. Ohio	742
7. Tennessee	517	32. Vermont	748
8. South Dakota	519	33. Pennsylvania	749
9. New Hampshire	520	34. Virginia	753
10. Louisiana	529	35. Illinois	785
10. New Mexico	529	36. Maine	812
12. Texas	544	37. Oregon	824
13. Kentucky	582	38. Colorado	871
14. South Carolina	588	39. Washington	940
15. Idaho	589	40. New Jersey	943
16. Oklahoma	594	41. Connecticut	948
17. Wyoming	608	42. Rhode Island	959
18. West Virginia	610	43. California	975
19. Nevada	620	44. Maryland	995
20. North Carolina	624	45. Michigan	1,002
21. Florida	640	46. Minnesota	1,028
22. Missouri	669	47. Wisconsin	1,060
23. Indiana	674	48. Massachusetts	1,073
24. Kansas	681	49. Hawaii	1,163
25. Nebraska	713	50. New York	1,266

Source: Advisory Commission on Intergovernmental Relations, *Tax Capacity of the States*, 1986.

The above figures are each state's total per capita tax collections on personal income, residential property, retail sales, gasoline, and automobile registration. The U.S. average is $805.

states tax income from out-of-state municipal bonds; of these, five states tax income from in-state municipal bonds as well. Only five states—Indiana, Nebraska, New Mexico, Utah, and Vermont—don't tax the income at all. Alaska, Florida, Nevada, South Dakota, Texas, Washington, and Wyoming do not tax personal income from any source.

Personal Income Taxes on Municipal Bonds

State	State's Own Bonds	Other States' Bonds
Alabama		•
Arizona		•
Arkansas		•
California		•
Colorado		•
Connecticut		•
Delaware		•
Georgia		•
Hawaii		•
Idaho		•
Illinois	•	•
Indiana		
Iowa	•	•
Kansas	•	•
Kentucky		
Louisiana		•
Maine		•
Maryland		•
Massachusetts		•
Michigan		•
Minnesota		•
Mississippi		•
Missouri		•
Montana		•
Nebraska		
New Hampshire		•
New Jersey		•
New Mexico		
New York		•
North Carolina		•
North Dakota		•
Ohio		•
Oklahoma	•	•
Oregon		•
Pennsylvania		•
Rhode Island		•
South Carolina		•
Tennessee		•
Utah		
Vermont		
Virginia		•
West Virginia		•
Wisconsin	•	•

Source: Commerce Clearing House, *State Tax Guide*, 1987.
A • indicates municipal bonds are taxable.

FEDERAL TAXES AREN'T DEDUCTIBLE EVERYWHERE

Of the 40 states with broad-based income taxes, 15 allow taxpayers to deduct federal income taxes. Is this an advantage? It is if you're deciding between two states with similar tax rates, but only one of them allows you to deduct. In the latter case, your effective tax rate would be less. The following states allow deductions of federal income taxes:

Alabama	Minnesota
Arizona	Missouri
Colorado	Montana
Delaware	North Dakota
Iowa	Oklahoma
Kansas	Oregon
Kentucky	Utah
Louisiana	

Source: Commerce Clearing House, *State Tax Guide,* 1987.

OVERCOMING THE "OVERQUALIFIED" OBJECTION

While job discrimination on the basis of age is against the law, you might still be a victim of what labor economists call "statistical discrimination," which happens when an employer assumes three things about an older person applying for a job:

- You want more money because you have more experience.
- Your fringe coverage—life insurance, health insurance, and pension benefits—will cost more than fringes for younger applicants.
- Your prospects for staying with a job and justifying the employer's investment in on-the-job training are less than those of a younger worker.

All of these factors fall under the catch-all word *overqualified;* it's the word most frequently used by an employer when turning down older people who've applied for a job.

Anyone who has worked 20, 30, or 40 years is overqualified by standard definition. Too often, older workers nod agreement, thank the employer for his or her time, and hit the pavement for more job hunting.

Why not ask the employer what is meant by "overqualified"? If you'll go to work at the going rate, plus bring experience and maturity to the job, won't that mean that the cost of your productivity will be less than or equal to a younger worker's? If you're already covered by Medicare and Social Security, won't the employer avoid the cost of health insurance and a pension plan if you're hired? If the average tenure of younger workers in certain jobs is less than the shelf life of hamburger or yogurt, mightn't you make a better bet for longevity?

SHOULD YOU RAID YOUR SAVINGS?

How long would your savings last if you dipped into them for regular income? Suppose you have a $20,000 savings account, earning 5.5 percent interest compounded quarterly, at a local savings and loan association. You could withdraw $136 each month for the next 20 years before your savings would be reduced to zero. Or you could take out $92 from the account each month for as long as you wanted and the $20,000 balance of your savings account would remain intact.

Whether or not you should raid your savings depends on how much you want to leave your heirs, how well insured you are against medical and other emergencies, how prudently you make other investments, and how the inflation rate fluctuates. Drawing from your savings isn't wrong; after all, it's your money. Some retired persons, however, spend too much of their savings too soon. Others never touch their savings; to their regret, they learn too late that they could easily have afforded more comforts in their retirement.

Drawing on a Savings Account

Starting with savings of . . .	. . . you can withdraw this much each month for the stated number of years, reducing the savings account to zero in,				OR, you can withdraw this much each month and leave the original amount intact
	10 years	15 years	20 years	25 years	
$10,000	$ 107	$ 81	$ 68	$ 61	$ 46
15,000	161	121	102	91	69
20,000	215	162	136	121	92
25,000	269	202	170	152	115
30,000	322	243	204	182	138
40,000	430	323	272	243	184
50,000	537	404	340	304	230
60,000	645	485	408	364	276
80,000	859	647	544	486	368
100,000	1,074	808	680	607	468

Climate:
Seasons,
Temperatures,
and Comfort

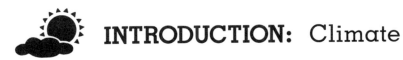 **INTRODUCTION:** Climate

"The fortunate people of the planet," John Kenneth Galbraith wrote years ago in *Harper's*, "are those who live by the seasons. There is far more difference between a Vermont farm in the summer and that farm in the winter than there is between San Diego and São Paulo. This means that people who live where the seasons are good and strong have no need to travel; they can stay at home and let change come to them. This simple truth will one day be recognized and then we will see a great reverse migration from Florida to Maine and on into Quebec."

Galbraith's forecast may still be too optimistic. The migration to the sun continues—and it won't let up, some experts predict, until well into the 21st century. Why should it? Americans say they prefer mild, sunny climates, and when asked where in the country these climates are, they point to the fast-growing lower half of the Pacific Coast, Florida, and anywhere along the South Atlantic and Gulf Coast Shore. Certainly this area, between 25 degrees and 35 degrees latitude, has been drawing older adults for decades.

But other places north of the Mason-Dixon line and hundreds of miles from ocean beaches benefit from retirement growth, and many of these enjoy mild climates, too. Some of these places might surprise you.

What has always been surprising is the enormous variety of global climates found right here at home. Northern maritime, extremely mild Mediterranean, southerly mountain, lowland desert, tropical "paradise," desert highland, rugged northern continental, windward slope, leeward slope, and humid subtropical climates—you name it, you'll meet up with it somewhere in the United States.

Climate is a part of your circumstances that can't be bought, built, remodeled, or relocated. A place's climate is there for keeps, and the weather events that make up a place's climate—rain, snow, heat, cold, drought, wind—will have a profound effect on the rest of your life.

WHAT FACTORS DETERMINE CLIMATE?

Five geographic factors are major determinants of the climate of any area: water, latitude, elevation, prevailing winds, and mountain ranges.

Large bodies of water, particularly oceans, take the edge off temperature. Water warms up slowly, holds much more heat than does land, and cools more slowly. Places near or surrounded by water tend to be cooler in summer and warmer in winter than others far from water. San Francisco, with water on three sides, experiences a marine climate that is one of the mildest and least changing in North America.

Places located in the middle of large landmasses, away from the moderating effects of water, experience wide swings of temperature. These continental climates tend to be more rigorous in the higher latitudes. The closer to the poles you get, the more exaggerated are the seasonal shifts, because polar (and very northerly) locations undergo the greatest seasonal variation in the amount and intensity of sunlight. In Fairbanks, Alaska, for example, the average "day" (the period between the sun's rising and setting) in December is only 4 hours long. But in late June, the day has lengthened to more than 18 hours, and the sun's heat is intense. Places in the North and Far North, then, can experience not only Siberian winters but also sun-baked summers. Elevation, or height above sea level, has the same effect as a higher latitude. Each 1,000 feet of elevation lowers the average temperature by 3.3 degrees Fahrenheit. In New Mexico, for example, there are just 3 degrees difference in annual average temperature between two weather stations at similar elevations, one in the extreme northeast and the other in the extreme southwest. However, at two weather stations just 15 miles apart, but differing in elevation by 4,700 feet, the average annual temperatures differ by 16 degrees.

In the United States, places that combine high altitudes with southerly latitudes seem to get the best of both North and South, enjoying the mild, short winters of the South and the cooler nights and crisp falls of the North. Asheville, North Carolina, in the southern Appalachian Mountains, and Santa Fe, New Mexico, in the mountains of the Southwest have long been known for their mild, four-season climates.

To understand how prevailing winds influence climate, consider a pair of retirement places: Port Angeles–Strait of Juan de Fuca, Washington, and Bar Harbor–Frenchman Bay, Maine. Both are at northerly latitudes. Both are situated on major oceans. You'd naturally suppose that the two retirement places

---

Behind Every Silver Lining . . .

The National Oceanic and Atmospheric Administration (NOAA), at each of its weather stations, measures local cloudiness during daylight hours only.

NOAA defines a day as . . .	if clouds form
Clear	0% to 30%
Partly cloudy	40% to 70%
Cloudy	80% to 100%
	of the sky cover.

would have roughly the same type of climate. Why, then, does Port Angeles have much milder temperatures? The answer lies in the prevailing winds that sweep across the continent. In the United States, prevailing winds blow from west to east. Places on the West Coast are landfalls for air that has moved thousands of miles over water; cities even hundreds of miles inland still feel some of the beneficial effects of the Pacific winds. But inland cities in the East feel few consequences of the Atlantic save on those rare occasions when the prevailing wind direction turns. Sad to say, this reversal of wind direction often means a storm.

Mountain ranges help determine climate and weather by acting as giant barriers that deflect and channel winds and weather. The weather—and also climate—on one side of a mountain range is often radically different from that on the other. In winter, for example, the Great Divide shields Missoula, Montana, from much of the bitter cold air that moves down the continent from the Arctic. Because of this, mountain ranges are natural dividing points between climate zones.

AMERICA'S MAJOR CLIMATIC REGIONS

Mountain ranges also mark the seven major climatic regions of the continental United States. The Pacific Coast is the mildest of these regions, and the northern portion of the Great Interior is the most rigorous. The Intermountain Plateau (also called the "Great Basin"), lying between the Sierra Nevada range to the west and the Rocky Mountains to the east, is noted primarily for its dryness. Some of the best climates for variety and mildness are found in the southern portion of this area. The southern half of the Appalachian Mountains region also offers climates that are both mild and variable.

Most Americans live in the large climatic zone that includes the Great Interior, Southern Plains, and Lowlands regions. Ironically, this zone also happens to be the least desirable for human comfort. Those who live in its northern part are plagued by severe winters and hot, humid summers with springs and autumns that are all too short. In the southern portion, winters are mild and springs and autumns are longer, but the steam-bath summers are uncomfortable. The climate of the East Coast (called the "Middle and North Atlantic Lowlands") is similar to that of the Great Interior, but milder and somewhat damper. Right on the coast, winters are milder and summers are noticeably cooler. Several retirement places with excellent climates can be found here, notably New Jersey's Cape May and Ocean counties, Ocean City–Assateague Island in Maryland, and Rehoboth Bay–Indian River Bay in Delaware.

Climatic Regions of the United States

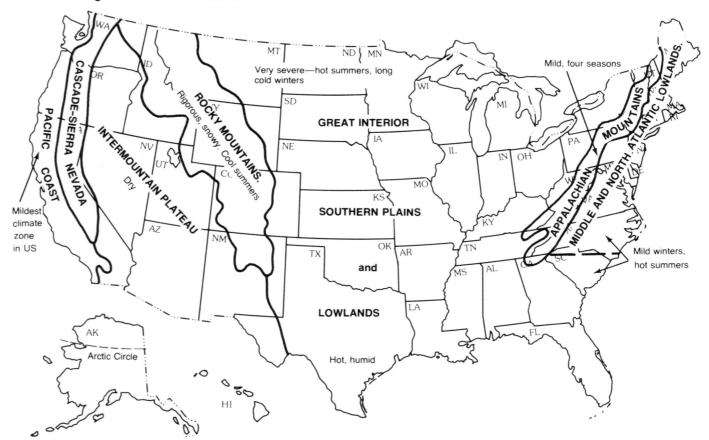

The high-altitude regions that include the Rocky Mountains, the Cascades and Sierra Nevada range, and the northern half of the Appalachian Mountains are resort areas because they all have cool, crisp, sunny summers with cold nights and winters that provide plenty of snow for outdoor sports. These places are popular with older adults who enjoy a stimulating yet not too mild climate.

The Alaskan climate varies from bitterly cold in the northern tundra area—one fifth of the state lies north of the Arctic Circle—to relatively mild temperatures in the interior and southern regions. The southern area experiences abundant rainfall, the Aleutian Islands chain being one of the stormiest regions in the world.

Hawaii is the only state situated in the tropical zone, officially defined as any area where temperatures don't drop below 64 degrees. These islands experience small temperature changes; summer temperatures average only 4 to 8 degrees higher than those in winter. Moisture-bearing trade winds from over the Pacific provide a system of natural ventilation for the heat associated with tropical climates.

SO, WHAT'S COMFORTABLE?

Mop the sweat from pulling a balky lawnmower's starter cord a dozen times on a July afternoon, hack away at the icy rime on the car's windshield one morning in January, or gaze out the window at a gray day, and you're forgiven for fantasizing about a place where it's never hot or cold and always bright.

It may be a fantasy, indeed. Not only might you become bored with endless dry sunny days and tepid temperatures, but you'll also find that none of the climates of the retirement places profiled here matches this pattern 365 days a year. Because the thermometer is the most useful instrument for telling how comfortable you might be outdoors, however, *Retirement Places Rated* considers air temperature in rating climate.

Temperature

Beware of chamber of commerce blandishments about a place's annual average temperature. San Francisco's is 57 degrees. So is St. Louis's. But San Francisco enjoys both a diurnal (24 hour) temperature range of 12 degrees and an annual range (the difference between January's and July's average temperatures) of 12 degrees. St Louis has a diurnal range of 17 degrees and an annual range of 47. The temperature swings in these two cities highlight the difference between a marine climate and a continental climate. San Francisco's climate is somewhat cool and remarkably stable year-round. St. Louis's is neither.

Among retirement regions, the greatest annual temperature ranges (up to 77 degrees) are found in the North Woods, the Rocky Mountains, and northern parts of the Yankee Belt. The greatest diurnal temperature swings (up to 37 degrees) are in high desert parts

Hottest Retirement Places

	Annual 90-Degree Days	Relative Humidity
McAllen–Edinburg–Mission, TX	117	55%
San Antonio, TX	111	55
Ocala, FL	110	60
Fort Myers–Cape Coral, FL	106	56
Orlando, FL	104	60
Canton–Lake Tawakoni, TX	103	55
Brownsville–Harlingen, TX	102	61
Austin, TX	101	56
Naples, FL	101	60
Athens–Cedar Creek Lake, TX	95	68
Hot Springs–Lake Ouachita, AR	90	55
Lakeland–Winter Haven, FL	83	60
Bradenton, FL	81	65
St. Petersburg–Clearwater, FL	81	57
Sarasota, FL	81	65
Fort Lauderdale–Hollywood–Pompano Beach, FL	76	65
Fort Walton Beach, FL	75	65
Panama City, FL	75	65

Listed above are those retirement places that combine 75 or more 90-degree days with relative humidities closest to noon of 55 percent or higher. Four retirement places have more than 130 ninety-degree days per year—Yuma (168), Phoenix (164), and Tucson (139), Arizona, and Las Vegas (131)—but all of them have summer noontime relative humidities of less than 30 percent; therefore, they are not included on the list.

Coldest Retirement Places

	Annual Freezing Days
Flagstaff, AZ	213
Kalispell, MT	191
Bend, OR	190
Missoula, MT	189
Reno, NV	189
Laconia–Lake Winnipesaukee, NH	187
North Conway–White Mountains, NH	187
Eagle River, WI	182
Rhinelander, WI	182

Source: National Oceanic and Atmospheric Administration, *Local Climatological Data,* and *Climatography of the United States.*

Listed above are those retirement places with six months or more of days when the temperature drops to 32 degrees Fahrenheit or below.

of the Rio Grande and Desert Southwest regions. The smallest diurnal *and* annual temperature swings are in Hawaii and along the Pacific Coast.

More than any other climate variable, temperature—and temperature changes—influence comfort and daily activities. Many older adults readily adapt to wide temperature swings. Others, even if they are in excellent health, need a much longer time. "In rapid weather changes," observed the late bioclimatologist H. E. Landsberg, the human body sometimes "lags behind the events in its attempts to keep all factors in equilibrium. Thus, a person may always be a bit out of balance and not feel well even though he has no specific disease."

Bioclimatologists—scientists who study the connection between weather and health—generally agree that temperatures that don't fall far below 65 degrees Fahrenheit are ideal for outdoor work and play. Under that point, the body's metabolism is pressed to maintain its normal warm core temperature. Eventually, you either put on extra clothing or you go indoors. *Retirement Places Rated* fixes 65 degrees as a standard for mildness at the low end of the thermometer.

At the thermometer's upper end, we stop at 80 degrees. Why? Under experimental conditions, a person lying nude in a dark room neither gains nor loses body heat if the dry air temperature is 86 degrees. At most locations in this country, however, an 80-degree air temperature marks the point above which humidity starts to increase "felt" heat up to and beyond normal 86-degree skin temperature. Just as the body works harder to maintain a warmer core temperature when the thermometer falls below 65 degrees, so also is it pressed to maintain a cooler core temperature when the temperature is above 80.

This 15-degree swing between a low of 65 and a high of 80 is a sufficiently stimulating daily temperature variation for many older adults. It marks a cool point at night (65 degrees) below which home heating may be necessary and a warm point during the day (80 degrees) above which the human body starts to gain heat.

None of the 131 retirement places *exactly* matches this cool night–warm day cycle throughout the year. However, if you count each degree of monthly mean temperature variation (from a low of 65 and a high of 80) during June, July, and August, the retirement places with the mildest summers may surprise you. San Diego and the Hawaiian twins aside, these places are on the Atlantic Coast above Chesapeake Bay and in the country's interior.

What would surprise no one are the retirement places that experience mild winters. They make up nearly an all-Florida list. Certainly, retirement places in the Sunshine State enjoy mild weather for most of the year. In the summer months, however, their weather turns hellish with high temperatures and humidity.

Humidity

After temperature, humidity—the amount of moisture in the air—is the major factor in climatic comfort. As anyone who has suffered a hot, humid summer knows, humidity intensifies heat. A hot day that is humid is uncomfortable because the body's natural cooling process of evaporation is retarded.

But there is another reason damp air increases felt heat in the summertime. Just as warm air holds more moisture, so damp air holds heat better and longer. Therefore, in hot, humid climates, heat is retained in the damp air even after the sun goes down, resulting in nights that are almost as hot as the days.

The Mildest Winters

Bradenton, FL
Brownsville–Harlingen, TX
Daytona Beach, FL
Fort Lauderdale–Hollywood–
  Pompano Beach, FL
Fort Myers–Cape Coral, FL
Kauai, HI
Lakeland–Winter Haven, FL
Maui, HI
McAllen–Edinburg–Mission, TX
Melbourne–Titusville–Palm Bay, FL
Miami–Hialeah, FL
Naples, FL
Ocala, FL
Orlando, FL
St. Petersburg–Clearwater, FL
San Diego, CA
Sarasota, FL
West Palm Beach–Boca Raton–
  Delray Beach, FL

Listed in alphabetical order are retirement places that experience fewer than 90 total monthly degrees of variation from a high of 80 degrees Fahrenheit and a low of 65 during December, January, and February.

The Mildest Summers

Ann Arbor, MI
Asheville, NC
Cape May, NJ
Crossville, TN
Easton–Chesapeake Bay, MD
Franklin County, TN
Gainesville–Lake Lanier, GA
Hendersonville–Brevard, NC
Iowa City, IA
Lexington, KY
Ocean City–Assateague Island, MD
Ocean County, NJ
Rehoboth Bay–Indian River Bay, DE
San Diego, CA
State College, PA

Listed in alphabetical order are the retirement places that experience fewer than 25 total monthly degrees of variation from a high of 80 degrees Fahrenheit and a low of 65 during June, July, and August.

Cloudiest Retirement Places

	Annual Cloudy Days
Port Angeles–Strait of Juan de Fuca, WA	246
Bellingham, WA	229
Friday Harbor–San Juan Islands, WA	229
Oak Harbor–Whidbey Island, WA	229
Olympia, WA	228
Hamilton–Bitterroot Valley, MT	213
Kalispell, MT	213
Missoula, MT	210
Newport–Lincoln City, OR	210
Petoskey–Straits of Mackinac, MI	209
Traverse City–Grand Traverse Bay, MI	209
Eugene–Springfield, OR	207
Bennington, VT	206
Burlington, VT	204
Canandaigua, NY	197
Houghton Lake, MI	197

Source: National Oceanic and Atmospheric Administration, *Local Climatological Data.*

Again You Ask, "What's Comfortable?"

Is all of this statistical searching for the ideal year-round retirement climate merely an illusion, much like the quest for perfect health, an honest man, or the Holy Grail? Perhaps. Consider the many retired persons living in Florida who vacate the Sunshine State's summers for a cottage on the Jersey Shore, the New England Coast, or a cabin in the southern Appalachians. Consider others in the Desert Southwest who shun a broiling summer by heading for Rocky Mountain foothills.

This migratory existence isn't just an American pattern. Older adults from northern Europe who live in Spain, southern Italy, Greece, or North Africa annually pack up and return to their native country for a summer that's milder than the one on the Mediterranean coast.

Having acknowledged this, we can still rate places that approach a climatic ideal by pointing to conditions that detract from maximum comfort. Read on.

The 16 Sunniest Retirement Places

	Annual Clear Days
Yuma, AZ	246
Chico–Paradise, CA	219
Las Vegas, NV	216
Phoenix, AZ	214
Tucson, AZ	198
Las Cruces, NM	194
Red Bluff–Sacramento Valley, CA	176
Roswell, NM	176
Santa Rosa–Petaluma, CA	176
Grass Valley–Truckee, CA	175
Albuquerque, NM	172
Santa Fe, NM	172
Flagstaff, AZ	168
Reno, NV	165
St. George–Zion, UT	153
San Diego, CA	150

Source: National Oceanic and Atmospheric Administration, *Local Climatological Data.*

Listed above are the retirement places, described in the Place Profiles, with 150 or more days of clear, sunny skies.

 SCORING: Climate

Because most people prefer (or say they prefer) mild climates, *Retirement Places Rated* compares 131 places on the basis of climate mildness, using a combination of monthly temperature factors. *Mild*, as we use the term, doesn't necessarily mean a winterless, perpetually Mediterranean climate; it simply refers to the absence of great variations or extremes of temperature. Older adults tend to be better off in comfortable, stable weather conditions than they are in climates that make large physiological demands and where radical weather changes come on quickly.

Retirement Places Rated defines the mildest climates as those whose monthly low temperatures remain closest to 65 degrees Fahrenheit coupled with monthly high temperatures of 80 degrees. Any deviations from this comfort zone are labeled negative indicators and are scored as such.

Each retirement place starts with a base score of 1,000 from which points are subtracted according to the following indicators:

1. *Variation from a monthly high of 80.* For each month of the year, 1 point is subtracted for each degree the average daily high temperature varies from 80 degrees. Miami–Hialeah, for example, loses 58 points for summer months where the average daily high exceeds 80 degrees. Burlington, Vermont, loses 364 points for an 11-month stretch when the daily high is *under* 80.

2. *Variation from a monthly low of 65.* The day's low temperature almost always occurs at night, usually in the early morning hours. For each month of the year, 1 point is subtracted for each degree the average daily low temperature varies from 65 degrees. Reno, Nevada, for example, loses 398 points; not only will you need blankets there most nights, you'll need to heat the bedroom, too. Fort Myers–Cape Coral, Florida, on the other hand, loses 88 points for uncomfortably warm summer nights.

SCORING EXAMPLES

Phoenix and all of Metropolitan South Florida experience two climate types favored by many footloose older adults: desert and subtropical.

Phoenix, Arizona (#37)

If Phoenix's summertime temperatures of 30 years ago were to have persisted to this day, the Arizona capital might be rated much higher than the ranking of 37 by *Retirement Places Rated*'s standards for climate mildness.

According to climatologists at Arizona State University, afternoon high temperatures during June, July, and August have remained constant over the years, but low temperatures during those months are now 8 degrees hotter than they were in 1948. These 8 degrees make the difference between formerly bearable warm nights and currently oppressive hot ones. The change is due to an extraordinary twelvefold increase in population since the end of World War II.

Long-time residents who recall the old desert-cowtown days blame the heat on humidity caused by evaporating surface water in swimming pools, fountains, and man-made lakes. Actually, atmospheric moisture hasn't changed much since the late 1940s.

According to the ASU scientists, modern Phoenix, with a population of 1.8 million persons, has classic "urban heat island" characteristics: (1) the ability of concrete and asphalt to absorb and store more radiant energy than natural vegetation and soil, (2) low winds, (3) man-made sources of heat, especially the automobile, and (4) a persistent high-pressure cell that traps air pollution, creating a "blanket" effect.

There can be no doubt that temperatures in the Valley of the Sun are mild most of the year. Catch a televised winter golf tournament from Scottsdale, and you may wish you were there. The biggest comfort liability here, however, is an intense period from mid-May through September when temperatures rarely drop to 65 degrees at night, and usually exceed 100 degrees during the day. The total monthly degrees of variation from a low of 65 and high of 80, particularly in June, July, and August, results in a loss of 336 points.

Metropolitan South Florida (13 Retirement Places)

Climate is arguably Florida's greatest natural resource. After all, it permits commercial crops from winter vegetables to tropical fruits and even gladioli and chrysanthemums to be grown almost all year, and it annually brings in millions of dollars from visitors fleeing a long, northern winter.

And it may well be the most important factor behind the Sunshine State's explosive population growth. Summers here are long, warm, and relatively humid; winters, though subject to periodic invasions of cool to occasionally cold air from the north, are mild because of the southern latitude and also because no point in the state is more than 70 miles from salt water.

Daily sea breezes temper the summer heat along the coast and as far inland as 30 miles. Afternoon thunderstorms occur about half of the days in summer everywhere but are frequently accompanied by a rapid 10 degree to 20 degree drop in temperature, resulting in comfortable weather for the rest of the day.

Though there may seem to be minuscule differences in climate scores among retirement places here, there is a geographic pattern: stations on the lower coasts are warmer in winter and cooler in summer than coastal stations at a higher latitude and stations in the interior. The three top-rated retirement places—Miami–Hialeah (867 points), Fort Lauderdale–Hollywood–Pompano Beach (861 points), and West Palm Beach–Boca Raton–Delray Beach (859 points)—are situated on the lower east coast where onshore winds passing over the Gulf Stream exert a warming influence in winter and a cooling influence in summer. The next two highest rated retirement places—Naples (846 points) and Fort Myers–Cape Coral (838 points)—are situated on the lower west coast.

 # RANKINGS: Climate

Just two criteria are used to determine a score for climate mildness: (1) variation from a monthly high of 80 degrees Fahrenheit and (2) variation from a monthly low of 65 degrees Fahrenheit. The source used for scoring data, the NOAA publication *Local Climatological Data*, does not provide information for 54 of the 131 retirement places; the scores for these places are determined from the NOAA *Series 20* publications.

Retirement places that receive tie scores are given the same rank and are listed in alphabetical order. The retirement places described in detail in the Place Profiles are shown in boldface type.

Retirement Places from First to Last

Rank	Score	Rank	Score	Rank	Score
1. **Maui, HI**	925	8. Melbourne–Titusville–Palm Bay, FL	837	16. Ocala, FL	796
2. **Kauai, HI**	915	9. **Lakeland–Winter Haven, FL**	828	17. McAllen–Edinburg–Mission, TX	793
3. **Miami–Hialeah, FL**	867	10. **Orlando, FL**	825	18. **San Diego, CA**	773
4. Fort Lauderdale–Hollywood–Pompano Beach, FL	861			19. Panama City, FL	757
5. **West Palm Beach–Boca Raton–Delray Beach, FL**	859	11. Bradenton, FL	816	20. Fort Walton Beach, FL	751
		11. **St. Petersburg–Clearwater, FL**	816	21. Fairhope–Gulf Shores, AL	750
6. Naples, FL	846	11. Sarasota, FL	816	22. **Brunswick–Golden Isles, GA**	747
7. **Fort Myers–Cape Coral, FL**	838	14. **Daytona Beach, FL**	814		
		15. **Brownsville–Harlingen, TX**	810	23. **Biloxi–Gulfport, MS**	742

Rank	Score	Rank	Score	Rank	Score
24. San Antonio, TX	730	59. Ocean City–		96. Litchfield County, CT	441
25. Hilton Head–Beaufort, SC	729	Assateague Island, MD	580	97. State College, PA	438
		59. St. George–Zion, UT	580	98. Ann Arbor, MI	437
26. Austin, TX	724			99. Iowa City, IA	431
27. Fredericksburg, TX	721	61. Fayetteville, AR	578	100. Carson City–Minden, NV	428
28. Athens–Cedar Creek		62. Asheville, NC	574		
Lake, TX	709	63. Roswell, NM	568	101. New Paltz–	
29. Charleston, SC	708	64. Rehoboth Bay–Indian River		Ulster County, NY	424
30. Myrtle Beach, SC	696	Bay, DE	564	102. Colorado Springs, CO	410
		65. Cape May, NJ	563	103. Amherst–Northampton, MA	406
30. Southport, NC	696			104. Fort Collins–	
32. Kerrville, TX	692	66. Easton–		Loveland, CO	405
32. Tucson, AZ	692	Chesapeake Bay, MD	561	105. Canandaigua, NY	404
32. Yuma, AZ	692	67. Deming, NM	560		
35. Burnet–Marble Falls–		68. Branson–Cassville–		106. Reno, NV	400
Llano, TX	685	Table Rock Lake, MO	558	107. Coeur d'Alene, ID	397
		68. Springfield, MO	558	108. Columbia County, NY	390
36. San Luis Obispo, CA	677	70. Lexington, KY	554	109. Bennington, VT	371
37. Phoenix, AZ	664			110. Bend, OR	354
38. Redding, CA	661	71. Albuquerque, NM	553		
39. Canton–Lake Tawakoni, TX	659	72. Las Cruces, NM	552	111. Bar Harbor–	
40. Red Bluff–		73. Clear Lake, CA	543	Frenchman Bay, ME	346
Sacramento Valley, CA	655	73. Twain Harte–Yosemite, CA	543	111. Camden–Penobscot Bay,	
		75. Front Royal, VA	536	ME	346
41. Hot Springs–				113. Hamilton–	
Lake Ouachita, AR	652	76. Crossville, TN	534	Bitterroot Valley, MT	343
42. Gainesville–Lake Lanier,		76. Winchester, VA	534	114. Flagstaff, AZ	341
GA	644	78. Ocean County, NJ	518	114. Monticello–Liberty, NY	341
43. Athens, GA	642	79. Eugene–Springfield, OR	515		
44. Virginia Beach–Norfolk, VA	634	80. Lancaster, PA	497	116. Madison, WI	337
45. Chico–Paradise, CA	629			117. Oscoda–Huron Shore, MI	334
		81. Medford–Ashland, OR	492	118. Hanover, NH	333
46. Las Vegas, NV	628	81. Prescott, AZ	492	118. Portsmouth–Dover–	
47. Chapel Hill, NC	626	83. Blacksburg, VA	487	Durham, NH	333
48. Santa Rosa–Petaluma, CA	625	83. Newport–Lincoln City, OR	487	120. Burlington, VT	324
49. Lake Havasu City–		85. Bloomington–			
Kingman, AZ	621	Brown County, IN	482	121. Door County, WI	320
50. Franklin County, TN	620			122. Petoskey–Straits of	
		86. Grand Junction, CO	469	Mackinac, MI	316
51. Salinas–Seaside–		87. Grass Valley–Truckee, CA	465	122. Traverse City–Grand	
Monterey, CA	616	88. Olympia, WA	460	Traverse Bay, MI	316
52. Hendersonville–Brevard,		89. Cape Cod, MA	459	124. Keene, NH	315
NC	615	90. Oak Harbor–		125. Laconia–	
53. Clayton–Clarkesville, GA	605	Whidbey Island, WA	452	Lake Winnipesaukee, NH	307
54. Grand Lake–					
Lake Tenkiller, OK	594	91. Bellingham, WA	449	125. North Conway–	
55. Mountain Home–		91. Friday Harbor–San Juan		White Mountains, NH	307
Bull Shoals, AR	592	Islands, WA	449	127. Missoula, MT	294
		93. Santa Fe, NM	447	128. Houghton Lake, MI	285
55. Murray–Kentucky Lake, KY	592	94. Boise, ID	446	129. Kalispell, MT	263
57. Charlottesville, VA	587	95. Port Angeles–Strait of		130. Eagle River, WI	261
58. Paris–Big Sandy, TN	581	Juan de Fuca, WA	444	130. Rhinelander, WI	261

Retirement Places Listed Alphabetically

Retirement Place	Rank	Retirement Place	Rank	Retirement Place	Rank
Albuquerque, NM	71	Bloomington–		Canton–Lake Tawakoni, TX	39
Amherst–Northampton, MA	103	Brown County, IN	85	Cape Cod, MA	89
Ann Arbor, MI	98	Boise, ID	94		
Asheville, NC	62			Cape May, NJ	65
Athens, GA	43	Bradenton, FL	11	Carson City–Minden, NV	100
		Branson–Cassville–		Chapel Hill, NC	47
Athens–Cedar Creek Lake, TX	28	Table Rock Lake, MO	68	Charleston, SC	29
Austin, TX	26	Brownsville–Harlingen, TX	15	Charlottesville, VA	57
Bar Harbor–Frenchman Bay, ME	111	Brunswick–Golden Isles, GA	22		
Bellingham, WA	91	Burlington, VT	120	Chico–Paradise, CA	45
Bend, OR	110			Clayton–	
		Burnet–Marble Falls–		Clarkesville, GA	53
Bennington, VT	109	Llano, TX	35	Clear Lake, CA	73
Biloxi–Gulfport, MS	23	Camden–Penobscot Bay, ME	111	Coeur d'Alene, ID	107
Blacksburg, VA	83	Canandaigua, NY	105	Colorado Springs, CO	102

Retirement Place	Rank	Retirement Place	Rank	Retirement Place	Rank
Columbia County, NY	108	**Kerrville, TX**	32	Paris–Big Sandy, TN	58
Crossville, TN	76	Laconia–		**Petoskey–Straits of Mackinac,**	
Daytona Beach, FL	14	Lake Winnipesaukee, NH	125	**MI**	122
Deming, NM	67			**Phoenix, AZ**	37
Door County, WI	121	Lake Havasu City–Kingman, AZ	49	**Port Angeles–Strait of**	
		Lakeland–Winter Haven, FL	9	**Juan de Fuca, WA**	95
Eagle River, WI	130	**Lancaster, PA**	80		
Easton–Chesapeake Bay, MD	66	**Las Cruces, NM**	72	Portsmouth–Dover–Durham, NH	118
Eugene–Springfield, OR	79	**Las Vegas, NV**	46	Prescott, AZ	81
Fairhope–Gulf Shores, AL	21			**Red Bluff–Sacramento Valley,**	
Fayetteville, AR	61	**Lexington, KY**	70	**CA**	40
		Litchfield County, CT	96	Redding, CA	38
Flagstaff, AZ	114	**Madison, WI**	116	Rehoboth Bay–Indian River	
Fort Collins–		**Maui, HI**	1	Bay, DE	64
Loveland, CO	104	McAllen–Edinburg–Mission, TX	17		
Fort Lauderdale–Hollywood–				**Reno, NV**	106
Pompano Beach, FL	4	**Medford–Ashland, OR**	81	**Rhinelander, WI**	130
Fort Myers–Cape Coral, FL	7	Melbourne–Titusville–		**Roswell, NM**	63
Fort Walton Beach, FL	20	Palm Bay, FL	8	**St. George–Zion, UT**	59
		Miami–Hialeah, FL	3	**St. Petersburg–Clearwater, FL**	11
Franklin County, TN	50	Missoula, MT	127		
Fredericksburg, TX	27	Monticello–Liberty, NY	114	Salinas–Seaside–Monterey, CA	51
Friday Harbor–San Juan Islands,				**San Antonio, TX**	24
WA	91	**Mountain Home–Bull Shoals, AR**	55	**San Diego, CA**	18
Front Royal, VA	75	**Murray–Kentucky Lake, KY**	55	San Luis Obispo, CA	36
Gainesville–Lake Lanier, GA	42	**Myrtle Beach, SC**	30	**Santa Fe, NM**	93
		Naples, FL	6		
Grand Junction, CO	86			**Santa Rosa–Petaluma, CA**	48
Grand Lake–Lake Tenkiller, OK	54	New Paltz–Ulster County, NY	101	Sarasota, FL	11
Grass Valley–Truckee, CA	87	**Newport–Lincoln City, OR**	83	Southport, NC	30
Hamilton–Bitterroot Valley, MT	113	**North Conway–**		**Springfield, MO**	68
Hanover, NH	118	**White Mountains, NH**	125	**State College, PA**	97
		Oak Harbor–Whidbey Island, WA	90		
Hendersonville–Brevard, NC	52	Ocala, FL	16	Traverse City–Grand Traverse	
Hilton Head–Beaufort, SC	25			Bay, MI	122
Hot Springs–		Ocean City–		**Tucson, AZ**	32
Lake Ouachita, AR	41	Assateague Island, MD	59	Twain Harte–Yosemite, CA	73
Houghton Lake, MI	128	Ocean County, NJ	78	**Virginia Beach–Norfolk, VA**	44
Iowa City, IA	99	**Olympia, WA**	88	**West Palm Beach–Boca Raton–**	
		Orlando, FL	10	**Delray Beach, FL**	5
Kalispell, MT	129	Oscoda–Huron Shore, MI	117		
Kauai, HI	2			**Winchester, VA**	76
Keene, NH	124	Panama City, FL	19	Yuma, AZ	32

PLACE PROFILES: Climate

Principally for reasons of space, the pages that follow describe climate at weather stations in 77 out of the 131 retirement places. The places were selected because they represent a distinct part of the country with a distinct climate type, or because they embrace large populations of retired persons, or both. Because most of the weather stations at these places are classified as "first order," many elements besides normal monthly temperatures are measured, thereby providing additional climate information.

The data come from the National Oceanic and Atmospheric Administration (NOAA) series of publications, *Local Climatological Data,* and *Climatography of the United States.* (Because the NOAA publication *Local Climatological Data* does not provide data for the 54 retirement places not included here, their scores are determined from temperature tables in the NOAA *Series 20* publications.)

The figures presented are referred to by the NOAA as 30-year normals—averages collected over 3 decades. Each 10 years, the data for the new decade are added into the normal, and the data for the earliest 10 years are dropped. Data are collected and averaged over this period to flatten out anomalies and weather extremes. Atypical events such as a freak blizzard in San Antonio or a heat wave that might occur once every 50 years in Coeur d'Alene, Idaho, have little effect on each place's 30-year normal.

These summaries describe each location and point out distinctive features of the climate and terrain. When terrain is described in the profiles, it is usually in connection with the effect it has on the climate in the immediate area. Few people would deny that terrain is an important element in its own right; to many it's as important as climate. Some people prefer mountain vistas or seacoasts, others rolling hills or flatwoods forests. Rather than judging, rating, or scoring terrain, *Retirement Places Rated* simply describes it briefly and lets you decide.

The table of average temperatures on the right-hand side of each profile gives a clear idea of the monthly temperature ranges for each place. For example, if you want to know how hot it gets in Albuquerque in July, look at the table in Albuquerque's profile. In July the daily high temperatures (which usually occur in mid-afternoon) average 92 degrees Fahrenheit. That sounds hot, and it is. But look at the average daily low temperature (a point reached in the early morning) for the same month. It is 65 degrees. Even a quick glance at these temperatures shows that July in Albuquerque means hot days and cool nights. This fits Albuquerque's dry, desert location and 5,314 foot elevation.

Rounding out each place's weather picture are data for relative humidity, wind speed, amount of snow and rain, clear and cloudy days, storms, very hot and very cold days, precipitation days (days on which there is at least .01 inch of precipitation), and storm days. To derive the greatest benefit from these assorted indicators, compare two or more retirement places. Which has more snow? More rain? More 90-degree days? Comparing two places you're interested in may lead to your deciding which to visit first. It can be enlightening to compare a place you've never been to with one you already know.

A unique visual device in each profile is the circular graph showing the length of each season. These graphs are prepared from a formula showing that seasonal change is defined and measured by weather conditions, human activities, and growth or dormancy of plant life rather than by the calendar. In *Retirement Places Rated*, the seasons are defined as follows: Summer begins when the mean monthly temperature rises above 60 degrees Fahrenheit; summer ends when it falls below 60. Winter begins when the average daily low falls below 32 degrees and ends when it rises above that mark. The remaining portions of the year constitute fall and spring. In the seasonal graphs, winter is shown by the black segments, spring and fall appear as gray, and summer is white.

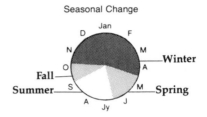

Seasonal Change

If you glance at several graphs you'll see that the length of a season varies. Winter is represented by a tiny sliver in Hot Springs, Arkansas, and a full semicircle in Colorado Springs. Some places don't have four distinct separate seasons. Places along the South Atlantic and Gulf shores usually have just two— spring and summer. Some, like Miami–Hialeah, have only one—perpetual summer.

A star preceding a retirement place's name highlights it as one of the top 15 places for climate mildness.

Albuquerque, NM

Terrain: Rests in the Rio Grande Valley 55 miles southwest of Santa Fe, and is surrounded by mountains, most of them to the east. These mountainous areas receive more precipitation than does the city proper. With an annual rainfall of 8 inches, only the most hardy desert flora can grow. However, successful farming—primarily fruit and produce—is carried out in the valley by irrigation.

Climate: Arid continental. No muggy days. Half the moisture falls between July and September in the form of brief but severe thunderstorms. Long drizzles are unknown. These storms do not greatly interfere with outdoor activities and they have a moderating effect on the heat. The hottest month is July, with temperatures reaching 90° F almost constantly. However, the low humidity and cool nights make the heat much less felt.

Pluses: Sunny and dry, with mild winters.　　**Minuses:** Dust storms.

Elevation: 5,314 feet

Relative Humidity: 37%
Wind Speed: 9 mph

Seasonal Change

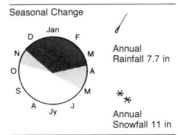

Annual Rainfall 7.7 in

Annual Snowfall 11 in

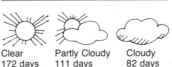

Clear 172 days　　Partly Cloudy 111 days　　Cloudy 82 days

Precipitation Days: 59　　Storm Days: 43

Average Temperatures		
	Daily High	Daily Low
January	47	24
February	53	27
March	59	32
April	70	41
May	80	51
June	90	60
July	92	65
August	90	63
September	83	57
October	72	45
November	57	32
December	48	25

Zero-Degree Days: 1
Freezing Days: 123
90-Degree Days: 61

Score: 553　　　　　**Rank: 71**

Asheville, NC

Terrain: Located on both banks of the French Broad River, near the center of the basin of the same name. Two miles upstream from Asheville, the Swannanoa River joins the French Broad River from the east. The entire valley is called the Asheville Plateau and is flanked on the east and west by mountain ranges. Thirty miles south, the Blue Ridge Mountains form an escarpment, with an average elevation of 2,700 feet. Tallest peaks near Asheville are Mount Mitchell (6,684 feet), 20 miles northeast, and Big Pisgah (5,721 feet), 16 miles southwest.

Climate: Temperate but invigorating. Considerable variation in temperature occurs from day to day throughout the year. The valley has a pronounced effect on wind direction, which is mostly from the northwest. Destructive weather events are rare. However, the French Broad Valley is subject to flooding, with especially high flooding occurring in 12-year cycles.

Pluses: Long spring, beginning early.

Minuses: Drizzly, flood-prone.

Score: 574   **Rank: 62**

Elevation: 2,207 feet

Relative Humidity: 59%
Wind Speed: 7.7 mph

Seasonal Change

Annual Rainfall 45 in

Annual Snowfall 18 in

Clear 102 days   Partly Cloudy 107 days   Cloudy 156 days

Precipitation Days: 128   Storm Days: 49

Average Temperatures		
	Daily High	Daily Low
January	48	27
February	51	28
March	58	34
April	69	42
May	77	51
June	83	59
July	84	63
August	84	62
September	78	55
October	69	45
November	58	34
December	49	28

Zero-Degree Days: 1
Freezing Days: 106
90-Degree Days: 5

Athens, GA

Terrain: Located in the Piedmont Plateau section of northeast Georgia. The land is rolling to hilly, with elevations ranging between 600 and 800 feet. The Atlantic Ocean 200 miles to the southeast, the Gulf of Mexico 275 miles to the south, and the southern Appalachian Mountains to the north and northwest, all exert some influence on the city's climate, resulting in moderate summer and winter weather.

Climate: Summers are warm and somewhat humid, but there is a noticeable absence of prolonged periods of extreme heat. The mountains to the north serve as a partial barrier to extremely cold airflows; as a result, the city's winters aren't severe. Cold spells are short-lived, interspersed with periods of warm southerly airflow, making normal outside activities possible throughout most of the year. Precipitation is evenly distributed during the year. Measurable amounts of snow occur infrequently.

Pluses: Mild winters.

Minuses: Humid summers, frequent serious dry spells.

Score: 642   **Rank: 43**

Elevation: 802 feet

Relative Humidity: 56%
Wind Speed: 7.4 mph

Seasonal Change

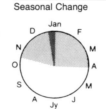

Annual Rainfall 50 in

Annual Snowfall 2 in

Clear 113 days   Partly Cloudy 105 days   Cloudy 147 days

Precipitation Days: 111   Storm Days: 52

Average Temperatures		
	Daily High	Daily Low
January	53	33
February	56	35
March	63	40
April	74	50
May	82	58
June	88	66
July	90	69
August	88	68
September	83	82
October	74	51
November	63	40
December	54	34

Zero-Degree Days: 0
Freezing Days: 54
90-Degree Days: 48

Athens–Cedar Creek Lake, TX

Terrain: Athens, seat of Henderson County, is located in the pine and post oak area of East Texas, about 70 air miles southeast of Dallas. The surrounding rolling to hilly terrain drains to the Neches River on the east and the Trinity River on the west. Cedar Creek Reservoir, 5 miles northwest, is one of the most popular recreation areas in the state. Nestled among the post oaks and pines, the lakes offer innumerable campsites, excellent fishing, swimming, and boating.

Climate: Humid subtropical, with hot summers. Rainfall is about 39 inches annually, evenly distributed. July and August, though, are somewhat dry. Winters are mild, with temperatures almost always rising above freezing in the daytime. No zero temperatures on record. Spring and fall are the best seasons, and are long. There are sufficient changes to make the weather interesting. The growing season is long (260 days); flowers bloom as late as December, as early as March.

Pluses: Mild winters, lovely springs and falls.

Minuses: Hot, humid summers.

Score: 709   **Rank: 28**

Elevation: 490 feet

Relative Humidity: 68%
Wind Speed: 10.8 mph

Seasonal Change

Annual Rainfall 39 in

Annual Snowfall 1 in

Clear 141 days   Partly Cloudy 93 days   Cloudy 131 days

Precipitation Days: 55   Storm Days: 52

Average Temperatures		
	Daily High	Daily Low
January	58	36
February	63	41
March	69	46
April	79	56
May	85	63
June	91	69
July	96	72
August	96	71
September	90	66
October	81	56
November	70	47
December	62	40

Zero-Degree Days: 0
Freezing Days: 33
90-Degree Days: 95

Austin, TX

Terrain: Located on the Colorado River where it crosses the Balcones escarpment, which separates the Texas hill country from the blackland prairies of East Texas. Elevations within the city limits vary from 400 feet to 900 feet above sea level. Native trees include cedar, oak, walnut, mesquite, and pecan.
Climate: Subtropical. Although summers are hot, the nights are a bit cooler, with temperatures usually dropping into the 70s. Winters are mild, with below-freezing temperatures on fewer than 25 days; strong northers may bring cold spells, but these rarely last more than a few days. Precipitation is well distributed, but heaviest in late spring, with a secondary rainfall peak in September. With summer come heavy thunderstorms; in winter, the rain tends to be slow and steady. Snowfall (1 inch per year) is inconsequential. Prevailing winds are southerly. Destructive weather infrequent. Freeze-free season: 270 days. Average date of last freeze: March 3. First freeze: November 28.

Pluses: Mild winters.   **Minuses:** Hot.

Score: 724   **Rank: 26**

Elevation: 570 feet

Relative Humidity: 56%
Wind Speed: 9.3 mph

Seasonal Change

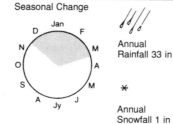

Annual Rainfall 33 in

Annual Snowfall 1 in

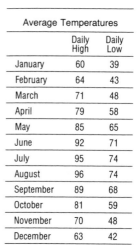

Clear 115 days   Partly Cloudy 116 days   Cloudy 134 days

Precipitation Days: 82   Storm Days: 41

Average Temperatures		
	Daily High	Daily Low
January	60	39
February	64	43
March	71	48
April	79	58
May	85	65
June	92	71
July	95	74
August	96	74
September	89	68
October	81	59
November	70	48
December	63	42

Zero-Degree Days: 0
Freezing Days: 23
90-Degree Days: 101

Bend, OR

Terrain: Located along the western border of the Great Basin, near the center of the state. The Cascade foothills rise immediately west of the city and terrace upwards to crests of 10,000 feet about 10 miles away. The rolling plateau extends south and east from Bend into California, Nevada, and Idaho. To the north, the plateau is cut by canyons and drainage streams that feed into the Columbia River.
Climate: Bend has primarily the continental climate of the Great Basin. The mountains moderate the more extreme temperatures of summer. Precipitation is generally light (12 inches of rain annually as opposed to 60 inches to 100 inches on the coast!) because the high Cascades block the moisture-laden Pacific winds. Moderate days and cool nights characterize the climate here. Even in July the temperature may drop to freezing one night. There is, on the average, only one day per year with rainfall of an inch or more.

Pluses: Scenic terrain. Dry and mild, with cool nights.

Minuses: Large temperature shifts. Too dry for some.

Score: 354   **Rank: 110**

Elevation: 3,599 feet

Relative Humidity: 45%
Wind Speed: 7 mph

Seasonal Change

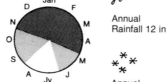

Annual Rainfall 12 in

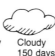

Annual Snowfall 36 in

Clear 123 days   Partly Cloudy 92 days   Cloudy 150 days

Precipitation Days: 33   Storm Days: 8

Average Temperatures		
	Daily High	Daily Low
January	41	21
February	46	24
March	50	24
April	57	28
May	65	34
June	73	40
July	82	44
August	80	43
September	74	37
October	63	31
November	49	26
December	43	23

Zero-Degree Days: 3
Freezing Days: 190
90-Degree Days: 11

Bennington, VT

Terrain: This historic city is nestled in the valley of the Walloomsac River, which is a part of the Hudson River drainage system. At 700 feet, it is surrounded by mountains. Mount Anthony (2,300 feet) is nearby to the southwest. A ridge of the Green Mountains, at a similar altitude, lies a few miles to the east. The terrain is more open to the west, though many hills rise to 1,000 feet between Bennington and the Hudson.
Climate: The surrounding mountains tend to modify the local climate, especially those to the east, which block some effects of the coastal storms, called "northeasters," which pass along the Atlantic Coast (125 miles distant). There are large differences of temperature, both daily and annually. Winters are cold and snowy, which accounts for the region's many fine ski resorts. Summers are very comfortable, with daytime temperatures in the 70s and low 80s and nighttime temperatures in the 50s.

Pluses: Beautiful summers. Scenic terrain. Great winter skiing.

Minuses: Long and fairly rigorous winters.

Score: 371   **Rank: 109**

Elevation: 670 feet

Relative Humidity: 55%
Wind Speed: 8.8 mph

Seasonal Change

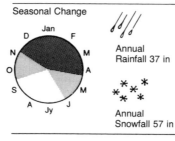

Annual Rainfall 37 in

Annual Snowfall 57 in

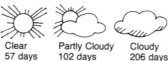

Clear 57 days   Partly Cloudy 102 days   Cloudy 206 days

Precipitation Days: 88   Storm Days: 25

Average Temperatures		
	Daily High	Daily Low
January	31	11
February	35	14
March	43	23
April	58	34
May	70	43
June	78	52
July	82	56
August	80	54
September	73	47
October	62	38
November	49	30
December	35	17

Zero-Degree Days: 17
Freezing Days: 166
90-Degree Days: 8

Biloxi–Gulfport, MS

Terrain: In speaking of the Mississippi Gulf Coast, one usually thinks of the thickly settled area stretching from St. Louis Bay at Pass Christian to Biloxi Bay and Ocean Springs. This area is climatologically homogeneous, and a summary of any town (in this case, Biloxi–Gulfport) is applicable to the others. The terrain is flat, consisting of low-lying delta floodplains sloping down to sand beaches and rather shallow harbors and bays.

Climate: The Gulf waters have a modifying effect on the local climate that is not felt farther inland. Temperatures of 90° F or higher occur only half as often here as they do in Hattiesburg, 60 miles north. However, there is no such reverse effect on cold air moving down from the north in winter. Rainfall is plentiful and is heaviest in July, with totals in March and September following close behind. Damage from hurricanes and tropical storms can occur six to seven times a year.

Pluses: Warm, mild beach climate.

Minuses: Relatively chilly winters; hurricane-prone.

Score: 742   **Rank:** 23

Elevation: 15 feet

Relative Humidity: 65%
Wind Speed: 9.1 mph

Seasonal Change

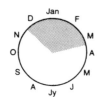

Annual Rainfall 59 in

Annual Snowfall 0 in

Clear 100 days   Partly Cloudy 119 days   Cloudy 146 days

Precipitation Days: 75   Storm Days: 94

Average Temperatures		
	Daily High	Daily Low
January	61	42
February	64	44
March	70	51
April	77	59
May	84	71
June	90	71
July	91	73
August	91	73
September	88	69
October	80	58
November	70	49
December	64	44

Zero-Degree Days: 0
Freezing Days: 11
90-Degree Days: 52

Boise, ID

Terrain: Cradled in the valley of the Boise River about 8 miles below the mouth of a mountain canyon, where this valley widens. The Boise Mountains rise to a height of 5,000 feet to 6,000 feet within 8 miles. Their slopes are partially mantled with sagebrush and chaparral, changing to stands of fir, spruce, and pine trees higher up.

Climate: Almost a typical upland continental climate in summer but one tempered by periods of cloudy or stormy and mild weather during almost every winter. The cause of this modification in the winter months is the flow of warm, moist Pacific air, called Chinook winds. While this air is considerably moderated by the time it reaches Boise, its effect is nonetheless felt. Summer hot spells rarely last longer than a few days, but temperatures may reach 100° F each year. However, due to the low humidity, the average 5:00 PM July temperature of 62° F is comfortable. In general, the climate is dry and temperate, with enough variation to be stimulating.

Pluses: Mild; low humidity.

Minuses: Stormy winters.

Score: 446   **Rank:** 94

Elevation: 2,868 feet

Relative Humidity: 52%
Wind Speed: 9 mph

Seasonal Change

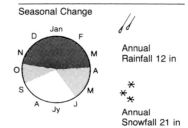

Annual Rainfall 12 in

Annual Snowfall 21 in

Clear 124 days   Partly Cloudy 90 days   Cloudy 151 days

Precipitation Days: 91   Storm Days: 15

Average Temperatures		
	Daily High	Daily Low
January	37	21
February	44	27
March	52	31
April	61	37
May	71	44
June	78	51
July	91	59
August	88	57
September	78	49
October	65	39
November	49	31
December	39	25

Zero-Degree Days: 2
Freezing Days: 124
90-Degree Days: 43

★ Brownsville–Harlingen, TX

Terrain: Situated at the extreme southern tip of Texas, on the Mexican border, and on the alluvial soils of the Rio Grande. The only more southerly city in America is Key West, Florida. The Gulf of Mexico is 18 miles to the east, and more than half the land toward the coast consists of tidal marshlands, which have the net effect of "moving" the coast 10 miles nearer to the city.

Climate: Humid subtropical. It's always summer here, accounting for the area's agricultural importance in growing citrus fruits, cotton, and warm-weather vegetables. Part of the climate is man-made: irrigation, used for all the crops, adds considerably to the humidity. Summer temperatures follow a predictable pattern of lower 90s in the day and middle 70s at night. Gulf breezes help temper the summer heat. This is a popular tourist spot in the winter months. The normal daily January minimum temperature is 51° F.

Pluses: Long growing season.

Minuses: Hot.

Score: 810   **Rank:** 15

Elevation: 20 feet

Relative Humidity: 61%
Wind Speed: 11.7 mph

Seasonal Change

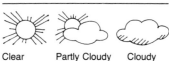

Annual Rainfall 25 in

Annual Snowfall 0 in

Clear 96 days   Partly Cloudy 138 days   Cloudy 131 days

Precipitation Days: 73   Storm Days: 24

Average Temperatures		
	Daily High	Daily Low
January	70	51
February	73	54
March	77	59
April	83	67
May	87	71
June	91	75
July	93	76
August	93	76
September	90	73
October	85	66
November	78	59
December	72	53

Zero-Degree Days: 0
Freezing Days: 2
90-Degree Days: 102

Brunswick–Golden Isles, GA

Terrain: The city of Brunswick, and neighboring St. Simons Island, which lies across the Intracoastal Waterway, are located on Georgia's southeast coast. Land surface is flat, and elevation averages from 10 feet to 15 feet. Much of the surrounding area is marshland. Fine beaches are plentiful. The low terrain and low latitude East Coast location of the area make it vulnerable to occasional tropical storms, though their full force is felt only infrequently.

Climate: The area enjoys mild and relatively short winters due to the moderating effect of coastal waters. There are only 11 days below freezing in the average winter, and no zero days. Summers are warm and humid, but very high temperatures are rare. Heat waves are usually interrupted by thundershowers, and even in the summer the nights are usually pleasant. Most of the annual 53 inches of rain falls in the summer and early autumn.

Pluses: Warm, mild climate with little temperature change.

Minuses: Can be hot and humid, with frequent rain.

Score: 747　　　　　　　　　　　　**Rank: 22**

Elevation: 13 feet

Relative Humidity: 60%
Wind Speed: 8 mph

Seasonal Change

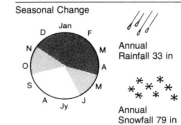

Annual
Rainfall 55 in

Annual
Snowfall 0 in

Clear
99 days

Partly Cloudy
113 days

Cloudy
153 days

Precipitation Days: 74　　Storm Days: 72

Average Temperatures		
	Daily High	Daily Low
January	61	42
February	62	44
March	69	50
April	76	58
May	82	66
June	87	72
July	90	74
August	89	74
September	85	71
October	77	61
November	69	51
December	63	44
Zero-Degree Days: 0		
Freezing Days: 11		
90-Degree Days: 75		

Burlington, VT

Terrain: Located on the eastern shore of Lake Champlain at the widest part of that lake. About 35 miles to the west lie the highest peaks of the Adirondacks; the foothills of the Green Mountains begin 10 miles to the east and southeast.

Climate: Burlington's northerly latitude assures the variety and vigor of a true New England climate. Lake Champlain, however, has a tempering effect; during the winter months, temperatures along the lakeshore often run from 5 degrees to 10 degrees warmer than those at the airport 3.5 miles away. The summer, while not long compared with most, is quite pleasant, with only four 90-degree days per year on the average. Fall is cool, extending through October. Winters are cold, with intense cold snaps (usually not lasting long) formed by high-pressure systems moving down from central Canada and Hudson Bay. Because of its location in the path of the St. Lawrence Valley storm track and the effects of the lake, Burlington is one of the cloudiest cities in the United States.

Pluses: Cool summers.

Minuses: Long, cold winters.

Score: 324　　　　　　　　　　　　**Rank: 120**

Elevation: 340 feet

Relative Humidity: 60%
Wind Speed: 8.8 mph

Seasonal Change

Annual
Rainfall 33 in

Annual
Snowfall 79 in

Clear
58 days

Partly Cloudy
103 days

Cloudy
204 days

Precipitation Days: 153　Storm Days: 25

Average Temperatures		
	Daily High	Daily Low
January	26	8
February	28	9
March	38	20
April	53	33
May	66	44
June	77	54
July	81	59
August	78	56
September	70	49
October	59	39
November	44	30
December	30	15
Zero-Degree Days: 28		
Freezing Days: 163		
90-Degree Days: 5		

Camden–Penobscot Bay, ME

Terrain: Penobscot Bay lies at the mouth of the Penobscot River in the middle of Maine's seacoast. Although low-lying, the coastal terrain is very rugged and rocky in most places, allowing for hundreds of bays, islands, peninsulas, and harbors. Just to the northeast of Penobscot Bay lies the smaller Frenchman Bay, containing Mount Desert Island and Acadia National Park. Vegetation consists of evergreen coniferous trees, maple, birch, and scrub oak, and many marshes and ponds with cranberry bogs. Fruit orchards, truck farming, and fishing are the predominant coastal industries.

Climate: The Atlantic Ocean has a considerable modifying effect on the local climate, resulting in cool summers and winters that are very mild for so northerly a location. Though fall is generally mild, spring comes late and the weather isn't really warm until July.

Pluses: Cool summers. Winters relatively mild.

Minuses: Long winters. Cold, damp springs.

Score: 346　　　　　　　　　　　　**Rank: 111**

Elevation: 49 feet

Relative Humidity: 60%
Wind Speed: 8.7 mph

Seasonal Change

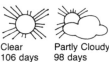

Annual
Rainfall 47 in

Annual
Snowfall 60 in

Clear
106 days

Partly Cloudy
98 days

Cloudy
161 days

Precipitation Days: 85　　Storm Days: 21

Average Temperatures		
	Daily High	Daily Low
January	32	14
February	34	14
March	41	24
April	52	33
May	63	42
June	72	50
July	78	56
August	77	55
September	69	48
October	60	39
November	48	31
December	36	18
Zero-Degree Days: 11		
Freezing Days: 152		
90-Degree Days: 4		

Cape Cod, MA

Terrain: Cape Cod is a crooked spit of land that juts out into the Atlantic Ocean from the southeastern corner of Massachusetts, stretching roughly 80 miles from the Cape Cod Canal (at Buzzards Bay) to its tip at Provincetown. The western end of the cape is higher and hillier than the eastern, or "outer cape," which is almost flat and treeless. The sandy soil, arranged in rolling hills and dunes, supports scrub oak and pine trees, while dune grasses and low trees grow on the outer cape.

Climate: Mild, cool, and maritime, with cool summers and cold, wet winters that are seldom severe. Summer temperatures are usually ideal for outdoor recreation. Both zero and 90° F days are very rare.

Pluses: Mild four-season climate, with long and pleasant falls.

Minuses: Winters wet and sleety. Summers can be damp and foggy.

Score: 459   **Rank:** 89

Elevation: 35 feet

Relative Humidity: 60%
Wind Speed: 13 mph

Seasonal Change

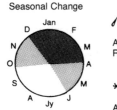

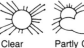

Annual Rainfall 43 in

Annual Snowfall 24 in

Clear 97 days   Partly Cloudy 114 days   Cloudy 154 days

Precipitation Days: 79   Storm Days: 14

Average Temperatures		
	Daily High	Daily Low
January	38	23
February	39	23
March	44	29
April	53	37
May	64	46
June	73	56
July	79	62
August	78	61
September	72	55
October	63	46
November	53	37
December	42	26

Zero-Degree Days: 1
Freezing Days: 115
90-Degree Days: 2

Cape May, NJ

Terrain: Located at New Jersey's southernmost point on a peninsula between the mouth of Delaware Bay and the Atlantic Ocean. The surrounding flat terrain is composed of tidal marshes and beach sand.

Climate: Continental, but the moderating influence of the Atlantic Ocean is apparent throughout the year. Summers are relatively cooler, winters warmer than those of other places at the same latitude. During the warm season, sea breezes in the late morning and afternoon prevent excessive heat. On occasion, sea breezes may lower the temperature between 15 degrees and 20 degrees within a half hour. Temperatures of 90° F or higher are recorded only about three times a year here. Fall is long, lasting until almost mid-November. On the other hand, warming is somewhat delayed in the spring. Ocean temperatures range from an average near 37° F in winter to 72° F in August. Precipitation is moderate and well distributed throughout the year, but great variation is seen from year to year in precipitation during the late summer and early fall (August, September, and October).

Pluses: Moderate temperatures.

Minuses: Late springs.

Score: 563   **Rank:** 65

Elevation: 10 feet

Relative Humidity: 60%
Wind Speed: 11.4 mph

Seasonal Change

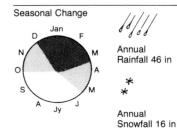

Annual Rainfall 46 in

Annual Snowfall 16 in

Clear 96 days   Partly Cloudy 108 days   Cloudy 161 days

Precipitation Days: 112   Storm Days: 25

Average Temperatures		
	Daily High	Daily Low
January	41	28
February	42	28
March	50	35
April	60	44
May	69	53
June	78	62
July	83	67
August	83	67
September	77	62
October	67	51
November	56	42
December	46	32

Zero-Degree Days: 1
Freezing Days: 15
90-Degree Days: 16

Chapel Hill, NC

Terrain: Situated in the transition zone between the Coastal Plain and the Piedmont Plateau of North Carolina. The surrounding topography is rolling, with elevations from 200 feet to 500 feet within a 10-mile radius.

Climate: Because it is located between mountains to the west and the Atlantic Coast to the east and south, the metro area enjoys a favorable climate. The mountains form a partial barrier to cold air masses moving eastward from the nation's interior, so that there are very few days in the heart of the winter when the temperature falls below 20° F. Tropical air is present over the eastern and central sections of North Carolina during much of the summer, bringing warm temperatures and high humidity. In midsummer, afternoon temperatures reach 90° F or higher on an average of every fourth day. Rainfall is well distributed throughout the year. July has, on the average, the greatest amount of rainfall, and November the least.

Pluses: Mild four-season climate.

Minuses: Long, humid summers.

Score: 626   **Rank:** 47

Elevation: 441 feet

Relative Humidity: 54%
Wind Speed: 7.9 mph

Seasonal Change

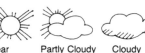

Annual Rainfall 43 in

Annual Snowfall 7 in

Clear 113 days   Partly Cloudy 107 days   Cloudy 145 days

Precipitation Days: 112   Storm Days: 46

Average Temperatures		
	Daily High	Daily Low
January	51	30
February	53	31
March	61	37
April	72	47
May	79	55
June	86	63
July	88	67
August	87	66
September	82	60
October	72	48
November	62	38
December	52	31

Zero-Degree Days: 0
Freezing Days: 82
90-Degree Days: 25

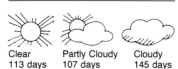

Charleston, SC

Terrain: Before the expansion begun in 1960, Charleston was limited to the peninsula bounded on the west and south by the Ashley River, on the east by the Cooper River, and on the southeast by a spacious harbor that contains historic Fort Sumter. The terrain is generally level and the soil sandy to sandy loam. Because of the low elevation, a portion of the city and nearby coastal islands are vulnerable to tidal flooding.

Climate: Generally temperate, modified considerably by the ocean. Summer is warm and humid, but temperatures over 100° F are infrequent. Most rain—41% of the annual total—occurs then. The fall passes from an Indian summer to the prewinter cold spells that begin in November. From late September to early November, the weather is very pleasant, being cool and sunny. Winters are mild; temperatures of 20° F or less are very unusual. Spring is warm, windy, and change-able. Most storms occur then.

Pluses: Pleasant falls, mild winters.

Minuses: Hot, humid, stormy.

Score: 708 **Rank: 29**

Elevation: 48 feet

Relative Humidity: 56%
Wind Speed: 8.8 mph

Seasonal Change

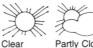

Annual Rainfall 52 in

Annual Snowfall .5 in

Clear 101 days | Partly Cloudy 113 days | Cloudy 151 days

Precipitation Days: 115 Storm Days: 56

Average Temperatures		
	Daily High	Daily Low
January	60	37
February	62	39
March	68	45
April	76	53
May	83	61
June	88	68
July	89	71
August	89	71
September	85	66
October	77	55
November	68	44
December	61	32

Zero-Degree Days: 0
Freezing Days: 36
90-Degree Days: 47

Charlottesville, VA

Terrain: Located in the center of Albemarle County, which is on the Central Piedmont Plateau. The Blue Ridge Mountains are on the western edge of the county. These and several smaller ranges make the topography vary from rolling to quite steep. Elevations range from 300 feet to 800 feet, with some points in the Blue Ridge as high as 3,200 feet.

Climate: Modified continental, with mild winters and warm, humid summers. The mountains produce various steering and blocking effects on storms and air masses. Chesapeake Bay to the east further modifies the climate, making it warmer in winter, cooler in summer. Precipitation is well distributed throughout the year, with the maximum in July, the minimum in January. Tornadoes and violent storms are rare, but severe thunderstorms occur each year.

Pluses: Scenic mountain ter-rain. Mild four-season climate.

Minuses: Summers can be hot and rainy.

Score: 587 **Rank: 57**

Elevation: 870 feet

Relative Humidity: 55%
Wind Speed: 8.3 mph

Seasonal Change

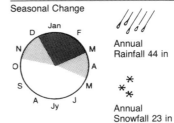

Annual Rainfall 44 in

Annual Snowfall 23 in

Clear 102 days | Partly Cloudy 114 days | Cloudy 149 days

Precipitation Days: 116 Storm Days: 45

Average Temperatures		
	Daily High	Daily Low
January	44	26
February	46	28
March	56	36
April	68	46
May	76	55
June	83	62
July	87	67
August	86	66
September	80	60
October	69	49
November	59	39
December	47	30

Zero-Degree Days: 0
Freezing Days: 87
90-Degree Days: 35

Chico–Paradise, CA

Terrain: Lies in the northern third of the Sacramento River valley in the foothills of the Sierra Nevada. Chico is about 6 miles east of the Sacramento River. The lower slopes of the nearby Sierra foothills are cut by well-defined canyons draining from northeast to southwest. To the west the Coast Ranges rise up to 7,000 feet; to the east, the peaks of the Sierra Nevada reach as high as 9,000 feet. Thus, the towns of the upper valley are sheltered from ocean breezes and the extreme dryness of the Great Basin.

Climate: As a result of its inland location, the Chico–Paradise region experiences a considerable range of temperature. However, even in winter the average low temperature is not below freezing, which enhances the region's agricultural productivity, particularly in fruit- and nut-growing. The Chico–Paradise area receives 26 inches of rain per year, most of it in the cooler winter months.

Pluses: Mild, sunny, variable.

Minuses: Hot summer days.

Score: 629 **Rank: 45**

Elevation: 230 feet

Relative Humidity: 35%
Wind Speed: 8 mph

Seasonal Change

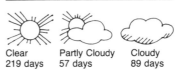

Annual Rainfall 26 in

Annual Snowfall .6 in

Clear 219 days | Partly Cloudy 57 days | Cloudy 89 days

Precipitation Days: 62   Storm Days: 7

Average Temperatures		
	Daily High	Daily Low
January	54	36
February	60	39
March	65	41
April	72	44
May	81	51
June	89	57
July	95	61
August	94	59
September	89	55
October	79	48
November	64	41
December	54	37

Zero-Degree Days: 0
Freezing Days: 36
90-Degree Days: 92

Clayton–Clarksville, GA

Terrain: Located in Habersham and Rabun counties is the Mountain and Intermountain Plateau Province of northeast Georgia. The terrain is hilly to mountainous, with elevations averaging 1,500 feet. To the north, some of the mountains rise above 3,000 feet.

Climate: Nearby mountains, and higher mountains farther north, have a marked influence. Summer heat is tempered by the higher elevations. The contrast of valley and hill exposures results in wide variations in winter low temperatures. Generally, places halfway up the mountain slopes remain warmer during winter nights than do places on the valley floor. Summers are quite pleasant, with warm days and cool nights. Winters are cold but not severe. Spring is changeable and sometimes stormy. Fall is clear and sunny, with chilly nights.

Pluses: Ideal mountain climate, with cool nights year round.

Minuses: Large daily temperature shifts. Stormy springs.

Elevation: 1,470 feet

Relative Humidity: 60%
Wind Speed: 6.8 mph

Seasonal Change

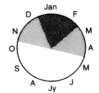

Annual Rainfall 58 in

Annual Snowfall 3.1 in

Clear 122 days   Partly Cloudy 100 days   Cloudy 143 days

Precipitation Days: 86   Storm Days: 70

Average Temperatures		
	Daily High	Daily Low
January	51	28
February	54	29
March	62	36
April	72	43
May	77	51
June	83	58
July	85	62
August	85	62
September	80	56
October	72	44
November	62	35
December	54	30

Zero-Degree Days: 0
Freezing Days: 73
90-Degree Days: 26

Score: 605   **Rank: 53**

Clear Lake, CA

Terrain: Clear Lake is located at an elevation of 1,347 feet in one of California's major recreational and agricultural areas. The rounded mountains of the Coast Range surround the lake on all sides, reaching heights of 3,000 feet to 4,000 feet. A broad valley extends from the lake southward, and the smaller Scott's Valley is directly northwest. Clear Lake is about 40 miles due east of the coast and Point Arena.

Climate: Winters here are cool and wet, and summers are warm and dry. The Pacific remains the dominant climatic influence, but it is modified by the lake's high, mountainous location. There are marked seasonal differences here, and greater temperature extremes than at coastal locations. About 60% of the 29 inches of rain annually falls in the winter months. Summers can be hot, but nights are cool.

Pluses: Scenic setting. Mild, warm climate with seasonal variations.

Minuses: A bit hot and dry.

Elevation: 1,347 feet

Relative Humidity: 55%
Wind Speed: 7.4 mph

Seasonal Change

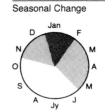

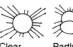
Annual Rainfall 29 in

Annual Snowfall 1.4 in

Clear 148 days   Partly Cloudy 112 days   Cloudy 105 days

Precipitation Days: 50   Storm Days: 9

Average Temperatures		
	Daily High	Daily Low
January	52	32
February	57	34
March	62	35
April	69	39
May	77	43
June	84	48
July	94	52
August	92	50
September	88	48
October	76	42
November	62	36
December	54	33

Zero-Degree Days: 0
Freezing Days: 74
90-Degree Days: 74

Score: 543   **Rank: 73**

Coeur d'Alene, ID

Terrain: The city lies north of Coeur d'Alene Lake, which is about 30 miles long and 2 miles wide. To the east and southwest the city is sheltered by forested hills or low mountains. To the north and northwest lies Rathdrum Prairie. The Coeur d'Alene, St. Joe, and St. Maries rivers drain the heavily forested mountains between the lake and the Bitterroot Mountains, which form the boundary between Idaho and Montana. Within a 10-mile radius of the city, quite a few mountain peaks rise over 4,000 feet.

Climate: Can be generally described as temperate, with dry summers and rainy winters. Though seasonal variation is large, it is less so than most other locations this far north. Rain is heaviest from autumn to early spring. Sunshine records haven't been kept here, but for nearby (and similar) Spokane, they reveal sun 20% of the time in January, 81% in July.

Pluses: Dry, warm summers.

Minuses: Long, rainy winters.

Elevation: 2,158 feet

Relative Humidity: 35%
Wind Speed: 8 mph

Seasonal Change

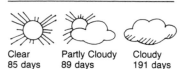

Annual Rainfall 26 in

Annual Snowfall 50 in

Clear 85 days   Partly Cloudy 89 days   Cloudy 191 days

Precipitation Days: 73   Storm Days: 14

Average Temperatures		
	Daily High	Daily Low
January	35	22
February	42	26
March	48	28
April	58	34
May	69	41
June	76	48
July	86	52
August	85	52
September	76	45
October	61	37
November	45	30
December	37	26

Zero-Degree Days: 4
Freezing Days: 141
90-Degree Days: 29

Score: 397   **Rank: 107**

Colorado Springs, CO

Terrain: At an elevation of more than 6,000 feet, Colorado Springs is located in relatively flat semiarid country on the eastern slope of the Rocky Mountains. Immediately to the west, the mountains rise abruptly to heights ranging from 10,000 feet to 14,000 feet. To the east lies the gently undulating prairie land of eastern Colorado. The land slopes upward to the north, reaching an average height of 8,000 feet within 20 miles, at the top of Palmer Lake Divide.

Climate: The terrain of the area, particularly its wide range of elevations, helps to give Colorado Springs the pleasant plains-and-mountain mixture of climate that has established it as a desirable place to live. Precipitation is generally light, with 80% of it falling between April 1 and September 30. Heavy downpours accompany summer thunderstorms. Temperatures are on the mild side for a city in this latitude and at this elevation.

Pluses: Dry, sunny, variable. **Minuses:** Long winters.

Score: 410 **Rank: 102**

Elevation: 6,170 feet

Relative Humidity: 38%
Wind Speed: 10.4 mph

Seasonal Change

Annual Rainfall 16 in

Annual Snowfall 40 in

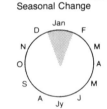

Clear 130 days Partly Cloudy 119 days Cloudy 116 days

Precipitation Days: 87 Storm Days: 59

Average Temperatures		
	Daily High	Daily Low
January	41	16
February	44	19
March	48	23
April	59	33
May	68	43
June	78	51
July	84	57
August	82	56
September	75	47
October	64	37
November	50	25
December	43	19

Zero-Degree Days: 7
Freezing Days: 162
90-Degree Days: 15

★ Daytona Beach, FL

Terrain: Located on the Atlantic Ocean, with the Halifax River, part of the Intracoastal Waterway, running through the city. The land is flat, with no elevations above 35 feet. Soil is mainly sandy.

Climate: Nearness to the ocean results in a climate tempered by land and sea breezes. In the summer, the number of hours of 90° F or more is relatively small due to the beginning of the sea breeze at midday and the occurrence of local afternoon thundershowers which lower the temperature to the more comfortable 80s. Winters, although subject to cold airflows from the north, are relatively mild because of the city's ocean setting and southerly latitude.

Pluses: Mild winters. **Minuses:** Hot, stormy summers.

Score: 814 **Rank: 14**

Elevation: 41 feet

Relative Humidity: 61%
Wind Speed: 9 mph

Seasonal Change

Annual Rainfall 48 in

Annual Snowfall 0 in

Clear 92 days Partly Cloudy 137 days Cloudy 136 days

Precipitation Days: 115 Storm Days: 78

Average Temperatures		
	Daily High	Daily Low
January	69	48
February	70	49
March	75	53
April	80	59
May	85	65
June	88	71
July	90	73
August	89	73
September	87	72
October	81	65
November	75	56
December	70	49

Zero-Degree Days: 0
Freezing Days: 6
90-Degree Days: 54

Eugene–Springfield, OR

Terrain: Situated at the southern end of the fertile Willamette Valley. This valley is bounded on both sides by mountain ranges: the Cascades to the east and the Coast Ranges to the west. To the north, the valley widens and levels out. Hills of the rolling, wooded Coast Ranges begin about 5 miles west of the airport and rise to between 1,500 feet and 2,000 feet midway between the city and the Pacific, 50 miles to the west. The Cascades, 75 miles east, reach heights of 10,000 feet. These sheltering ranges and the proximity of the ocean contribute heavily to Eugene's extremely mild climate. This is one of the nation's most important agricultural and lumbering areas.

Climate: Very mild maritime climate. Temperature minima below 20° F occur only five times a year. The temperature rarely reaches the mid-90s. Seasonal change is gradual, with intermediate seasons being as long as summer and winter.

Pluses: Mild; gradual change of seasons. **Minuses:** Cloudy, damp.

Score: 515 **Rank: 79**

Elevation: 373 feet

Relative Humidity: 73%
Wind Speed: 7.6 mph

Seasonal Change

Annual Rainfall 43 in

Annual Snowfall 7 in

Clear 77 days Partly Cloudy 81 days Cloudy 207 days

Precipitation Days: 137 Storm Days: 5

Average Temperatures		
	Daily High	Daily Low
January	46	33
February	52	35
March	55	37
April	61	39
May	68	44
June	74	49
July	83	51
August	81	51
September	77	47
October	64	42
November	53	38
December	47	36

Zero-Degree Days: 0
Freezing Days: 54
90-Degree Days: 15

Flagstaff, AZ

Terrain: Flagstaff, elevation 7,000 feet, is situated on the volcanic Mogollon plateau at the base of the San Francisco Mountains, the highest in Arizona. The city is entirely surrounded by national forests.
Climate: Classified as vigorous, with cold winters, mild, pleasantly cool summers, and moderate humidity. The stormy months are January, February, March, July, and August. Temperatures in Flagstaff are characteristic of high-altitude climates. The average daily range of temperature is relatively high, especially in winter when extensive snow cover and clear skies cause maximum radiation.

Pluses: Cool, dry summers; snow conditions in winter provide excellent skiing.

Minuses: Extremely high elevation; cold winters, heavy snowfalls.

Elevation: 7,018 feet

Relative Humidity: 39%
Wind Speed: 7.5 mph

Seasonal Change

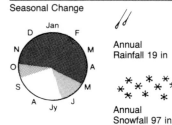

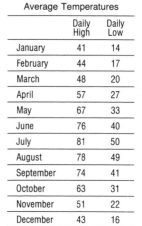

Annual Rainfall 19 in

Annual Snowfall 97 in

Clear 168 days   Partly Cloudy 97 days   Cloudy 100 days

Precipitation Days: 80   Storm Days: 50

Average Temperatures		
	Daily High	Daily Low
January	41	14
February	44	17
March	48	20
April	57	27
May	67	33
June	76	40
July	81	50
August	78	49
September	74	41
October	63	31
November	51	22
December	43	16
Zero-Degree Days: 9		
Freezing Days: 213		
90-Degree Days: 3		

Score: 341   **Rank: 114**

Fort Collins–Loveland, Co

Terrain: Located on the eastern slope of the Rocky Mountains between Denver and Cheyenne, Wyoming, the Fort Collins-Loveland area lies in some of the most spectacular mountain terrain in the country. Steep cliffs (some nearly vertical), high waterfalls, and forested mountain slopes cut by swift rivers are all found to the west. Within 30 miles to the east, the landscape settles into grassland prairies of the Great Plains.
Climate: Near the center of the continent, Fort Collins and Loveland are removed from any major source of airborne moisture and are further shielded from rainfall by the high Rockies to the west. In wintertime, cold air masses from Canada may bring temperatures well below zero at night. In summer, hot, dry air from the desert to the southwest brings with it daytime temperatures of 90° F. However, felt heat is low because of dryness.

Pluses: Semirigorous four-season climate. Spectacular terrain.

Minuses: Cold winters. Hot, dry summers.

Elevation: 5,004 feet

Relative Humidity: 35%
Wind Speed: 9 mph

Seasonal Change

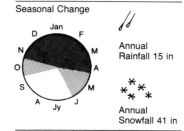

Annual Rainfall 15 in

Annual Snowfall 41 in

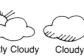

Clear 118 days   Partly Cloudy 128 days   Cloudy 119 days

Precipitation Days: 37   Storm Days: 50

Average Temperatures		
	Daily High	Daily Low
January	41	13
February	45	19
March	50	23
April	60	33
May	70	43
June	80	51
July	86	57
August	83	55
September	75	45
October	65	35
November	50	23
December	44	17
Zero-Degree Days: 15		
Freezing Days: 175		
90-Degree Days: 17		

Score: 405   **Rank: 104**

★ Fort Myers–Cape Coral, FL

Terrain: Located on the Caloosahatchee River, about 15 miles from the Gulf of Mexico, Fort Myers and Cape Coral sit on land that is level and low, with lush greenery.
Climate: Subtropical, with temperature extremes of both summer and winter checked by the influence of the Gulf. The average annual mean temperature is a warm 74° F, with averages ranging from the low 60s in January to the low 80s in the summer months. Winters are mild, with many bright, warm days and moderately cool nights. Maximum temperatures average in the low 90s from June through the first part of September, with daily highs of 90° F or greater on 80% of the days. Rainfall averages more than 50 inches annually, with two-thirds of this total coming between June and September. Most rain falls as late afternoon or early evening thunderstorms, which in the summer bring welcome relief from the heat and occur almost every day.

Pluses: Mild, sunny winters.

Minuses: Hot, humid, stormy.

Elevation: 15 feet

Relative Humidity: 56%
Wind Speed: 8.2 mph

Seasonal Change

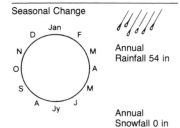

Annual Rainfall 54 in

Annual Snowfall 0 in

Clear 103 days   Partly Cloudy 161 days   Cloudy 101 days

Precipitation Days: 112   Storm Days: 93

Average Temperatures		
	Daily High	Daily Low
January	75	52
February	76	53
March	80	57
April	85	62
May	89	66
June	91	72
July	91	72
August	92	74
September	90	73
October	85	66
November	80	59
December	76	54
Zero-Degree Days: 0		
Freezing Days: 1		
90-Degree Days: 106		

Score: 838   **Rank: 7**

Gainesville–Lake Lanier, GA

Terrain: Gainesville is located in central Hall County, where the Piedmont Plateau Province joins the foothills of the Blue Ridge Mountains. The soil is sandy clay loam and the terrain is rolling to hilly. Elevation in Gainesville is around 1,200 feet, but varies considerably over the county. The city is on the eastern shore of Lake Sidney Lanier, a huge reservoir noted for its fishing, recreational facilities, and beauty.

Climate: Due to its elevation and proximity to the higher elevation of the mountains to the north and northwest, Gainesville has a comparatively mild summer climate. Some hot days can be expected, but fewer than half the days in summer reach 90° F, and summer nights are almost always comfortable. Winters are not severe, though cold weather can be expected. There is usually snow every year, but accumulations are rare.

Pluses: Mild yet variable, with seasonal changes.

Minuses: Rainy. Tornado danger. Can be hot.

Score: 644　　　　　　　　**Rank: 42**

Elevation: 1,170 feet

Relative Humidity: 60%
Wind Speed: 9.1 mph

Seasonal Change

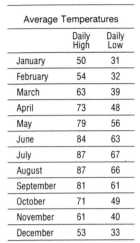

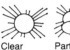
Annual Rainfall 53 in

Annual Snowfall 3 in

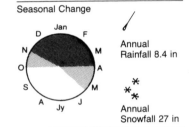

Clear 112 days　Partly Cloudy 105 days　Cloudy 148 days

Precipitation Days: 84　Storm Days: 70

Average Temperatures		
	Daily High	Daily Low
January	50	31
February	54	32
March	63	39
April	73	48
May	79	56
June	84	63
July	87	67
August	87	66
September	81	61
October	71	49
November	61	40
December	53	33
Zero-Degree Days: 0		
Freezing Days: 63		
90-Degree Days: 48		

Grand Junction, CO

Terrain: Situated in a large mountain valley at the junction of the Colorado and Gunnison rivers, Grand Junction lies on the western slope of the Rocky Mountains. The city's climate is marked by wide seasonal temperature changes, but thanks to the protection of the surrounding mountains, sudden and severe weather changes are infrequent. Elevations on the valley floor average about 4,600 feet above sea level, with mountains on all sides reaching as high as 12,000 feet.

Climate: The interior location, coupled with the ring of high mountains, results in low rainfall, and agriculture depends heavily on irrigation, derived from mountain streams and runoff. Winter snows are frequent but light, and do not remain long. In the summer, relative humidity is very low, making the region as dry as parts of Arizona. Sunny days predominate in all seasons.

Pluses: Four-season climate milder than others in comparable latitudes.

Minuses: Low rainfall. Some hot weather.

Score: 469　　　　　　　　**Rank: 86**

Elevation: 4,843 feet

Relative Humidity: 40%
Wind Speed: 8.1 mph

Seasonal Change

Annual Rainfall 8.4 in

Annual Snowfall 27 in

Clear 139 days　Partly Cloudy 107 days　Cloudy 119 days

Precipitation Days: 70　Storm Days: 33

Average Temperatures		
	Daily High	Daily Low
January	37	17
February	44	23
March	53	30
April	65	39
May	76	49
June	86	57
July	93	64
August	89	62
September	81	53
October	68	42
November	51	29
December	39	20
Zero-Degree Days: 7		
Freezing Days: 137		
90-Degree Days: 66		

Grass Valley–Truckee, CA

Terrain: Located on the western slope of the Sierra Nevada. The climate is primarily that of a mountainous region, in this instance modified by the proximity of the Sacramento Valley to the west. The temperature and snowfall can vary greatly from one town to the next in Nevada County, due to the high peaks and ridges of the Sierra Nevada, which serve to block air masses from the coast and the Great Basin, and to channel warm, moist air to high elevations where the moisture is extracted in the form of rain or snow.

Climate: The average annual temperature for the area is about 50° F, with the mean wintertime low being around 29° F and the mean high temperature in the summertime about 76° F. The temperature range during the year is great, with occasional lows at zero and highs in the low 90s. Though the climate is generally mild during most of the year, blizzard conditions and very deep snows (245 inches at Blue Canyon) may prevail during the winter.

Pluses: Spectacular scenery. Pleasant summers and falls.

Minuses: High elevations have blizzard conditions in winter.

Score: 465　　　　　　　　**Rank: 87**

Elevation: 5,280 feet

Relative Humidity: 35%
Wind Speed: 8 mph

Seasonal Change

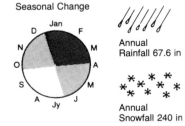
Annual Rainfall 67.6 in

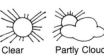
Annual Snowfall 240 in

Clear 175 days　Partly Cloudy 64 days　Cloudy 126 days

Precipitation Days: 89　Storm Days: 12

Average Temperatures		
	Daily High	Daily Low
January	43	30
February	44	31
March	45	31
April	52	36
May	60	43
June	68	50
July	78	59
August	76	57
September	73	53
October	63	45
November	52	37
December	46	33
Zero-Degree Days: 0		
Freezing Days: 100		
90-Degree Days: 1		

Hendersonville–Brevard, NC

Terrain: Hendersonville and Brevard are located in the mountainous southwestern part of the state, just above the South Carolina border. The relief is mostly broken, mountainous, and rugged, with some very steep slopes and high waterfalls. There is a large intermountain valley, with rolling to strongly rolling mountain meadows. The cool climate favors the growth of pasture grasses, potatoes, apples and tree fruits, cabbage, and late truck crops.

Climate: Mildly continental, with considerable differences in temperature between winter and summer. It is mild and pleasant from late spring to late fall, and summer nights are always cool, even following hot afternoons. Hendersonville, Brevard and the cities surrounding them have long been famous as recreational and health resorts.

Pluses: Ideal mild four-season climate.

Minuses: Pronounced temperature shifts possible.

Score: 615   **Rank: 52**

Elevation: 2,153 feet

Relative Humidity: 60%
Wind Speed: 7 mph

Seasonal Change

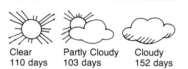

Annual Rainfall 50 in

Annual Snowfall 8.6 in

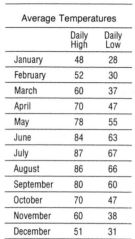

	Average Temperatures	
	Daily High	Daily Low
January	48	28
February	52	30
March	60	37
April	70	47
May	78	55
June	84	63
July	87	67
August	86	66
September	80	60
October	70	47
November	60	38
December	51	31

Zero-Degree Days: 0
Freezing Days: 80
90-Degree days: 8

Clear 110 days   Partly Cloudy 103 days   Cloudy 152 days

Precipitation Days: 132   Storm Days: 47

Hilton Head–Beaufort, SC

Terrain: This area comprises a group of islands in the southern tip of the state. The land is low and flat with elevations mostly under 25 feet. There are dozens of islands of various shapes and sizes, and on them are fresh and saltwater streams, inlets, rivers, and sounds. Most of the islands (except Hilton Head and Port Royal) contain much swampy area. The best beaches are found on Hilton Head, Fripps, and Hunting islands.

Climate: The island group is just on the edge of the balmy subtropical climate enjoyed by Florida and the Caribbean islands. The surrounding water produces a maritime climate, with mild winters, hot summers, and temperatures that shift slowly. The inland Appalachian Mountains block much cold air from the northern interior, and the Gulf Stream moderates the climate considerably.

Pluses: Mild, yet with more seasonal change than places to the south.

Minuses: Summers can be uncomfortably hot and humid.

Score: 729   **Rank: 25**

Elevation: 25 feet

Relative Humidity: 65%
Wind Speed: 7.2 mph

Seasonal Change

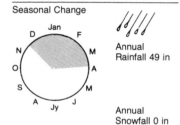

Annual Rainfall 49 in

Annual Snowfall 0 in

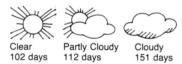

	Average Temperatures	
	Daily High	Daily Low
January	59	38
February	61	42
March	67	46
April	76	55
May	82	62
June	86	68
July	89	71
August	89	71
September	84	67
October	77	57
November	69	47
December	61	39

Clear 102 days   Partly Cloudy 112 days   Cloudy 151 days

Precipitation Days: 115   Storm Days: 77

Zero-Degree Days: 0
Freezing Days: 31
90-Degree Days: 39

Hot Springs–Lake Ouachita, AR

Terrain: This region, famous for its fishing and thermal springs, is located in Garland County in south-central Arkansas. The city of Hot Springs is adjacent to Hot Springs National Park and is in the eastern part of the Ouachita Mountain system. It is near the boundary between the highland (Ozark) and delta regions of the state.

Climate: The irregular topography, with elevations varying from 400 feet to 1,000 feet, has considerable effect on the microclimate of the area, particularly with regard to temperature extremes, ground fog, and precipitation. The climate is generally mild, and favors outdoor activities almost year round. However, the area is subject to storms, flash floods, and extreme heat and cold. Winter temperatures fall below freezing only half the time. Summers are warm and long, springs changeable. The freeze-free growing period is long: 225 days.

Pluses: Long, warm summers. Mild winters.

Minuses: Hot, muggy spells in summer.

Score: 652   **Rank: 41**

Elevation: 630 feet

Relative Humidity: 55%
Wind Speed: 8.1 mph

Seasonal Change

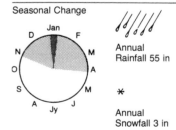

Annual Rainfall 55 in

Annual Snowfall 3 in

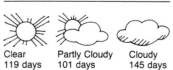

	Average Temperatures	
	Daily High	Daily Low
January	52	31
February	57	34
March	65	41
April	75	52
May	82	59
June	89	67
July	93	71
August	93	70
September	87	63
October	77	53
November	63	42
December	55	35

Zero-Degree Days: 0
Freezing Days: 47
90-Degree Days: 90

Clear 119 days   Partly Cloudy 101 days   Cloudy 145 days

Precipitation Days: 72   Storm Days: 79

Houghton Lake, MI

Terrain: This resort area is located in north-central Lower Michigan. Houghton Lake, the largest inland lake in the state, lies within Michigan's central plateau, which is 1,000 feet above sea level. The land around the lake is level to rolling, gradually dropping off toward the east and, more rapidly, to the south; to the north are hills and ridges 100 feet to 300 feet higher. However, the region's thick woods and abundant streams and lakes make it a natural tourist and recreation area.

Climate: The daily and seasonal temperature range is greater here than along Michigan's shorelines, where the modifying effects of the various Great Lakes can be felt. Rainfall is heaviest in the summer, with 60% of it falling between April and September. Winters here are cold and snowy, though not as snowy as those in locations to the north and west. Cloudiness is greatest in late fall and winter. The growing season is only 90 days.

Pluses: Excellent fishing, hunting, water sports.

Minuses: Long, cold winters. Cloudy.

Score: 285   **Rank: 128**

Elevation: 1,149 feet

Relative Humidity: 64%
Wind Speed: 8.9 mph

Seasonal Change

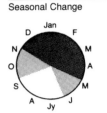

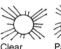
Annual Rainfall 28 in

Annual Snowfall 83 in

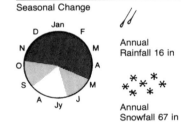

Clear 70 days   Partly Cloudy 98 days   Cloudy 197 days

Precipitation Days: 144   Storm Days: 36

Average Temperatures		
	Daily High	Daily Low
January	26	9
February	28	8
March	37	16
April	53	31
May	65	40
June	75	50
July	79	54
August	77	53
September	68	46
October	58	37
November	42	27
December	30	16

Zero-Degree Days: 25
Freezing Days: 175
90-Degree Days: 2

Kalispell, MT

Terrain: Kalispell, the seat of Flathead County, is located 8 miles northwest of the north end of Flathead Lake, in the valley of the same name. The climate of Flathead Valley differs from that found east of the Continental Divide (40 miles east of Kalispell), largely because of the high mountains to the east, which block cold air from Alberta in the wintertime. These rise 4,500 feet above the valley floor, and assure frequent and beneficial rains by cooling the moist ocean air arriving from the west. In addition to Flathead, the valley contains four smaller lakes and numerous streams and sloughs.

Climate: There is more precipitation on the eastern side of the valley than the western. In winter, the eastern portion receives 68 inches of snow, the western only 49 inches. Kalispell is windy, with intense winds often reaching 30 mph to 40 mph. Winter is cold; summers are pleasant and dry.

Pluses: Beautiful, rugged northern mountain country.

Minuses: Can be cold, cloudy, windy.

Score: 263   **Rank: 129**

Elevation: 2,965 feet

Relative Humidity: 51%
Wind Speed: 6.8 mph

Seasonal Change

Annual Rainfall 16 in

Annual Snowfall 67 in

Clear 71 days   Partly Cloudy 81 days   Cloudy 213 days

Precipitation Days: 131   Storm Days: 23

Average Temperatures		
	Daily High	Daily Low
January	27	11
February	34	16
March	41	20
April	54	30
May	64	38
June	70	44
July	81	48
August	79	46
September	68	39
October	54	31
November	39	23
December	31	17

Zero-Degree Days: 17
Freezing Days: 191
90-Degree Days: 15

★ Kauai, HI

Terrain: Kauai is an island 33 miles long and 25 miles wide. The eastern third consists of broadly eroded valley lands; the western two-thirds is mountainous. Mt. Waialeale, the highest elevation on the island (5,075 feet above sea level) lies near the center of Kauai.

Climate: Marked by extremely equable temperature conditions from day to day and from season to season, the persistent trade-wind airflow from the northeasterly quadrant, and the marked variation in rainfall from the wet to the dry season. Completely cloudless skies are quite rare. Three-fourths of Kauai's precipitation falls during the seven-month wet season which extends from October to April. Relative humidity, moderate to high in all seasons, is slightly higher in the wet season than in the dry. However, even during periods when the temperature and humidity are both high, trade winds provide natural ventilation.

Pluses: Extremely mild.

Minuses: A bit monotonous.

Score: 915   **Rank: 2**

Elevation: 148 feet

Relative Humidity: 67%
Wind Speed: 11.7 mph

Seasonal Change

Annual Rainfall 44 in

Annual Snowfall 0 in

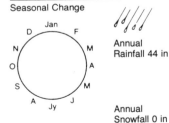

Clear 51 days   Partly Cloudy 176 days   Cloudy 138 days

Precipitation Days: 202   Storm Days: 9

Average Temperatures		
	Daily High	Daily Low
January	78	64
February	78	64
March	78	65
April	79	67
May	81	70
June	83	72
July	84	73
August	85	74
September	85	73
October	83	71
November	81	70
December	78	67

Zero-Degree Days: 0
Freezing Days: 0
90-Degree Days: 0

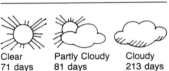

Keene, NH

Terrain: Located in southwestern New Hampshire, in the relatively flat Ashuelot River Valley, which is about 2 miles wide near the city. The valley is about 500 feet above sea level and is surrounded by hills. Peaks of 1,300 feet to 1,500 feet are within 5 miles of Keene. High peaks of the White Mountains lie 80 miles north northwest, while the main ridge of the Green Mountains lies 40 miles west.

Climate: Semirigorous continental, characterized by changeable weather, large annual and daily temperature ranges, and great differences between the same seasons in different years. In common with most of New England, there is no "rainy" or "dry" season, but rather, abundant rainfall year round. Summers are delightful but short, winters moderately cold and fairly long, and springs and falls pleasant, changeable, and brief.

Pluses: Fine four-season climate, a bit on the rugged side.

Minuses: Brief summers.

Score: 315

Rank: 124

Elevation: 490 feet

Relative Humidity: 60%
Wind Speed: 10.4 mph

Seasonal Change

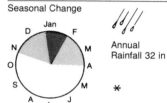

Annual Rainfall 41 in

Annual Snowfall 60 in

Clear 90 days   Partly Cloudy 109 days   Cloudy 166 days

Precipitation Days: 83   Storm Days: 24

Average Temperatures		
	Daily High	Daily Low
January	29	6
February	32	8
March	41	20
April	55	31
May	68	41
June	77	51
July	81	56
August	79	54
September	70	46
October	59	36
November	45	27
December	32	13

Zero-Degree Days: 16
Freezing Days: 167
90-Degree Days: 11

Kerrville, TX

Terrain: Kerr County lies across the hills, valleys, and uplands of the rolling Hill Country of southwest Texas, at the edge of the Edwards Plateau. The western part of the county is on a rolling plain covered with cedars and live oak trees. The eastern part breaks into the deep valleys of the Guadalupe River and its tributaries. Kerr County is an outstanding tourist resort area for hunting deer, turkey, and other game.

Climate: Mainly continental in character, especially in the winter, with wide swings of temperature both daily and seasonally. Rainfall tapers off from east to west rather sharply, from annual totals of 32 inches in the east to only 24 inches in the west. Winter precipitation is mostly slow, steady, light rain. Summer months are dry and hot. Falls are pleasant but can be stormy due to "northers" and Gulf storms moving north.

Pluses: Minimal winter. Warm.

Minuses: Summers can be hot.

Score: 692

Rank: 32

Elevation: 1,650 feet

Relative Humidity: 50%
Wind Speed: 9.3 mph

Seasonal Change

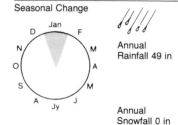

Annual Rainfall 32 in

Annual Snowfall 1.1 in

Clear 116 days   Partly Cloudy 114 days   Cloudy 135 days

Precipitation Days: 50   Storm Days: 51

Average Temperatures		
	Daily High	Daily Low
January	61	33
February	64	37
March	71	42
April	78	51
May	84	59
June	90	66
July	94	68
August	95	67
September	89	62
October	80	52
November	68	40
December	63	34

Zero-Degree Days: 0
Freezing Days: 60
90-Degree days: 101

★ Lakeland–Winter Haven, FL

Terrain: Located slightly west of the center of the Florida peninsula in the rolling lake-ridge section, 50 miles from the Gulf of Mexico and 70 miles from the Atlantic Ocean. Lakeland's elevation of 236 feet above sea level is the highest of any town or city in the Florida peninsula.

Climate: Classified as subtropical because of its low latitude and the proximity of the Gulf of Mexico and the Atlantic Ocean. Winters are pleasant, characterized by bright warm days, cool nights, and moderately light rainfall. Occasionally, major cold waves overspread the area, bringing temperatures down to the low 30s and mid-20s. Summers are long with high temperatures moderated in the afternoon by thundershowers.

Pluses: Mild, pleasant winters.

Minuses: Hot summers; frequent thundershowers.

Score: 828

Rank: 9

Elevation: 236 feet

Relative Humidity: 60%
Wind Speed: 6.9 mph

Seasonal Change

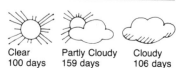

Annual Rainfall 49 in

Annual Snowfall 0 in

Clear 100 days   Partly Cloudy 159 days   Cloudy 106 days

Precipitation Days: 120   Storm Days: 100

Average Temperatures		
	Daily High	Daily Low
January	71	51
February	72	52
March	76	56
April	82	62
May	87	67
June	90	71
July	90	73
August	90	73
September	88	72
October	82	66
November	76	58
December	72	53

Zero-Degree Days: 0
Freezing Days: 2
90-Degree Days: 83

Lancaster, PA

Terrain: Situated in the heart of Pennsylvania Dutch country in the southeastern part of the state, Lancaster lies about 100 miles northwest of the Atlantic and 30 miles southeast of the Blue Ridge Mountains. All around the city, the rich farmland—flat to gently rolling—is extensively cultivated.

Climate: Because of its proximity to the ocean and the protection afforded by the mountains of central Pennsylvania, Lancaster enjoys a comparatively moderate climate. Conditions range from relatively mild in winter to warm and humid in summer, with weather changes every few days throughout the year. Cold air outbreaks in winter can result in zero or near zero temperatures, but these are rare. Hot spells occur each summer, during which afternoons are uncomfortable. However, nights are generally cooler—in the 70s—and the heat spells don't last more than a few days.

Pluses: Mild four-season climate.

Minuses: Humid, can be muggy.

Score: 497 **Rank: 80**

Elevation: 255 feet

Relative Humidity: 55%
Wind Speed: 7.7 mph

Seasonal Change

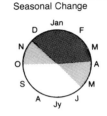

Annual Rainfall 43 in

Annual Snowfall 24 in

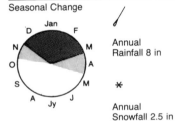

Clear 86 days Partly Cloudy 107 days Cloudy 172 days

Precipitation Days: 77   Storm Days: 46

Average Temperatures		
	Daily High	Daily Low
January	41	23
February	43	22
March	52	29
April	65	38
May	76	49
June	83	58
July	87	62
August	84	61
September	78	53
October	67	42
November	54	32
December	42	24

Zero-Degree Days: 2
Freezing Days: 135
90-Degree Days: 27

Las Cruces, NM

Terrain: The seat of Dona Ana County, Las Cruces is located in the Rio Grande River Valley, about 25 miles north of the Texas border. The wide, level valley runs northwest to southeast through this area, with rolling desert bordering it to the southwest and west. About 12 miles to the east the Organ Mountains, with peaks above 8,500 feet, form a rugged backdrop for the city. The northwest portion of the valley narrows, and is bordered by low hills and buttes.

Climate: Arid continental, characterized by low rainfall, moderately warm summers, and mild, pleasant winters. The rainfall, at 8 inches per year, is light. But since almost all of it falls during the summer growing months, considerable forage is available on nearby grazing lands. The rain falls in brief showers; drizzles are unknown. Summers are hot, but the nights are cool. Winters tend to be mild and sunny.

Pluses: Warm and sunny, even in winter.

Minuses: Summer afternoons can be hot and dusty.

Score: 552 **Rank: 72**

Elevation: 3,881 feet

Relative Humidity: 40%
Wind Speed: 9.5 mph

Seasonal Change

Annual Rainfall 8 in

Annual Snowfall 2.5 in

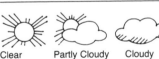

Clear 194 days Partly Cloudy 99 days Cloudy 72 days

Precipitation Days: 21   Storm Days: 58

Average Temperatures		
	Daily High	Daily Low
January	56	25
February	62	28
March	27	34
April	77	41
May	85	49
June	94	59
July	94	65
August	92	64
September	87	56
October	78	44
November	65	30
December	58	26

Zero-Degree Days: 0
Freezing Days: 111
90-Degree Days: 101

Las Vegas, NV

Terrain: Situated near the center of a broad desert valley surrounded by mountains ranging from 2,000 feet to 10,000 feet higher than the valley's floor. These mountains act as effective barriers to moisture-laden storms moving eastward from the Pacific Ocean, so that Las Vegas sees very few overcast or rainy days.

Climate: Summers are typical of a desert climate—low humidity with maximum temperatures in the 100-degree levels. Nearby mountains contribute to relatively cool nights, with minimums between 70° F and 75° F. Springs and falls are ideal: Outdoor activities are rarely interrupted by adverse weather conditions. Winters, too, are mild, with daytime averages of 60° F, clear skies, and warm sunshine.

Pluses: Mild year-round climate with especially pleasant springs and falls.

Minuses: High winds, though infrequent, bring dust and sand.

Score: 628 **Rank: 46**

Relative Humidity: 20%
Wind Speed: 9 mph

Seasonal Change

Annual Rainfall 4 in

Annual Snowfall 1.5 in

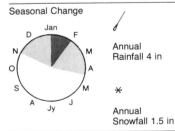

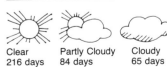

Clear 216 days Partly Cloudy 84 days Cloudy 65 days

Precipitation Days: 24   Storm Days: 15

Average Temperatures		
	Daily High	Daily Low
January	56	33
February	61	37
March	68	42
April	78	50
May	88	59
June	97	67
July	104	75
August	102	73
September	95	65
October	81	53
November	66	41
December	57	34

Zero-Degree Days: 0
Freezing Days: 41
90-Degree Days: 131

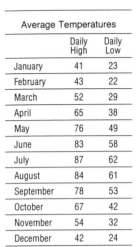

Lexington, KY

Terrain: Located in the heart of the Kentucky Bluegrass region on a gently rolling plateau with varying elevations of 900 feet to 1,050 feet. The surrounding country is noted for its beauty, fertile soil, excellent grass, stock farms, and burley tobacco. There are no bodies of water nearby that are large enough to have an effect on climate.
Climate: Decidedly continental, temperate, yet subject to sudden large but brief changes in temperature. Precipitation is evenly distributed throughout the winter, spring, and summer, with an average of 12 inches falling in each of these seasons. Snowfall is variable, but the ground does not retain snow for more than a few days at a time. The months of September and October are the most pleasant of the year; they have the least precipitation, the most clear days, and generally comfortable temperatures.

Pluses: Temperate four-season climate with pleasant falls.

Minuses: Large diurnal temperature range.

Score: 554   **Rank: 70**

Elevation: 989 feet

Relative Humidity: 60%
Wind Speed: 9.6 mph

Seasonal Change

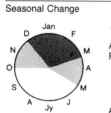

Annual Rainfall 50 in

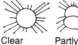

Annual Snowfall 16 in

Clear 95 days   Partly Cloudy 102 days   Cloudy 168 days

Precipitation Days: 130   Storm Days: 47

Average Temperatures		
	Daily High	Daily Low
January	42	25
February	44	26
March	53	34
April	66	45
May	76	54
June	84	63
July	86	66
August	86	64
September	80	58
October	69	47
November	54	35
December	44	27

Zero-Degree Days: 2
Freezing Days: 97
90-Degree Days: 16

Madison, WI

Terrain: Madison sits on a narrow isthmus of land between Lakes Mendota (15 square miles) and Monona (5 square miles). Normally these lakes are frozen from December 17 to April 5. Most farming is dairying, with field crops mainly of corn, oats, and alfalfa. The majority of fruits grown are apples, strawberries, and raspberries.
Climate: Continental, typical of interior North America, with a large annual temperature range and frequent short periods of temperature changes. Winter temperatures average 20° F and summer ones 68° F. The most common air masses are of polar origin, with occasional outbreaks of arctic air during the winter. Much of the precipitation falls between May and September. Lighter winter precipitation falls over a longer period of time.

Pluses: Pleasant summers with moderate growing season; even precipitation.

Minuses: Long, severe winters.

Score: 337   **Rank: 116**

Elevation: 866 feet

Relative Humidity: 61%
Wind Speed: 9.9 mph

Seasonal Change

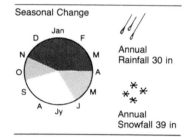

Annual Rainfall 30 in

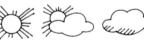

Annual Snowfall 39 in

Clear 94 days   Partly Cloudy 96 days   Cloudy 175 days

Precipitation Days: 117   Storm Days: 40

Average Temperatures		
	Daily High	Daily Low
January	25	8
February	30	11
March	39	21
April	56	35
May	67	45
June	77	55
July	81	59
August	80	57
September	71	49
October	61	39
November	43	26
December	30	14

Zero-Degree Days: 25
Freezing Days: 164
90-Degree Days: 12

★ Maui, HI

Terrain: The most centrally located of Hawaii's major islands, Maui lies between Oahu and the Big Island of Hawaii. The island is mountainous, with the peaks of west Maui rising to almost 6,000 feet, and those to the southeast rising to over 10,000 feet.
Climate: The outstanding features of Maui's climate are the equable temperatures from day to day and season to season; the marked variation in rainfall on the island from season to season and place to place; the persistence of winds from the northeast quadrant; and the rarity of severe storms. For a visitor from the mainland, the steady, mild temperature is probably the biggest surprise. The normal temperature range between the warmest month (August) and the coldest (February) is only eight degrees! At Kahului, where these data were recorded, the average mean humidity is fairly high (72%) and the rainfall is low, averaging under 30 inches.

Pluses: Very mild maritime climate.

Minuses: Monotonous.

Score: 925   **Rank: 1**

Elevation: 103 feet

Relative Humidity: 58%
Wind Speed: 12.9 mph

Seasonal Change

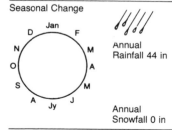

Annual Rainfall 44 in

Annual Snowfall 0 in

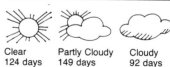

Clear 124 days   Partly Cloudy 149 days   Cloudy 92 days

Precipitation Days: 202   Storm Days: 8

Average Temperatures		
	Daily High	Daily Low
January	80	64
February	79	64
March	80	64
April	82	66
May	84	67
June	85	69
July	86	70
August	87	71
September	87	70
October	86	69
November	83	68
December	80	66

Zero-Degree Days: 0
Freezing Days: 0
90-Degree Days: 0

Medford–Ashland, OR

Terrain: Located in a mountain valley formed by the famous Rogue River and one of its tributaries, Bear Creek. Most of the valley ranges in elevation from 1,300 feet to 1,400 feet above sea level. The valley's outlet to the ocean 80 miles west is the narrow canyon of the Rogue.
Climate: Moderate, with marked seasonal characteristics. Late fall, winter, and early spring are cloudy, damp, and cool. The remainder of the year is warm, dry, and sunny. The rain shadow afforded by the Siskiyous and the Coast Range results in relatively light rainfall, most of which falls in the wintertime. Snowfalls are very light and seldom remain on the ground more than 24 hours. Winters are mild, with the temperatures just dipping below freezing during December and January. Summer days can reach 90° F, but nights are cool. The climate is ideal for truck and fruit farming, and the area is dotted with orchards.

Pluses: Very mild four-season climate. Sunny summers.

Minuses: Half the year is damp and cloudy.

Score: 492　　　　　**Rank: 81**

Elevation: 1,298 feet

Relative Humidity: 67%
Wind Speed: 4.8 mph

Seasonal Change

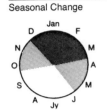

Annual Rainfall 21 in

Annual Snowfall 8 in

Clear 117 days　Partly Cloudy 79 days　Cloudy 169 days

Precipitation Days: 101　Storm Days: 9

Average Temperatures	Daily High	Daily Low
January	44	29
February	52	31
March	57	33
April	64	37
May	72	43
June	79	49
July	90	54
August	88	53
September	82	47
October	67	39
November	53	34
December	44	31

Zero-Degree Days: 0
Freezing Days: 90
90-Degree Days: 54

★ Miami–Hialeah, FL

Terrain: Located on the lower east coast of Florida. To the east lies Biscayne Bay, and east of it Miami Beach. The surrounding country-side is level and sparsely wooded.
Climate: Essentially subtropical marine, characterized by a long, warm summer with abundant rainfall and a mild, dry winter. The Atlantic Ocean greatly influences the city's small range of daily temperature and aids the rapid warming of colder air masses that pass to the east of the state. During the early morning hours, more rainfall occurs at Miami Beach than at the airport (9 miles inland), while during the afternoon the reverse is true. Even more striking is the difference in the annual number of days over 90° F: at Miami Beach, 15 days; at the airport, 60. Freezing temperatures occur occasionally in surrounding farming districts but almost never near the ocean. In 1977, for the first time in Miami's history, traces of snow were reported. Tropical hurricanes affect the area and are the most frequent in early fall.

Pluses: Single-season, sub-tropical marine climate.

Minuses: Hurricanes. Frequent thunderstorms.

Score: 867　　　　　**Rank: 3**

Elevation: 12 feet

Relative Humidity: 62%
Wind Speed: 9.2 mph

Seasonal Change

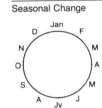

Annual Rainfall 60 in

Annual Snowfall 0 in

Clear 76 days　Partly Cloudy 172 days　Cloudy 117 days

Precipitation Days: 129　Storm Days: 75

Average Temperatures	Daily High	Daily Low
January	76	59
February	77	59
March	80	63
April	83	68
May	85	71
June	88	74
July	89	76
August	90	76
September	88	75
October	85	71
November	80	65
December	77	60

Zero-Degree Days: 0
Freezing Days: 0
90-Degree Days: 30

Missoula, MT

Terrain: Located in the heart of the Montana Rocky Mountains in the extreme north portion of the Bitterroot Valley. The Great Divide is 70 miles east of the city, and the Bitterroot Range is 20 miles to the southwest. These two mountain ranges have a marked effect on Missoula's climate.
Climate: Rigorous, semiarid continental. Missoula receives just 12 to 15 inches of precipitation annually. Generally the spring months are cool and a little damp, with almost daily shower activity during May and June. The summer months are dry with moderate temperatures. Oppressively warm nighttime temperatures are unknown. In the winter, the Great Divide shields Missoula from much of the severely cold air that sweeps down the continent from the arctic regions. Occasionally, the arctic air breaks over the mountains and moves with force into the Bitterroot Valley. When this happens, Missoula experiences severe blizzard conditions.

Pluses: Cool, dry summers.

Minuses: Cold winters with occasional blizzards.

Score: 294　　　　　**Rank: 127**

Elevation: 3,200 feet

Relative Humidity: 50%
Wind Speed: 5.2 mph

Seasonal Change

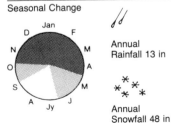

Annual Rainfall 13 in

Annual Snowfall 48 in

Clear 75 days　Partly Cloudy 82 days　Cloudy 210 days

Precipitation Days: 124　Storm Days: 24

Average Temperatures	Daily High	Daily Low
January	28	13
February	35	19
March	43	23
April	57	31
May	66	39
June	73	45
July	84	49
August	83	48
September	71	40
October	57	31
November	40	24
December	31	18

Zero-Degree Days: 11
Freezing Days: 189
90-Degree Days: 32

Mountain Home–Bull Shoals, AR

Terrain: Bull Shoals Dam and the White River lakes (Beaver, Table Rock, Bull Shoals, and Norfork) are located in the Arkansas–Missouri Ozark Mountain country. These lakes are really reservoirs, with a water surface area of 290 square miles. Elevations in the area vary from 500 feet to 1,400 feet. The most rugged terrain is near Beaver Dam. Gently rolling hills surround Lake Norfork. The country is rugged and wooded, with farms small and scattered. This area is one of the most famous fishing spots in the country. In addition, the woods are full of game such as deer, turkey, duck, and quail.
Climate: Primarily modified continental, with warm summers and mild winters. Each year it can vary from warm and humid maritime to cold and dry continental, but it is relatively free from climatic extremes.

Pluses: Scenic. Great recreational opportunities. Mild winters.

Minuses: Some winter cold snaps and summer heat waves. Subject to ice and sleet.

Score: 592　　　　　**Rank: 55**

Elevation: 900 feet

Relative Humidity: 55%
Wind Speed: 11 mph

Seasonal Change

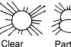

Annual Rainfall 42 in

Annual Snowfall 7.6 in

Clear 119 days　　Partly Cloudy 96 days　　Cloudy 150 days

Precipitation Days: 68　　Storm Days: 81

Average Temperatures		
	Daily High	Daily Low
January	46	24
February	51	28
March	60	36
April	72	47
May	79	55
June	86	63
July	91	67
August	90	66
September	84	59
October	74	47
November	60	36
December	50	29

Zero-Degree Days: 0
Freezing Days: 88
90-Degree Days: 69

Murray–Kentucky Lake, KY

Terrain: The Two Rivers Breaks area covers several hundred square miles in western Kentucky. Elevations vary from 350 feet to 600 feet. Lakes Barkley and Kentucky were formed by damming the Tennessee and Cumberland rivers. The thin finger of land between them is called Land Between the Lakes recreation area. The entire area, both in Kentucky and Tennessee, is famous for fishing.
Climate: Temperate, with moderately cold winters and warm, humid summers. Precipitation is ample and well-distributed throughout the year. Most days, even those in winter, are suitable for outdoor activity, with temperatures in winter reaching 50° F or more 11 to 16 days per month. Spring and fall are the most comfortable seasons, with fall being remarkably free from storms or cold. There are about 52 thunderstorms per year. The sunniest months are September and October; the cloudiest is January.

Pluses: Milder than many locations farther north. Scenic.

Minuses: Fairly damp. Summers can be uncomfortable.

Score: 592　　　　　**Rank: 55**

Elevation: 450 feet

Relative Humidity: 60%
Wind Speed: 8 mph

Seasonal Change

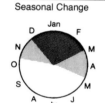

Annual Rainfall 49 in

Annual Snowfall 8 in

Clear 102 days　　Partly Cloudy 108 days　　Cloudy 155 days

Precipitation Days: 76　　Storm Days: 53

Average Temperatures		
	Daily High	Daily Low
January	44	26
February	49	29
March	59	37
April	71	48
May	79	56
June	87	64
July	90	68
August	89	66
September	83	59
October	72	47
November	59	37
December	49	30

Zero-Degree Days: 1
Freezing Days: 87
90-Degree Days: 67

Myrtle Beach, SC

Terrain: Located in the center of the long coastal area known as the Grand Strand, which extends for 43 miles and has a populated area only a few blocks wide. The land is low and swampy inland, and the entire area is quite flat, with no elevations greater than 50 feet above sea level. There are many more trees and wooded areas than are usually found in a beach area. The beaches themselves are of white sand, and the water is quite clean, as there are no harbors, shipping, or major industries nearby. Also, no rivers or streams empty into the sea for a distance of almost 30 miles.
Climate: Mild winters and warm summers are the rule. The ocean has a pronounced modifying effect on temperatures, and the Blue Ridge Mountains inland block much cold air from the interior. Some tropical storms reach the area every few years.

Pluses: Warm, mild, steady.

Minuses: Can be hot and muggy. Tropical storms.

Score: 696　　　　　**Rank: 30**

Elevation: 25 feet

Relative Humidity: 65%
Wind Speed: 8.8 mph

Seasonal Change

Annual Rainfall 48 in

Annual Snowfall 0 in

Clear 102 days　　Partly Cloudy 110 days　　Cloudy 153 days

Precipitation Days: 112　　Storm Days: 76

Average Temperatures		
	Daily High	Daily Low
January	57	35
February	59	36
March	64	42
April	73	52
May	80	61
June	84	67
July	88	70
August	89	70
September	83	65
October	75	53
November	68	44
December	58	35

Zero-Degree Days: 0
Freezing Days: 54
90-Degree Days: 28

Newport–Lincoln City, OR

Terrain: These places lie directly on the Pacific Coast, with marine climates typical of Oregon's coastal area. Although this climate summary describes Newport, it is applicable to Lincoln City, 25 miles north. Just to the east of Newport's city limits, the foothills of the Coast Range begin their fairly steep ascent to ridges which are 2,000 feet to 3,000 feet high 12 miles east of the city. Though part of the city sits at the water's edge, a considerable portion of it is built on level bench land about 150 feet above sea level.

Climate: Newport receives warm, moist air from the Pacific. Accordingly, summers are mild and pleasant. In the winter, the air releases its moisture over the cold landmass, resulting in frequent clouds and rain from November through March. Some 70% of the annual rainfall occurs during these winter months. Very high and very low temperatures are almost nonexistent.

Pluses: Very mild maritime climate, with cool summers, mild winters.

Minuses: Cloudy, wet winters with little sun or snow.

Score: 487   **Rank: 83**

Elevation: 136 ft

Relative Humidity: 60%
Wind Speed: 7.6 mph

Seasonal Change

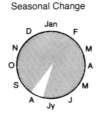

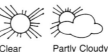
Annual Rainfall 63 in

Annual Snowfall 1.2 in

Clear 75 days   Partly Cloudy 80 days   Cloudy 210 days

Precipitation Days: 122   Storm Days: 3

Average Temperatures		
	Daily High	Daily Low
January	50	39
February	51	39
March	53	40
April	56	42
May	59	46
June	62	49
July	64	51
August	65	51
September	65	49
October	61	46
November	56	42
December	51	40

Zero-Degree Days: 0
Freezing Days: 17
90-Degree Days: 0

North Conway–White Mountains, NH

Terrain: North Conway, long famous as a recreation and resort area for both winter and summer sports and summer recreation, lies nestled in the White Mountains. About 20 miles south is Lake Winnipesaukee, the state's largest, noted for year-round recreation and fine fishing. From the lake to the ski resorts around North Conway, the terrain rises dramatically from elevations of about 2,000 feet to more than 6,000 feet in the Presidential Range. The area is generally rugged, scenic, and heavily forested. Interspersed between ranges and peaks are broad valleys suitable for dairy and truck farming.

Climate: Semirigorous continental, with delightful summers that aren't too hot. Summer nights are cool, and the days usually sunny. Falls are pleasant, and famous throughout the region for the bright colors of the foliage. Winters are long, snowy, and sometimes very cold for periods of several days to a week. Springs changeable.

Pluses: Scenic. Pleasant summers.

Minuses: Winters are long and snowy.

Score: 307   **Rank: 125**

Elevation: 720 feet

Relative Humidity: 60%
Wind Speed: 6.8 mph

Seasonal Change

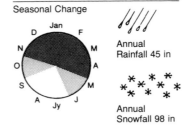

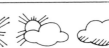
Annual Rainfall 45 in

Annual Snowfall 98 in

Clear 93 days   Partly Cloudy 111 days   Cloudy 161 days

Precipitation Days: 90   Storm Days: 46

Average Temperatures		
	Daily High	Daily Low
January	30	8
February	33	10
March	41	19
April	54	30
May	66	40
June	76	49
July	81	53
August	78	52
September	71	45
October	61	35
November	45	27
December	32	13

Zero-Degree Days: 25
Freezing Days: 187
90-Degree Days: 7

Olympia, WA

Terrain: The capital of the state of Washington, Olympia lies at the southernmost end of Puget Sound, some 60 miles south-southwest of Seattle. The Olympic Peninsula, with its fine remnants of the Pacific Northwest rain forests, active glaciers, and alpine meadows, lies to the northwest. The city and vicinity are quite well protected by the Coast Range from the strong south and southwest winds accompanying many Pacific storms during the fall and winter.

Climate: Characterized by warm, generally dry summers and wet, mild winters. Fall rains begin in October and continue with few interruptions until spring. During the rainy season there is little variation in temperature, with days in the 40s and 50s and nights in the 30s, and constant cloud cover. The summer highs are between 60° F and 80° F, with up to 20 days without rain. The summer is marked by clear skies at night and frequent morning fog.

Pluses: Mild winters, dry summers.

Minuses: Cloudy, damp, rainy.

Score: 460   **Rank: 88**

Elevation: 195 feet

Relative Humidity: 70%
Wind Speed: 6.7 mph

Seasonal Change

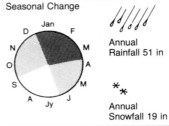

Annual Rainfall 51 in

Annual Snowfall 19 in

Clear 49 days   Partly Cloudy 88 days   Cloudy 228 days

Precipitation Days: 163   Storm Days: 5

Average Temperatures		
	Daily High	Daily Low
January	44	30
February	49	32
March	54	33
April	60	37
May	67	41
June	72	46
July	78	49
August	77	48
September	72	45
October	61	40
November	51	35
December	46	33

Zero-Degree Days: 0
Freezing Days: 89
90-Degree Days: 6

★ Orlando, FL

Terrain: Located in the central section of the Florida peninsula, almost surrounded by lakes. The countryside is flat, with no natural barriers to exterior weather systems.

Climate: Because of the surrounding water, relative humidity remains high year-round, hovering near 90% at night and dipping to 50% in the afternoon. The rainy season extends from June through September; afternoon thundershowers occur daily. Rain is light during the winter, and snow and sleet are rare. Winter temperatures may drop to freezing at night, but days are usually pleasant, with brilliant sunshine.

Pluses: Mild.

Minuses: Humid year-round; hot summers with daily thundershowers.

Score: 825   **Rank: 10**

Elevation: 106 feet

Relative Humidity: 60%
Wind Speed: 8.7 mph

Seasonal Change

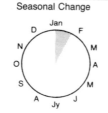

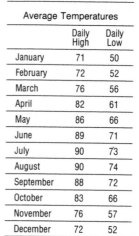

Annual Rainfall 51 in

Annual Snowfall 0 in

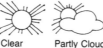

Clear 94 days   Partly Cloudy 148 days   Cloudy 123 days

Precipitation Days: 116   Storm Days: 81

Average Temperatures		
	Daily High	Daily Low
January	71	50
February	72	52
March	76	56
April	82	61
May	86	66
June	89	71
July	90	73
August	90	74
September	88	72
October	83	66
November	76	57
December	72	52
Zero-Degree Days: 0		
Freezing Days: 2		
90-Degree Days: 104		

Oscoda–Huron Shore, MI

Terrain: Located on the shore of Lake Huron at the northern edge of Saginaw Bay. The land is level and the soil is sandy. Most of the surrounding area is heavily forested with conifers, maple, oak, and birch.

Climate: Definitely influenced by the lake, especially when the winds are from the south or east. As in other parts of Michigan's Lower Peninsula, the climate is also modified by the westerly winds that have passed over Lake Michigan, picking up warmth and moisture in winter and being cooled in summer. The wettest month is June; the driest is February. Cloudiness is most pronounced in late fall and early winter. Winter comes early (in mid-to-late October) and does not cease until late April or early May. Thick ice extends over all the inland lakes during most of this period and oftentimes does not melt away until late May. Summers are delightful but rather short.

Pluses: Ideal summer weather, with warm days and cool nights.

Minuses: Winters are long and cold.

Score: 334   **Rank: 117**

Elevation: 590 feet

Relative Humidity: 60%
Wind Speed: 7.6 mph

Seasonal Change

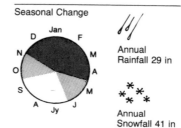

Annual Rainfall 29 in

Annual Snowfall 41 in

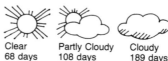

Clear 68 days   Partly Cloudy 108 days   Cloudy 189 days

Precipitation Days: 65   Storm Days: 39

Average Temperatures		
	Daily High	Daily Low
January	30	14
February	31	13
March	39	21
April	52	31
May	64	41
June	75	51
July	81	56
August	79	55
September	70	48
October	59	39
November	44	29
December	34	20
Zero-Degree Days: 13		
Freezing Days: 171		
90-Degree Days: 6		

Petoskey–Straits of Mackinac, MI

Terrain: The Straits of Mackinac are located in the northernmost part of Lower Michigan, where the waters of Lake Michigan meet those of Lake Huron. The land north of the straits forms Michigan's Upper Peninsula. The town of Petoskey is located some 30 miles south of the straits, on the south shore of Little Traverse Bay on the Lake Michigan shore. The terrain is generally level or gently undulating, with sandy and gravelly soils. The region abounds with lakes ideal for fishing and summer recreation.

Climate: Though rigorous because of its interior and northerly location, the climate is modified by the presence of the lakes on either side. Consequently, summertime temperatures average at least 5 degrees cooler than locations in the southern part of the state. However, winters are quite severe, with cold spells that may last for a week and snowfall that averages almost 75 inches.

Pluses: Pleasant summers with cool nights. Crisp falls.

Minuses: Long, cold, snowy winters.

Score: 316   **Rank: 122**

Elevation: 586 feet

Relative Humidity: 60%
Wind Speed: 8 mph

Seasonal Change

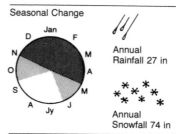

Annual Rainfall 27 in

Annual Snowfall 74 in

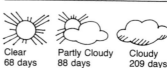

Clear 68 days   Partly Cloudy 88 days   Cloudy 209 days

Precipitation Days: 67   Storm Days: 33

Average Temperatures		
	Daily High	Daily Low
January	28	13
February	30	11
March	37	18
April	51	30
May	64	40
June	74	50
July	80	57
August	78	56
September	69	49
October	58	40
November	43	29
December	32	19
Zero-Degree Days: 14		
Freezing Days: 147		
90-Degree Days: 9		

Phoenix, AZ

Terrain: Located in the center of the Salt River Valley, on a broad, oval, nearly flat plain. To the south, west, and north are nearby mountain ranges, and 35 miles to the east are the famous Superstition Mountains, which rise to an elevation of 5,000 feet.
Climate: Typical desert, with low annual rainfall and low humidity. Daytime temperatures are high throughout the summer. Winters are mild, but nighttime temperatures frequently drop below freezing during December, January, and February. The valley floor is generally free of wind except during the thunderstorm season in July and August, when local gusts flow from the east. The majority of days are clear and sunny, except for July and August; then, considerable afternoon cloudiness builds up over nearby mountains.

Pluses: Dry, two-season desert climate.

Minuses: Hot summers.

Elevation: 1,107 feet

Relative Humidity: 32%
Wind Speed: 6.3 mph

Seasonal Change

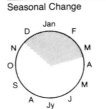

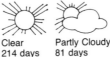

Annual Rainfall 7 in

Annual Snowfall 0 in

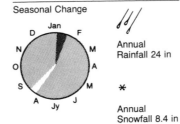

Clear 214 days   Partly Cloudy 81 days   Cloudy 70 days

Precipitation Days: 34   Storm Days: 23

Average Temperatures		
	Daily High	Daily Low
January	65	38
February	69	41
March	75	45
April	84	52
May	93	60
June	102	68
July	105	78
August	102	76
September	98	69
October	88	57
November	75	45
December	66	39
Zero-Degree Days: 0		
Freezing Days: 32		
90-Degree Days: 164		

Score: 664   **Rank: 37**

Port Angeles–Strait of Juan de Fuca, WA

Terrain: Located in the northeastern section of the Olympic Peninsula between the Strait of Juan de Fuca and the Olympic Mountains, which begin rising near the southern edge of the city and reach elevations of 6,000 feet within 15 miles. There are several glaciers on Mount Olympus, at 7,965 feet the highest point in the Olympic Range.
Climate: Predominantly marine, with cool summers, mild winters, moist air, and small daily temperature variation. Summers are cool and rather dry. The average summertime temperature is 65° F to 70° F during the day and about 55° F at night. The temperature seldom exceeds 75° F. The water temperature of the strait is 44° F in winter and 52° F in summer, which is an indication of the temperature stability of the climate. In winter, the daily temperatures are in the 40s in the daytime, dropping to the 30s at night. Like most other places in this region, the area is often foggy and cloudy.

Pluses: Cool, mild, maritime climate.

Minuses: Beach and sunbathing weather very scarce.

Elevation: 99 feet

Relative Humidity: 70%
Wind Speed: 8.6 mph

Seasonal Change

Annual Rainfall 24 in

Annual Snowfall 8.4 in

Clear 47 days   Partly Cloudy 72 days   Cloudy 246 days

Precipitation Days: 64   Storm Days: 8

Average Temperatures		
	Daily High	Daily Low
January	45	33
February	48	36
March	50	36
April	55	39
May	61	44
June	65	48
July	69	51
August	68	51
September	66	49
October	58	43
November	50	38
December	46	35
Zero-Degree Days: 0		
Freezing Days: 40		
90-Degree Days: 0		

Score: 444   **Rank: 95**

Red Bluff–Sacramento Valley, CA

Terrain: Located at the northern end of the Sacramento Valley, which is the northern half of the great Central Valley of California. Mountains surround the city on three sides, forming a huge horseshoe: The Coast Range is located 30 miles west, the Sierra Nevada system 40 miles east, and the Cascade Range about 50 miles north-northeast. The western part of the valley floor is mostly rolling hills with scrub oak trees. The Sacramento River flows in a north-south direction through the eastern portion of the valley, through fertile orchards and grain lands.
Climate: Precipitation is confined mostly to rain during the winter and spring months. Snowfall is infrequent and light. In the hot months (June through September), temperatures often exceed 100° F, but nighttime temperatures are almost always comfortable. The summer and fall are nearly cloudless, and the resulting warm days are ideal for fruit drying.

Pluses: Warm, dry, sunny.

Minuses: Hot summer days.

Elevation: 342 feet

Relative Humidity: 49%
Wind Speed: 8.7 mph

Seasonal Change

Annual Rainfall 22 in

Annual Snowfall 2.3 in

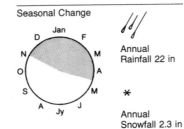

Clear 176 days   Partly Cloudy 70 days   Cloudy 119 days

Precipitation Days: 70   Storm Days: 10

Average Temperatures		
	Daily High	Daily Low
January	54	37
February	60	40
March	64	43
April	72	47
May	81	54
June	89	62
July	98	67
August	96	64
September	91	60
October	78	52
November	64	43
December	55	38
Zero-Degree Days: 0		
Freezing Days: 21		
90-Degree Days: 99		

Score: 655   **Rank: 40**

Reno, NV

Terrain: Located at the west edge of Truckee Meadows in a semiarid plateau lying in the lee of the Sierra Nevada. To the west, this range rises to elevations of 9,000 feet to 10,000 feet, and hills to the east reach 6,000 feet to 7,000 feet. The Truckee River, flowing from the Sierra Nevada eastward through Reno, drains into Pyramid Lake to the northeast.

Climate: Sunshine is abundant throughout the year. Temperatures are mild, but the daily range may exceed 45 degrees. Even when afternoons reach the upper 90s, a light jacket is needed shortly after sunset. Nights with a minimum temperature over 60° F are rare. Afternoon temperatures are moderate, and only about ten days a year fail to reach a level above freezing. Humidity is very low during the summer months and moderately low during winter.

Pluses: Mild, sunny climate in alpine setting.

Minuses: Considerable daily temperature variation. Little precipitation.

Score: 400　　　　　　　　　**Rank: 106**

Elevation: 4,400 feet

Relative Humidity: 44%
Wind Speed: 6.4 mph

Seasonal Change

Annual Rainfall 7 in

Annual Snowfall 27 in

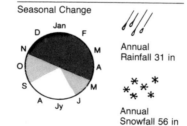

| Clear 165 days | Partly Cloudy 90 days | Cloudy 110 days |

Precipitation Days: 49　　Storm Days: 13

Average Temperatures		
	Daily High	Daily Low
January	45	18
February	51	23
March	56	25
April	64	30
May	72	37
June	80	43
July	91	47
August	89	45
September	82	39
October	70	31
November	56	24
December	46	20

Zero-Degree Days: 3
Freezing Days: 189
90-Degree Days: 52

Rhinelander, WI

Terrain: Rhinelander, seat of Oneida County, is located on the Wisconsin River in the northern part of the state. The area was once part of a great white pine forest, but it is now covered with second growth. Within a 12-mile radius of the city there are more than 200 lakes. The area is known for its fishing, particularly for smallmouth bass, walleye, and muskie.

Climate: Continental, and largely determined by the movement and interaction of large air masses. Winters are long and cold, while summers are warm and pleasant, with cool nights. Weather changes can be expected every few days in winter and spring. Spring and fall are short, with rapid transition from winter to summer and vice versa. The average number of thunderstorms per year is 30. With a mean of 39 days when the temperature falls below zero, this should be considered a rigorous climate.

Pluses: Warm, pleasant summers.

Minuses: Long, cold winters.

Score: 261　　　　　　　　　**Rank: 130**

Elevation: 1,560 feet

Relative Humidity: 55%
Wind Speed: 8.5 mph

Seasonal Change

Annual Rainfall 31 in

Annual Snowfall 56 in

| Clear 89 days | Partly Cloudy 102 days | Cloudy 174 days |

Precipitation Days: 66　　Storm Days: 30

Average Temperatures		
	Daily High	Daily Low
January	23	3
February	26	4
March	36	15
April	53	30
May	67	42
June	75	52
July	80	57
August	78	54
September	68	46
October	57	37
November	38	24
December	26	10

Zero-Degree Days: 39
Freezing Days: 182
90-Degree Days: 6

Roswell, NM

Terrain: Located in a valley in southern New Mexico amid higher land masses that modify air masses, especially the cold outbreaks in winter.

Climate: Conforms to the basic trend of four seasons. Summers are warm and dry. Half of the annual precipitation falls then. In the fall, frosty nights alternate with warm days of extremely low humidity. Winter is the season of least precipitation and is characterized by subfreezing temperatures at night followed by considerable warming in the day. The wind speed is in excess of 25 mph on some 60 days a year, usually between February and May.

Pluses: Low humidity year round. Long summers. Abundance of clear days.

Minuses: Cold nights. High winds.

Score: 568　　　　　　　　　**Rank: 63**

Elevation: 3,669 feet

Relative Humidity: 42%
Wind Speed: 8.9 mph

Seasonal Change

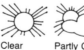

Annual Rainfall 11 in

Annual Snowfall 11 in

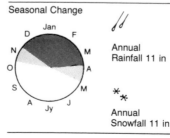

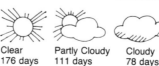

| Clear 176 days | Partly Cloudy 111 days | Cloudy 78 days |

Precipitation Days: 47　　Storm Days: 31

Average Temperatures		
	Daily High	Daily Low
January	55	21
February	61	25
March	68	31
April	78	41
May	86	51
June	94	60
July	95	64
August	93	62
September	87	54
October	77	42
November	65	29
December	57	22

Zero-Degree Days: 0
Freezing Days: 94
90-Degree Days: 75

St. George–Zion, UT

Terrain: St. George, at an elevation of 2,700 feet, is located 2 miles north of the junction of the Virgin and Santa Clara rivers in the fairly broad Virgin River Valley of southwestern Utah. Fifteen miles north the Pine Valley Mountains rise to over 10,000 feet. The same distance west are the Beaver Dam Mountains, rising to 7,000 feet. To the east and south is principally high plateau land. Nearby Zion National Park is noted for its spectacular canyons and rock formations.
Climate: Semiarid (steppe) type, with the most striking features being bright sunshine, small annual precipitation, dryness and purity of air, and large daily variations in temperature. Summers are characterized by hot, dry weather, with temperatures over 100° F occurring frequently during July and August. However, the low humidity makes these high temperatures somewhat bearable. Winters are short and mild, with the Rocky Mountains blocking cold air masses from the north and east.

Pluses: Very sunny, dry, and warm.

Minuses: Can be very hot and dry in summer.

Score: 580   **Rank: 59**

Elevation: 2,880 feet

Relative Humidity: 25%
Wind Speed: 8.7 mph

Seasonal Change

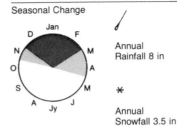

Annual Rainfall 8 in

Annual Snowfall 3.5 in

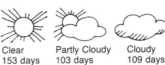

Clear 153 days   Partly Cloudy 103 days   Cloudy 109 days

Precipitation Days: 24   Storm Days: 48

Average Temperatures		
	Daily High	Daily Low
January	53	26
February	61	32
March	67	37
April	76	44
May	86	52
June	96	61
July	102	68
August	99	66
September	94	57
October	81	45
November	65	34
December	55	27

Zero-Degree Days: 0
Freezing Days: 95
90-Degree Days: 117

★ St. Petersburg–Clearwater, FL

Terrain: Located in flat topography on the Gulf coast of Florida.
Climate: An outstanding feature is the summer thunderstorm season. On the average, there are 88 days of thundershowers per year, occurring mostly in the afternoons in July, August, and September. The resulting temperature drop from 90° F to 70° F produces an agreeable physiologic reaction. Temperature throughout the year is modified by the waters of the Gulf of Mexico and surrounding bays. Snowfall is negligible, and freezing temperatures are rare; during the cooling season, however, night ground fogs occur frequently because of the flat terrain.

Pluses: Mild Gulf climate.

Minuses: Gulf hurricanes, regular summer thundershowers.

Score: 816   **Rank: 11**

Elevation: 11 feet

Relative Humidity: 57%
Wind Speed: 8.7 mph

Seasonal Change

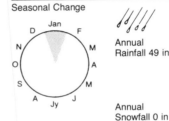

Annual Rainfall 49 in

Annual Snowfall 0 in

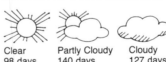

Clear 98 days   Partly Cloudy 140 days   Cloudy 127 days

Precipitation Days: 107   Storm Days: 88

Average Temperatures		
	Daily High	Daily Low
January	71	50
February	72	52
March	76	56
April	82	62
May	88	67
June	90	72
July	90	74
August	90	74
September	89	73
October	84	66
November	77	56
December	72	51

Zero-Degree Days: 0
Freezing Days: 4
90-Degree Days: 81

San Antonio, TX

Terrain: Located between the Edwards Plateau and the Gulf Coastal Plain of south-central Texas. Terrain is rolling. Vegetation consists of grasses and live oak trees, along with mesquite and cacti. Soils are blackland clay and silty loam.
Climate: Two-season, with mild weather during normal winter months and a long, hot summer. Though 140 miles from the Gulf of Mexico, the city feels the influence of its hot moist air. Thunderstorms and rains have occurred in every month of the year, but they are most common during the summer, with most rain falling in May and September. The winds during the winter are from the north, and from the south in the summer. Skies are clear more than 30% of the time, and cloudy about 30%.

Pluses: No winter; attractive terrain.

Minuses: Hot, muggy summers.

Score: 730   **Rank: 24**

Elevation: 794 feet

Relative Humidity: 55%
Wind Speed: 9.3 mph

Seasonal Change

Annual Rainfall 28 in

Annual Snowfall .5 in

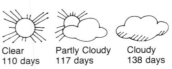

Clear 110 days   Partly Cloudy 117 days   Cloudy 138 days

Precipitation Days: 81   Storm Days: 36

Average Temperatures		
	Daily High	Daily Low
January	62	40
February	66	43
March	73	49
April	80	59
May	86	66
June	92	72
July	96	74
August	96	73
September	90	69
October	82	59
November	71	48
December	64	42

Zero-Degree Days: 0
Freezing Days: 22
90-Degree Days: 111

San Diego, CA

Terrain: Located on San Diego Bay in the southwest corner of California near the Mexican border. Its coastal location is backed by coastal foothills and mountains to the east.

Climate: One of the mildest in North America: typically marine, sometimes called Mediterranean. There are no freezing days and an average of only three 90-degree days each year. San Diego has abundant sunshine and mild sea breezes. Only two seasons occur here: a dry, mild summer and a spring that is cooler, with some rain. Storms are practically unknown, though there is considerable fog along the coast, and many low clouds in early morning and evening during the summer.

Pluses: One of the best climates for sun and mildness.

Minuses: Paradise climate lacking variety and seasonal contrasts.

Elevation: 28 feet

Relative Humidity: 61%
Wind Speed: 6.7 mph

Seasonal Change

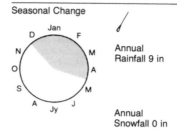

Annual Rainfall 9 in

Annual Snowfall 0 in

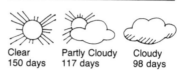

Clear 150 days Partly Cloudy 117 days Cloudy 98 days

Precipitation Days: 41   Storm Days: 3

Average Temperatures		
	Daily High	Daily Low
January	65	46
February	66	48
March	66	50
April	68	54
May	69	57
June	71	60
July	75	64
August	75	65
September	77	63
October	74	58
November	70	52
December	66	54

Zero-Degree Days: 0
Freezing Days: 0
90-Degree Days: 3

Score: 773   **Rank: 18**

Santa Fe, NM

Terrain: This historic city, the capital of New Mexico and seat of Santa Fe County, sits in the Rio Grande Valley in the north-central section of the state. It is situated amid the rolling foothills of the Sangre de Cristo Mountains, which rise to peaks of 10,000 feet. Westward the terrain slopes downward to the Rio Grande River, some 20 miles away. The high mountains to the east protect the city from much of the cold air of winter. The city's historic legacy, cultural facilities, and fine climate have long attracted tourists and retired people.

Climate: Semiarid continental, with cool and pleasant summers. Days are in the 80s, but nights in the 50s. Long cloudy periods are unknown. Winters are crisp, clear, and sunny, with considerable daytime warming.

Pluses: Beautiful scenery. Mild, sunny, four-season climate.

Minuses: Wide temperature range and high altitude may present health problems for some persons.

Elevation: 7,200 feet

Relative Humidity: 30%
Wind Speed: 9 mph

Seasonal Change

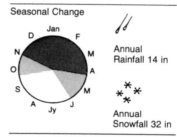

Annual Rainfall 14 in

Annual Snowfall 32 in

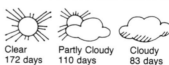

Clear 172 days Partly Cloudy 110 days Cloudy 83 days

Precipitation Days: 37   Storm Days: 54

Average Temperatures		
	Daily High	Daily Low
January	41	19
February	45	23
March	52	27
April	62	35
May	71	43
June	81	52
July	84	57
August	82	55
September	77	49
October	65	38
November	52	27
December	43	21

Zero-Degree Days: 1
Freezing Days: 152
90-Degree Days: 7

Score: 447   **Rank: 93**

Santa Rosa–Petaluma, CA

Terrain: Located in the east-central portion of the Petaluma–Santa Rosa–Russian River valley, which extends northwestward from San Pablo Bay, about 45 miles from the Golden Gate Bridge. This valley runs parallel to the Pacific Coast, with only low hills (300 feet to 500 feet) between it and the ocean 25 miles southwest. Higher hills rise to the east of the metro area, with greater elevations about 10 miles farther east, in the foothills of the Coast Ranges.

Climate: The nearness of the ocean and the surrounding topography join with the prevailing westerly circulation to produce a predominantly southerly air flow year-round. However, the area is sufficiently far inland to assure it a more varied climate than San Francisco's. Summers are warmer, winters cooler, and there is more daily temperature shift, as well as less fog and drizzle.

Pluses: Mild, yet sunnier and warmer than coastal locations.

Minuses: Some hot weather.

Elevation: 167 feet

Relative Humidity: 55%
Wind Speed: 7 mph

Seasonal Change

Annual Rainfall 30 in

Annual Snowfall 0 in

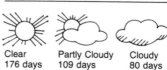

Clear 176 days Partly Cloudy 109 days Cloudy 80 days

Precipitation Days: 47   Storm Days: 4

Average Temperatures		
	Daily High	Daily Low
January	57	36
February	63	39
March	66	39
April	70	41
May	75	45
June	81	49
July	84	51
August	84	51
September	84	50
October	78	45
November	66	40
December	60	37

Zero-Degree Days: 0
Freezing Days: 43
90-Degree Days: 33

Score: 625   **Rank: 48**

Springfield, MO

Terrain: Located on very gently rolling tableland, almost atop the crest of the Missouri Ozark Plateau. The average elevation of the city proper is just over 1,300 feet above sea level.

Climate: As a result of this advantageous position, the city and surrounding countryside enjoy what is described as a plateau climate. The area possesses the mild and changeable climate often associated with high places in southerly latitudes, with warmer winters and cooler summers than other parts of the state at lower elevations. The city sits astride two major drainage systems: the Missouri River system to the north and the White-Mississippi system to the south.

Pluses: Mild, changeable.   **Minuses:** Short springs and falls.

Score: 558   **Rank:** 68

Elevation: 1,270 feet

Relative Humidity: 57%
Wind Speed: 11.1 mph

Seasonal Change

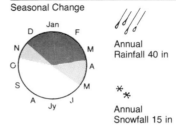

Annual Rainfall 40 in

Annual Snowfall 15 in

Clear 117 days   Partly Cloudy 99 days   Cloudy 149 days

Precipitation Days: 107   Storm Days: 58

Average Temperatures	Daily High	Daily Low
January	43	23
February	48	27
March	55	33
April	68	45
May	76	54
June	84	63
July	89	67
August	89	65
September	81	57
October	71	47
November	56	35
December	46	26

Zero-Degree Days: 3
Freezing Days: 105
90-Degree Days: 40

State College, PA

Terrain: Located in Centre County, the geographic center of Pennsylvania. The orientation of the ridges and valleys of the Appalachian Mountains is northeast to southwest. Elevations within Centre County vary from 977 feet to 2,400 feet. The largest valley in the area is Nittany Valley, much of which is under cultivation. The surrounding higher elevations are covered with second-growth forests.

Climate: A composite of the relatively dry midwestern continental climate and the more humid climate characteristic of the eastern seaboard. Prevailing westerly winds carry weather disturbances from the interior of the country into the area. Coastal storms occasionally affect the local weather as they move toward the northeast, but generally, the Atlantic is too distant to have a noticeable effect on the climate. Winters are cold and relatively dry, with thick cloud cover. Summer and fall are the most pleasant seasons of the year.

Pluses: Nice falls, summers.   **Minuses:** Humid, lots of cloudy days.

Score: 438   **Rank:** 97

Elevation: 1,200 feet

Relative Humidity: 55%
Wind Speed: 7.8 mph

Seasonal Change

Annual Rainfall 37 in

Annual Snowfall 48 in

Clear 66 days   Partly Cloudy 114 days   Cloudy 185 days

Precipitation Days: 122   Storm Days: 35

Average Temperatures	Daily High	Daily Low
January	33	18
February	36	19
March	45	27
April	59	38
May	70	48
June	79	57
July	82	61
August	81	60
September	74	52
October	62	41
November	49	33
December	37	23

Zero-Degree Days: 4
Freezing Days: 132
90-Degree Days: 8

Tucson, AZ

Terrain: Lies at the foot of the Catalina Mountains in a flat to gently rolling valley floor in southern Arizona.

Climate: Desert, characterized by a long, hot season beginning in April and ending in October. Temperature maxima above 90° F are the rule during this period; on 41 days each year, on the average, the temperature reaches 100° F. These high temperatures are modified by low humidity, reducing discomfort. Tucson lies in the zone receiving more sunshine than any other in the United States. Clear skies or very thin, high clouds permit intense surface heating during the day and active radiational cooling at night, a process enhanced by the characteristic atmospheric dryness.

Pluses: Clear, warm, dry.   **Minuses:** Intense summer heat.

Score: 692   **Rank:** 32

Elevation: 2,555 feet

Relative Humidity: 30%
Wind Speed: 8.2 mph

Seasonal Change

Annual Rainfall 11 in

Annual Snowfall 2 in

Clear 198 days   Partly Cloudy 89 days   Cloudy 78 days

Precipitation Days: 50   Storm Days: 40

Average Temperatures	Daily High	Daily Low
January	64	38
February	67	40
March	72	44
April	81	50
May	90	58
June	98	66
July	98	74
August	95	72
September	93	67
October	84	56
November	72	45
December	65	39

Zero-Degree Days: 0
Freezing Days: 21
90-Degree Days: 139

Virginia Beach–Norfolk, VA

Terrain: Located on low level land, with Chesapeake Bay immediately to the north, Hampton Roads to the west, and the Atlantic Ocean to the east.

Climate: The metro area is in a favorable geographic position, being north of the track of hurricanes and tropical storms and south of high-latitude storm systems. Winters are mild. Springs and falls are especially pleasant. Summers, though, are warm, humid, and long. A temperature of zero has never been recorded here, although there is occasional snow.

Pluses: Four-season climate suited for year-round outdoor activities.

Minuses: Long, humid summers.

Elevation: 30 feet

Relative Humidity: 58%
Wind Speed: 10.6 mph

Seasonal Change

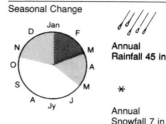

Annual Rainfall 45 in

Annual Snowfall 7 in

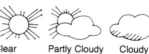

Clear 110 days   Partly Cloudy 102 days   Cloudy 153 days

Precipitation Days: 115 Storm Days: 37

Average Temperatures		
	Daily High	Daily Low
January	49	32
February	50	33
March	57	39
April	68	48
May	76	57
June	84	66
July	87	70
August	85	69
September	80	64
October	70	53
November	61	43
December	51	34

Zero-Degree Days: 0
Freezing Days: 54
90-Degree Days: 30

Score: 634   **Rank: 44**

★ West Palm Beach–Boca Raton–Delray Beach, FL

Terrain: Located on the coastal sand ridge of southeastern Florida. The entire coastal ridge is only about 5 miles wide and in early times the Everglades reached to its western edge. Now most of the swampland has been drained for development. The Atlantic Ocean forms the eastern edge, and the Gulf Stream flows northward 2 miles offshore, its nearest approach to the Florida coast.

Climate: Because of its southerly location near the ocean, the area has an equable climate. Winters are pleasantly warm. Summer daytime temperatures are high but are tempered by the ocean breeze, and by the frequent formation of cumulus clouds which shade the land without completely obscuring the sun. Rarely does the thermometer climb beyond 95° F. The moist, unstable air in this area results in frequent showers, usually of short duration.

Pluses: Single season, sub-tropical climate.

Minuses: Hurricanes, frequent summer thunderstorms.

Elevation: 21 feet

Relative Humidity: 60%
Wind Speed: 9.4 mph

Seasonal Change

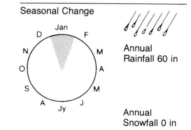

Annual Rainfall 60 in

Annual Snowfall 0 in

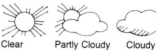

Clear 73 days   Partly Cloudy 155 days   Cloudy 137 days

Precipitation Days: 132 Storm Days: 79

Average Temperatures		
	Daily High	Daily Low
January	75	56
February	76	56
March	79	60
April	83	65
May	86	69
June	88	73
July	90	74
August	90	74
September	88	75
October	84	70
November	80	63
December	76	57

Zero-Degree Days: 0
Freezing Days: 1
90-Degree Days: 55

Score: 859   **Rank: 5**

Winchester, VA

Terrain: Located in central Frederick County, which is at the northern tip of the Shenandoah Valley and shares a common border with West Virginia on the north and west. The western part of the county is in the Allegheny Mountains, with Little North Mountain dividing it into two essentially different agricultural regions: warmer-weather truck and farm crops to the east and more rugged, cold-weather farming and pasture to the west. The terrain varies from rolling–hilly to rugged in the mountains. Elevations range from 600 feet to 1,800 feet in the county.

Climate: Modified continental, with mild winters and warm, humid summers. The mountains produce various steering, blocking, and modifying effects on storms and air masses. High elevations near the city promote the downward flow of cool mountain air tempering otherwise hot summer nights. All seasons are pleasant, except that summer (especially July) can be hot.

Pluses: Scenic. Mild.

Minuses: Can be hot and humid.

Elevation: 760 feet

Relative Humidity: 55%
Wind Speed: 8.3 mph

Seasonal Change

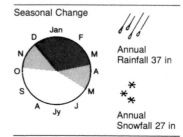

Annual Rainfall 37 in

Annual Snowfall 27 in

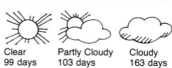

Clear 99 days   Partly Cloudy 103 days   Cloudy 163 days

Precipitation Days: 115 Storm Days: 47

Average Temperatures		
	Daily High	Daily Low
January	41	23
February	44	25
March	54	33
April	66	43
May	75	52
June	83	59
July	87	64
August	86	62
September	79	56
October	67	45
November	55	36
December	44	27

Zero-Degree Days: 0
Freezing Days: 103
90-Degree Days: 30

Score: 534   **Rank: 76**

Yuma, AZ

Terrain: Yuma is located in the extreme southwest corner of Arizona, near the California and Mexican borders. The land is typical desert-steppe, with dry, sandy, and dusty soil, scant vegetation, and craggy buttes and mountains that take their characteristic texture from wind erosion rather than water erosion. The various mountain ranges that surround Yuma are perhaps the dominant geologic features. They include the Trigo, Chocolate, Castle Dome, Mohawk, and Gila ranges.
Climate: Yuma's climate is definitely a desert product. Home heating is necessary from late October to mid-April. However, outdoor activities can be conducted comfortably during this period from 10:00 AM to 5:00 PM. It is very dry, with many places in the world receiving more rain in a year than has fallen in Yuma in the past 90 years. Yuma is officially the sunniest place in America.

Pluses: America's sunniest spot.

Minuses: Hot, dry, dusty.

Score: 692

Rank: 32

Elevation: 194 feet

Relative Humidity: 32%
Wind Speed: 7.8 mph

Seasonal Change

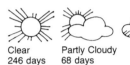

Annual Rainfall 2.7 in

Annual Snowfall 0 in

Clear 246 days | Partly Cloudy 68 days | Cloudy 51 days

Precipitation Days: 16   Storm Days: 7

Average Temperatures		
	Daily High	Daily Low
January	67	43
February	73	46
March	78	50
April	86	57
May	93	64
June	101	71
July	106	81
August	104	81
September	100	74
October	90	62
November	77	50
December	68	44

Zero-Degree Days: 0
Freezing Days: 2
90-Degree Days: 168

 ET CETERA: Climate

CLIMATE AND HEALTH

Most of us find that weather profoundly affects moods and emotions. Long snowy winters that confine people indoors can have adverse emotional effects; at the other extreme, many people become irritable when the weather gets so hot they cannot sleep.

Relative humidity, barometric pressure, and altitude are just a few factors related to climate or terrain that can influence your physical well-being. There is no proven link between longevity and climate, although the three places on the globe whose populations have the highest percentage of centenarians—the Caucasus Mountains of the Soviet Union, the mountains of Bolivia, and northwestern India—are all in southerly latitudes at high elevations. But in America, where careful records have been kept for generations, a similar situation does not exist. In fact, most of the longest average life spans have been recorded in states with severe climates—Minnesota, North Dakota, and Iowa, for example.

It has been shown, however, that people with certain chronic diseases or disorders are far more comfortable in some climates than others. Asthmatics generally do best in warm, dry places that have a minimum of airborne allergens and no molds. People with rheumatism or arthritis find comfort in warm, moist southerly climates where the weather is constant and the atmospheric pressure undergoes the least daily change. Those who suffer from tuberculosis or emphysema seem to do best in the lower elevations of mountainous locales with lots of clear air and sunshine.

A brief classic in the field of bioclimatology is H. E. Landsberg's *Weather and Health* (1969). Landsberg details some of the relationships that have been observed between climate and the aggravation of (or relief from) various physical afflictions. Drawing on this and other sources, *Retirement Places Rated* describes some basic weather phenomena and suggests how they can affect the way you feel.

Weather Stages: Beware of 3 and 4

The weather changes that cause the human body to react have been carefully studied by meteorologists and classified into six basic stages, which make up the clear-stormy–clear cycle that is constantly repeated all over the planet. The stages in the cycle have been linked to some of the joys and tragedies of human existence.

Stage 1. Cool, high-pressure air, with few clouds and moderate winds, followed by . . .
Stage 2. Perfectly clear, dry air, high pressure, and little wind, leading to . . .
Stage 3. Considerable warming, steady or slightly falling pressure, and some high clouds, until . . .
Stage 4. The warm, moist air gets into the lower

layers; pressure falls, clouds thicken, precipitation is common, and the wind picks up speed; then . . .

Stage 5. An abrupt change takes place; showery precipitation is accompanied by cold, gusty winds, rapidly rising pressure, and falling humidity as the moisture in the air is released.

Stage 6. Gradually, the pressure rises still farther and the clouds diminish; temperatures reach low levels and the humidity continues to drop, leading back to . . .

Stage 1. Cool, high-pressure air . . .

Of course, these phases aren't equally long, either in any given sequence or in the course of a year. During winter, all six stages may follow one another within three days, while in the summer two weeks may pass before the cycle is completed.

Obviously, the "beautiful weather" stages 1 and 2 stimulate the body very little. They make few demands that cannot be met by adequate clothing and housing. In contrast, weather stages 4 and 5 are often violent; they stir us up, both mentally and physically.

That weather phases affect the human body is beyond question; the records of hospital births and deaths prove it. For example, in the case of human pregnancy, in far more cases than statistical accident would permit, labor begins on days that are in weather stage 3. Coronary thrombosis—"heart attack"— shows a strong peak of frequency in weather stages 3 and 4, and a definite low in stages 1 and 6. Bleeding ulcers and migraine attacks peak in stage 4, too.

Weather events affect moods and behavior. There is a strong correlation between weather stage 3 and suicide, behavior problems in schoolchildren, and street riots. A study in Poland over a five-year period (1966–70) showed that accident rates in factory workers doubled during cyclonic weather conditions (stages 3 and 4: periods of falling pressure, rising tempera-

tures and humidity, which signal the onset of stormy weather) and returned to normal low levels in fair weather. Animals as well as humans are affected. Dogcatchers are invariably busiest during stages 3, 4, and 5 because dogs become restless, stray from their homes, and wander through the streets.

The Three Determinants of Human Comfort

As the six weather stages suggest, everyday human comfort is influenced by three basic climatic factors: humidity, temperature, and barometric pressure.

Humidity. Humidity, or the amount of moisture in the air, is closely related to air temperature in determining the comfort level of the atmosphere. Much of the discomfort and nervous tension experienced at the approach of stormy weather (weather stage 4), for example, is the result of rising temperatures and humidity. These atmospheric conditions are also related, at least in part, to the behavioral problems and medical emergencies described previously.

Extremely high levels of atmospheric moisture, such as those experienced most of the time in the Pacific Northwest and around the Gulf of Mexico and southern Atlantic Coast, aren't usually the cause of direct discomfort except in persons suffering from certain types of arthritis or rheumatism. But even in these cases, the mild temperatures found in these maritime locations usually do much to offset discomfort. In fact, the stability of the barometric pressure (which means small or gradual shifts in the air pressure) in these areas makes them ideal for people with muscle and joint pain.

But damp air coupled with low temperatures can be uncomfortable. Most people who've experienced damp winters, especially in places with high winds, complain that the cold, wet wind seems to go right through them. And the harmful effect of cold, damp air on pulmonary diseases, particularly tuberculosis, has long been known. With this in mind, it's wise to

Temperature, Humidity, and Apparent Temperature

Apparent Temperature

Air Temperature (°F)	0	5	10	15	20	25	30	35	40	45	50	55	60	65	70	75	80	85	90	95	100
110	99	102	105	108	112	117	123	130	137	143	150										
105	95	97	100	102	105	109	113	118	123	129	135	142	149								
100	91	93	95	97	99	101	104	107	110	115	120	126	132	138	144						
95	87	88	90	91	93	94	96	98	101	104	107	110	114	119	124	130	136				
90	83	84	85	86	87	88	90	91	93	95	96	98	100	102	106	109	113	117	122		
85	78	79	80	81	82	83	84	85	86	87	88	89	90	91	93	95	97	99	102	105	108
80	73	74	75	76	77	77	78	79	79	80	81	81	82	83	85	86	86	87	88	89	91
75	69	69	70	71	72	72	73	73	74	74	75	75	76	76	77	77	78	78	79	79	80
70	64	64	65	65	66	66	67	67	68	68	69	69	70	70	70	70	71	71	71	71	72

Relative Humidity (%)

Locate the air temperature at the left and the relative humidity along the bottom. The intersection of the horizontal row of figures opposite the temperature with the vertical row of figures above the relative humidity is the apparent temperature. For example, an air temperature of 85 degrees feels like 89 degrees at 55 percent relative humidity; but when the humidity is 90 percent, 85 degrees feels like 102.

Apparent Temperatures (July)

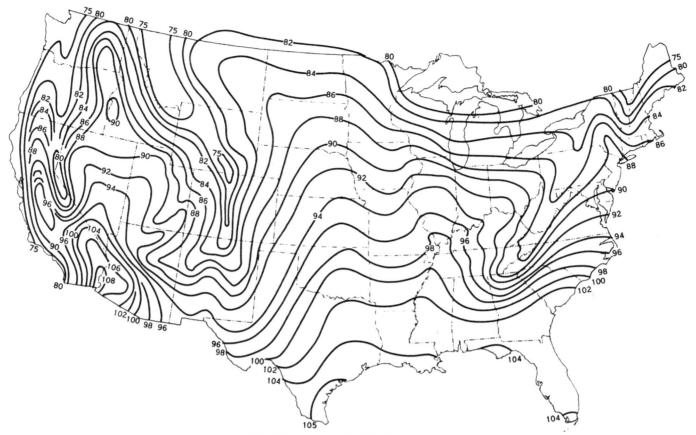

Source: National Oceanic and Atmospheric Administration, National Climatic Center, Asheville, North Carolina.

consider carefully before moving to the northerly coastal locations on the Eastern Seaboard—Cape Cod and the coast of Maine, for example—where these conditions will be common during the winter months.

Perhaps the most noticeable drawback to very moist air is the wide variety of organisms it supports. Bacteria, and the spores of fungi and molds, thrive in moist air but are almost absent in dry air. If the air is moist and also warm, the problem is multiplied. Therefore, people prone to bacterial skin infections, fungal infections such as athlete's foot, or mold allergies should carefully check out places with high humidities before moving there.

On the other end of the spectrum, very dry air produces effects on our bodies that are perceptible almost immediately and can cause discomfort within a day. When the relative humidity falls below 50 percent, most of us experience dry nasal passages and perhaps a dry, tickling throat. In the dry areas of the Southwest, where the humidity can drop to 20 percent or less, many people experience nosebleeds, flaking skin, and constant sore throats.

Temperature. Many bioclimatologists maintain that the human body (or most human bodies) is most comfortable and productive at "65–65," meaning an air temperature of 65 degrees with 65 percent humidity. High relative humidity intensifies the felt effect of high temperatures (see the table "Temperature, Humidity, and Apparent Temperature") because it impairs the evaporative cooling effect of sweating. At apparent temperatures as low as 80 to 90 degrees Fahrenheit, a person may begin to suffer symptoms of heat stress. The degree of heat stress experienced will vary depending on age, health, and body characteristics; generally speaking, infants, young children, and older adults are most likely to be affected by high temperature/humidity combinations. In the summer of 1980, record heat waves, often accompanied by high humidity, swept the Southwest, leaving hundreds dead.

The map "Apparent Temperatures (July)" shows how felt temperatures vary across the country. The places in America where the highest temperatures are constantly recorded are mostly in the desert areas of the Great Basin (the southern half of the plateau between the Sierra Nevada to the west and the Rocky Mountains to the east), the Great Interior Valley of California, and parts of the High Plains regions of New Mexico, Oklahoma, and Texas. However, these areas are generally dry, so the effects of the high temperatures on the human body are not particularly noticeable or damaging. This is particularly true of locations west of eastern New Mexico.

America's southeastern quadrant (which includes those states that border the Gulf of Mexico and the southern half of the Atlantic Coast) has temperatures that are less spectacularly high but humidity that can be oppressive. Most people would find a 90-degree day in Biloxi–Gulfport or Orlando far more uncomfortable than they would the same temperature in Las Vegas or Yuma, Arizona.

What about cold temperatures? In the past, most older adults have shunned cold weather in favor of the hot and sunny "beach" climates of the Sun Belt. Now, however, many are discovering the benefits of seasonal change and some cold weather, particularly around the holiday season. Therefore *Retirement Places Rated* includes many retirement places that have cold weather. Some of these—most notably in Michigan, Wisconsin, and Montana—have winters that can be rigorous and are not for the faint of heart.

Cold weather can have an adverse effect on persons with heart or circulatory ailments. According to the late bioclimatologist, H. E. Landsberg, these diseases follow a seasonal pattern, with a peak of deaths occurring in January and February. The cooling of the extremities can place greater stress on the heart as it tries to maintain a safe body temperature; breathing

very cold air can tax the heart-lung system, and some persons who have hardening of the coronary arteries may get chest pains when outdoors in a cold wind. Cold weather can also increase blood pressure, with adverse consequences for those with circulatory problems. Although extremely cold (polar) weather inhibits the survival of respiratory germs, these microbes thrive in a damp, cloudy, cool climate and contribute to high incidence of influenza, bronchitis, and colds.

As the body gets older, its circulatory system loses effectiveness. Add to this another natural consequence of aging—the decreased rate of the metabolic system (which keeps the body warm)—and you have partially explained older adults' need for higher household temperatures. Therefore, the expense of heating costs in a cool climate may offset the appeal of seasonal changes and winter weather.

But despite the dangers of extremes of heat or cold, sudden wide shifts of temperature in either direction constitute the gravest threat to human health. When the weather (and especially the temperature) changes suddenly and dramatically, the rates of cardiac arrest, respiratory distress, stroke, and other medical emergencies skyrocket.

Sudden atmospheric cooling can bring on attacks of asthma, bronchitis, and stroke. Heart attacks and other associated symptoms are also more frequent following these periods of rapid cooling. Often these are produced by changing air masses during autumn, particularly by the passage of a cold frontal system following a quickly falling barometer.

A sudden rise in the temperature may precipitate its own assortment of medical emergencies, among them heat stroke, heart attack, and stroke. It has been found that during a heat wave, the nighttime maximum air temperature is far more significant than the daytime maximum. This is because the body recuperates during the night. A hot night prevents the body from reestablishing its thermal equilibrium and tends to lessen the amount of sleep a person gets, thus increasing fatigue. Hospital employees call these sudden temperature shifts, which cause so much discomfort and harm, especially to older adults, "ambulance weather." It's a term that proves to be accurate, if unseemly. A study of the New York City heat wave of July 1966 revealed that the death rate more than doubled during the period of record temperature. The number of deaths from flu and pneumonia rose 315 percent, from strokes more than 176 percent, from heart attacks 161 percent, and from cancer 128 percent.

Barometric pressure. Even though most people may be unaware of the source of their discomfort, barometric pressure and its wide and rapid fluctuations are extremely powerful influences on human performance, comfort, and health. Pressure changes are felt even more keenly by older adults, whose bodies are generally more sensitive to change. As previously stated, the rapid fall of pressure that signals

---

RELOCATION RESOURCES

If climate is a factor in your decision about where to retire, these publications may be helpful.

How does your climate compare? Meteorologists at the National Climatic Data Center can take your order for comparative data the center publishes for any of thousands of locations in this country.

The Center's best-seller is the annual *Comparative Climatic Data for the United States*, a collection of month-by-month and annual summaries for normal daily maximum and minimum temperature, average and maximum wind speed, percentage of possible sunshine, rainfall, snowfall, and morning and afternoon humidity at each of 300 "first order" weather stations in this country. The cost is $3, plus $5 handling and shipping.

If the place you have in mind doesn't have a first order weather station, it may yet be one of 1,063 locations with a "cooperative" weather station. Their data are in *Climatography of the United States, Series 20*, a two-page publication for each location containing freeze and precipitation probability data; tables of long-term monthly and annual mean maximum, mean minimum, and average temperature; and tables of monthly and annual total precipitation and total snowfall. The cost is $1 per location, plus $5 handling and shipping.

All orders must be prepaid by check, Mastercard, Visa, or American Express. Call or write

National Climatic Data Center
Federal Building
Asheville, NC 28801
(704) 259-0682

the arrival of storms and advancing cold fronts can trigger episodes of asthma, heart disease, stroke, and pain in the joints. People with rheumatism or arthritis may suffer unduly if they live in places where pressure changes are continual and rapid. The map "Pressure Changes from Day to Day (February)" shows the regions with greatest and least pressure changes during an average day in February, when joint pain and other discomforts reach their peak.

As the map shows, the northern and eastern sections of the country experience the greatest variance, averaging a barometric change of .20 inch to .25 inch from one day to the next. (In summer, when pressure changes are relatively small, the average change in these regions is approximately .10 inch.) States in the southern latitudes, particularly Florida and southern California, show the least change, only about .10 inch in February (and less than .05 inch in summer). Of course, these figures are averages, and along the Gulf and Atlantic coasts, large and rapid pressure changes are caused on occasion by hurricanes.

The map, and the phenomenon it depicts, explain perhaps more than any other single reason why so many older adults have chosen to move to Florida and the Gulf Coast. Additionally, due to the stabilizing and modifying effects that large bodies of water have on temperature and pressure, weather conditions by seacoasts are steadier than those of most inland, desert, or mountain locations.

Although the climates found in Florida and the other Gulf states are not as pleasant year-round as they are advertised to be, there is no denying that the semitropical climate—hot, humid, monotonous, and even depressing as it might be to some—is just about perfect for people with severe rheumatoid joint pain or those who cannot tolerate sudden changes in the weather.

Questing for Relief

People with heart conditions should definitely avoid extreme heat and cold, rapid temperature variations, and extreme and sudden pressure changes. This can rule out most interior regions as well as northerly ones, even those on coastal locations. Recommended are places that have warm, mild, and steady weather. Mountains and high altitude should be avoided on two counts: less oxygen and strain caused by steep grades. Best bets are southerly coastal locations where sea-level, oxygen-rich air and stable pressures and temperatures predominate most of the year. Look along the coast of the Mid-Atlantic Metro Belt southward all the way around the Florida peninsula and westward along the Gulf. Also look along the southern third of the Pacific coastline.

Emphysema brings a completely different set of problems and solutions. In general, excessive dampness, coupled with cool or cold weather, is harmful. This eliminates all northerly locations, particularly the

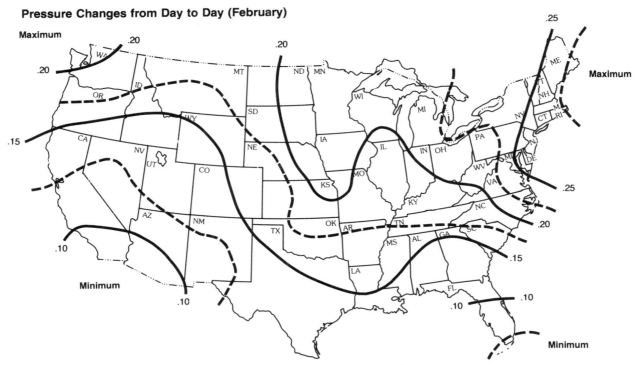

Pressure Changes from Day to Day (February)

Source: National Oceanic and Atmospheric Administration, National Climatic Center, Asheville, North Carolina.

Pacific Northwest Cloud Belt, the Yankee Belt, and the North Woods. Southerly coastal locations are better, but the air is perhaps still too damp. Seek out warm, sunny, dry climates such as those found in Arizona, New Mexico, Utah, Nevada, and the interior valleys of California. Remember to avoid high elevations.

Asthma is a complex disorder that is not yet completely understood. While it is believed to be an autoimmune disorder similar to allergies, it may be precipitated or worsened by different things in different individuals. Your wisest course is to consult medical specialists first to determine the specific cause of your attacks. Asthmatics seem to do best in the pollen-free, dry, warm air found in greatest abundance in the Desert Southwest. Because the air on the desert floor can be dusty, seeking a moderate altitude there may be beneficial.

Tuberculosis, recently considered a waning disease, is on the rise. It generally strikes people who have weakened resistance to infection, making older adults more susceptible than the rest of the population. Treatment is multifaceted, but an area that is mild, dry, sunny, and has clear air helps a great deal. Mountain locations have always been popular and can provide relief if the altitude isn't excessive. Because dampness isn't recommended, the dry, sunny places in the southern mountains of the West are preferable to locations in the southern Appalachians. Ocean breezes are thought to be beneficial, too, and may be better for people who cannot tolerate the more rugged climate of the interior mountains. Hawaii or the coast of southern California would be ideal.

For people with rheumatic pains, and discomfort in amputated limbs (called "phantom pains" because the limbs are missing) or in old scar tissue, the warm and steady climates of the subtropics are perfect. Here the surrounding water keeps temperatures and pressures from shifting quickly, and the prevailing warmth is soothing. It would be hard to miss with any seafront location from Myrtle Beach, South Carolina, south to the Florida Keys, around and up the west coast of the Florida peninsula, westward along the Gulf and down all the way to the mouth of the Rio Grande. Southern California and Hawaii, of course, shouldn't be overlooked.

Life at the Top

Many mountain resort areas got their start as 19th-century health retreats. Back then, "night air" and "bad air" were seen as causes for chronic respiratory diseases. The antidote demanded by well-to-do patients (and prescribed by their doctors) was "pine air" and a high altitude.

While most mountain air is clear and relatively free from pollutants, it is also less dense and contains less oxygen. A rapid change to a high altitude is risky for people with heart diseases and arteriosclerosis. If you suffer from asthma, emphysema, or anemia, you should consult local physicians before moving to any place more than 2,000 feet above sea level. Even if all indications point to a positive reaction on your part, it would be wise to take up residence for at least several months before making a permanent move.

For those who can tolerate the high country, the advantages of such locations are well known. Because atmospheric temperature decreases with increasing elevation (about 3.3 degrees Fahrenheit per 1,000 feet), places at high elevations in southerly locales (such as Santa Fe, New Mexico, or Asheville and Hendersonville–Brevard in North Carolina) enjoy the long summers and mild winters typical of the South, and also the cool summers, crisp autumns, and absence of mugginess usually associated with more northerly areas.

Since altitude puts a certain amount of stress on the body's circulatory system and lungs, becoming acclimated to high places is conducive to general good health. A higher altitude accelerates respiration and increases the lung capacity, strengthens the heart, increases the metabolic rate, and boosts the number and proportion of red blood cells.

In the United States, the highest town with a post office is Climax, Colorado. At 11,350 feet, Climax is beyond the comfort range of many older adults. Up there, a 3-minute egg takes 7 minutes to boil, corn on the cob needs to be on the fire 45 minutes, and home-brewed beer matures in half the expected time. Yet many of the 1,500 residents love it. The incidence of infection is amazingly low, and insects are practically unknown. In the East, the highest town of any size

The Highest Retirement Places

	Elevation Above Sea Level
Santa Fe, NM	7,200 feet
Flagstaff, AZ	7,018
Colorado Springs, CO	6,170
Prescott, AZ	5,368
Albuquerque, NM	5,314
Grass Valley–Truckee, CA	5,280
Fort Collins–Loveland, CO	5,004
Grand Junction, CO	4,843
Carson City–Minden, NV	4,687
Reno, NV	4,400
Deming, NM	4,336
Las Cruces, NM	3,881
Roswell, NM	3,669
Bend, OR	3,599
Hamilton–Bitterroot Valley, MT	3,572
Missoula, MT	3,200
Kalispell, MT	2,965
St. George–Zion, UT	2,880
Boise, ID	2,868
Twain Harte–Yosemite, CA	2,577
Tucson, AZ	2,555
Front Royal, VA	2,500

Source: National Oceanic and Atmospheric Administration, *Local Climatological Data*, and *Climatography of the United States*.

is Highlands, North Carolina, near the Great Smoky Mountains. Though less than half as high as Climax, Highlands and the neighboring towns offer the cool, clear air and invigorating climate that have long drawn people to the mountains.

NATURAL HAZARDS

We're all familiar—even if only through television or newspapers—with the awesome destruction that nature can unleash. Perhaps no sight in recent memory was more dramatic than the 1980 eruption of Mount St. Helens, with an initial blast equivalent to that of 10 million tons of TNT, that blew off the topmost 1,300 feet of the mountain. Volcanic eruptions can wipe out lives and property in an instant. Fortunately, however, volcanoes usually give warning of impending activity, as did Mount St. Helens. Even more fortunately, the places where volcanic activity is a potential hazard are very few. A number of violent natural events are much more common and widespread, and although they may be less cataclysmic than a full-blown volcanic eruption, they can cause great damage and present life-threatening conditions. Many of these natural hazards follow definite geographic patterns within the United States, and some retirement places are at much greater risk than others.

The Sun Belt Is Also a Storm Belt

Many, if not most, severe storms occur in the southern half of the nation. For this reason, you might say that the Sun Belt is also a storm belt.

Thunderstorms and Lightning. Thunderstorms are common and don't usually cause death. But lightning kills 200 Americans a year. It remains the most common and frequent natural danger. At any given moment there are about 2,000 thunderstorms in progress around the globe; in the time it takes you to read this paragraph, lightning will have struck the earth 700 times.

Florida, the Sunshine State, is actually the country's stormiest state, with three times as much thunder and lightning as any other. California, on the other hand, is one of the three most storm-free states (the other two are Oregon and Washington). In a typical year, coastal California towns will average between 2 and 5 thunderstorm episodes. Most American towns average between 35 and 50. Fort Myers, Florida, averages 128. (A thunderstorm episode represents the presence of a single storm cell; a place like Fort Myers can register 4 or 5 episodes in a single day.)

The Place Profiles earlier in this chapter tell how many thunderstorm days each place can expect in an average year. The southeastern quadrant of our country generally receives more rain and thunderstorms than the rest, although the thunderstorms of the Great Plains are awesome spectacles.

Tornadoes. While they are not nearly as large or long-lived as hurricanes and release much less total force, tornadoes have more destructive and killing power concentrated in a small area than any other storm known. For absolute ferocity and wind speed, a tornado has no rival.

The hallmark of this vicious inland storm is the huge, snakelike funnel cloud that sweeps and bounces along the ground, destroying buildings, sweeping up cars, trains, livestock, and trees, and sucking them up hundreds of feet into the whirling vortex. Wind speeds close to 300 miles per hour have been recorded.

Although no one can tell for certain just where particular tornadoes might touch down, their season, origin, and direction of travel are fairly predictable. Tornado season reaches its peak in late spring and early summer, and most storms originate in the central and southern Great Plains, in the states of Oklahoma, Texas, Arkansas, Kansas, and Missouri. After forming in the intense heat and rising air of the plains, these storms proceed toward the northeast at speeds averaging 25–40 miles per hour. Most tornadoes do not last very long or travel very far. Half of all tornadoes reported travel less than 5 miles on the ground; a few have been tracked for more than 200 miles.

Of our retirement places, the lake locations in Oklahoma, any location in Texas or Arkansas, and even the locations in Kentucky and Tennessee, have a high potential for tornado damage and danger (see map "Tornado and Hurricane Risk Areas" on the following page). Nearly one third of all tornadoes ever reported in the United States have occurred within the boundaries of Kansas, Oklahoma, and Texas.

Hurricanes. Giant tropical cyclonic storms that originate at sea, hurricanes are unmatched for sheer power over a very large area. Hurricanes last for days, measure hundreds of miles across, and release tremendous energy in the form of high winds, torrential rains, lightning, and tidal surges. They occur in late summer and fall, and strike the Gulf states and southern segments of the Atlantic Coast primarily, though they will also strike locations farther north (see map "Tornado and Hurricane Risk Areas" on the following page). Like thunderstorms, hurricanes are much less frequent, and less severe, on the Pacific Coast.

Hurricanes usually originate in the tropical waters of the Atlantic Ocean. They occur toward summer's end because it takes that long for the water temperature and evaporation rate to rise sufficiently to begin the cyclonic, counterclockwise rotation of a wind system around a low-pressure system. When the wind velocities are less than 39 miles per hour, this cyclone is called a "tropical depression"; when wind velocities are between 39 and 74 miles per hour, the cyclone is called a "tropical storm." And when the winds reach 74 miles per hour, the storm becomes a hurricane.

Often the greatest danger and destruction from hurricanes aren't due to the winds but to the tidal surges that sweep ashore with seas 15 feet or more

Tornado and Hurricane Risk Areas

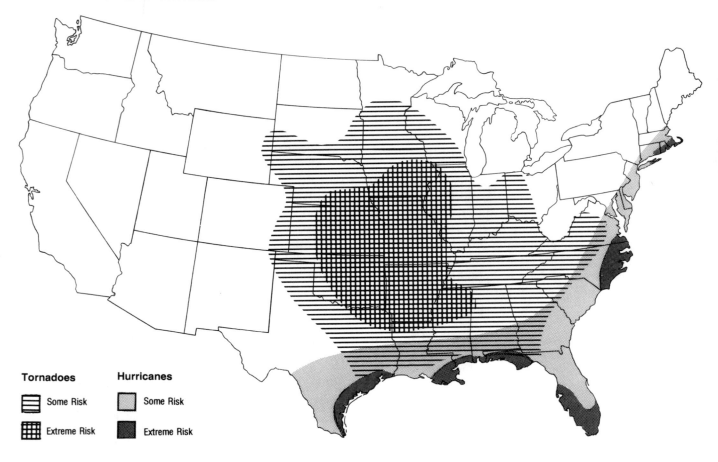

Tornadoes

⊟ Some Risk

▦ Extreme Risk

Hurricanes

▢ Some Risk

■ Extreme Risk

higher than normal high tides. Although Florida and the southern coasts are most vulnerable to hurricanes, locations as far north as Cape Cod and the coast of Maine are by no means immune.

Earthquake Hazard

California and the states of the Pacific Northwest may be relatively free of the thunderstorms, tornadoes, and hurricanes that buffet other parts of the country. But these states are in the area of the country most prone to earthquake damage. A glance at the map "Earthquake Hazard Zones," which predicts not only the probability of earthquakes but also their severity, confirms this.

All retirement places in California, Nevada, and Utah have the potential for substantial earthquake damage. Some locations in Oregon (such as Bend, Medford–Ashland, and Newport–Lincoln City) are relatively safe, but the Puget Sound area of Washington has experienced two major shocks in the past 35 years, both causing considerable damage. Portions of Montana and Idaho also are very vulnerable to earthquakes.

Other pockets of earthquake risk might surprise

you. Albuquerque is situated in a danger area, and so is Deming, New Mexico. The resorts of the South Carolina and Georgia coasts sit in the middle of a quake-sensitive zone that was the site of the strongest quake ever measured east of the Mississippi (it happened in Charleston, South Carolina, in 1886). The entire New England region shares a danger roughly comparable to this area; Boston has suffered a severe quake and remains earthquake prone today. A series of quakes occurred in southeastern Missouri in 1811–12, changing the course of the Mississippi River and creating a major lake. There is still some risk in this area, which includes the retirement places in western Kentucky and Tennessee and part of the Ozarks.

When It Comes to Natural Hazards, Can Anyone Win?

After studying the maps for a while, you may come to the dismal conclusion that you cannot win: where one natural disaster area stops, another begins. Some areas, like the coasts of South Carolina and Georgia, appear to contain a "triple threat" combination of earthquake, tornado, and hurricane possibilities.

Studying the map more closely, you might begin to

Earthquake Hazard Zones

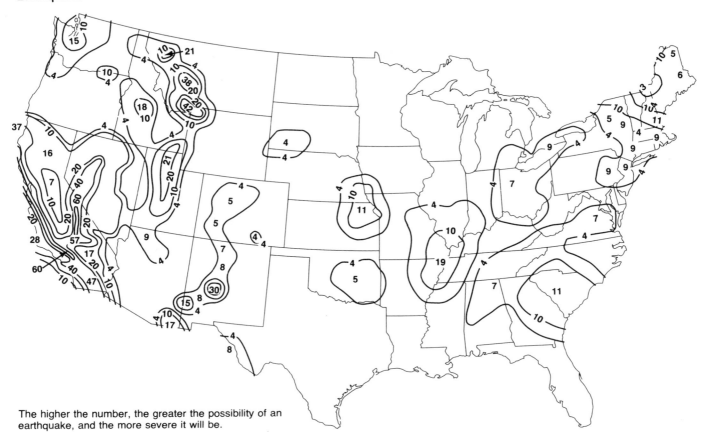

The higher the number, the greater the possibility of an earthquake, and the more severe it will be.

Source: U.S. Geological Survey Open-File Report 76-416, 1976.

detect retirement areas that seem safer than others. One such area is the Pacific Northwest, with the exception of the significant earthquake risk around Puget Sound. Parts of Arizona, Utah, and New Mexico, too, are relatively free from disaster risk. The southern Appalachians, despite a moderate earthquake risk, do not experience many storms, due to the protection of the mountains. But some parts of the region are flood-prone. And moderate earthquake risk seems almost unavoidable anywhere but the frigid North Central Plains or the steamy, tornado-ridden flatlands of Texas and the Gulf states.

So, as with most things in life, when it comes to avoiding natural disasters, you can only pay your money and take your chances.

HAY FEVER SUFFERERS, TAKE NOTE

It doesn't come from hay, and it doesn't cause a fever, but that's not much consolation to the 18 million Americans afflicted with hay fever.

Hay fever is any allergic reaction of the eyes, nose, or throat to certain airborne particles. These particles may be any of pollen from seed-bearing trees, grasses,

and weeds, or spores from certain molds. The term originated in Britain 150 years ago, when people assumed its feverlike symptoms had something to do with the fall haying. Most individuals might think that once they're into adulthood, they already know whether they have hay fever. But if you were to relocate, would you suddenly and mysteriously develop a continual runny nose and minor sore throat? Allergy problems aren't always alleviated by relocation, and sometimes a new allergen—absent where you used to live—can turn up to cause you problems with hay fever.

The incidence of hay fever varies around the world. In the Arctic, for example, it doesn't exist. Because of low temperatures and poor soil, arctic plants are small and primitive. In the tropics and subtropics, there is very little hay fever because the plants are generally flowered and produce pollen that is so heavy it cannot become airborne.

It is in the temperate regions that one finds the greatest amounts of irritating pollen. The worst places in America for hay fever are the middle regions, where grasses and trees without flowers predominate. Because farming continually disrupts the soil and there-

Counting All Those Pollen Grains

The American Academy of Allergy and Immunology has devised the Ragweed Pollen Index to indicate the local severity of the pollen problem. The index is derived from (1) length of the ragweed season, (2) concentration of pollen grains in the air at the season's peak, and (3) total pollen catch throughout the season. The table below lists Ragweed Pollen Index readings for reporting stations within retirement regions. The higher the index number, the worse the problem; an index greater than 10 means lots of discomfort.

Big Ten Country

119.0	Ann Arbor, MI
93.0	Madison, WI

Desert Southwest

2.0	Tucson, AZ
0.7	St. George–Zion, UT
0.2	Phoenix, AZ

Metropolitan South Florida

21.0	Melbourne–Titusville–Palm Bay, FL
9.0	Fort Lauderdale–Hollywood–Pompano Beach, FL
6.0	St. Petersburg–Clearwater, FL (Station: Tampa, FL)
5.0	West Palm Beach–Boca Raton–Delray Beach, FL
4.0	Bradenton, FL
3.0	Daytona Beach, FL
3.0	Orlando, FL
2.0	Miami–Hialeah, FL
0.2	Fort Myers–Cape Coral, FL

Mid-Atlantic Metro Belt

54.0	Virginia Beach–Norfolk, VA
48.0	Columbia County, NY (Station: Albany, NY)
35.0	Charlottesville, VA
30.0	Cape May, NJ (Station: Atlantic City, NJ)

Mid-South

151.0	Lexington, KY
28.0	Chapel Hill, NC (Station: Raleigh, NC)

New Appalachia

85.0	Blacksburg, VA (Station: Roanoke, VA)
57.0	Asheville, NC

North Woods

21.0	Petoskey–Straits of Mackinac, MI (Station: Charlevoix, MI)
13.0	Rhinelander, WI

Pacific Beaches

11.0	San Diego, CA

Rio Grande Country

24.0	Brownsville–Harlingen, TX
7.0	Albuquerque, NM
4.0	Roswell, NM

Rocky Mountains

5.0	Boise, ID
4.0	Colorado Springs, CO

South Atlantic and Gulf Coast Shore

32.0	Panama City, FL
11.0	Charleston, SC
8.0	Fairhope–Gulf Shores, AL (Station: Mobile, AL)
7.0	Biloxi–Gulfport, MS

Tahoe Basin and the Other California

3.0	Twain Harte–Yosemite, CA (Station: Alpine, CA)

Texas Interior

16.0	San Antonio, TX

Yankee Belt

47.0	Burlington, VT
27.0	Litchfield County, CT (Station: Waterbury, CT)
25.0	Northampton–Amherst, MA
5.0	Cape Cod, MA (Station: Nantucket, MA)
3.0	North Conway–White Mountains, NH (Station: Conway, NH)

Source: American Academy of Allergy, 1977

fore encourages the growth of weeds (especially the most troublesome of them all, ragweed), America's heartland is the most hay fever-ridden area. It extends from the Rockies to the Appalachian chain, and from the Canadian border down to the Mid-South.

Yet no areas of the country, except Alaska and the southern half of Florida, are free from hay fever—it's simply a question of degree.

Some retirement places that were once havens for asthmatics and hay fever sufferers are now less free of allergens. Examples are many of the fast-growing areas of the Desert Southwest. In the 1950s, Tucson was virtually free of ragweed pollen. Its desert location precluded the growth of weeds, grasses, and trees that cause hay fever. But as more and more people moved into the area, more trees were planted and lawns seeded. The result? A pollen index that's still good but not nearly as good as it used to be.

Personal Safety:
Violent and Property Crime Rates

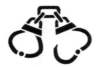 **INTRODUCTION:** Personal Safety

In Asheville, North Carolina, a drug dealer is kidnapped from a fleabag motel, murdered, and his body thrown down a mine shaft outside of town. In Coeur d'Alene, high in the Idaho panhandle, bombs explode in several public buildings. If you were passing through either of these retirement places and heard reports of these actual incidents, you might wonder whether you'd blundered into danger in the midst of spectacular mountain scenery.

The truth is, neither Asheville nor Coeur d'Alene has crime rates anywhere near the national average. The raw odds of your being a crime victim in either place are much below what they would be elsewhere. Indeed, of the 131 places profiled in *Retirement Places Rated*, some are so safe you could hardly pay someone to assault you; others, by comparison, seem just plain dangerous.

If you decide on retirement in Clayton–Clarkesville, Georgia, for example, the raw odds of your meeting up with violent crime—murder, rape, robbery, or assault—in a year's residence are 1 in 3,448. Should you opt for Miami, on the other hand, the raw chances are 1 in 61. One could say that retirement in heavily urbanized southern Florida is more than 50 times more dangerous than it is in rural northeastern Georgia.

But quoting raw odds distorts the local crime picture. Older adults most often are victims of "personal larceny with contact" (translation: purse-snatching and pocket-picking). For other crimes, they are the least victimized of all adult age groups, in spite of the popular belief that they are the preferred targets of crooks. So why a chapter on personal safety if your retirement years are statistically safer than all the years preceding?

The answer is that you are a crime "victim" whenever you must trim back shrubbery along your home's foundation to limit a burglar's potential hiding places, or must get rid of the mailbox and install a mail slot in your front door, or must keep your hand on your wallet at street festivals, or must avoid walking darkened streets, must use only empty elevators, or must stay indoors evenings more than you really care to. In some retirement places, such tactics are advised, in others they are merely prudent, and in still others, they may not be necessary at all.

CRIME RISK: SEVEN CONNECTIONS

Why are some places safer than others? Criminologists have pinned down several factors that are linked to local crime rates.

Population size is closely tied to crime rates. Retirement places with the lowest rates—Fredericksburg, Texas, and Door County, Wisconsin, for example—are rural. Retirement places with the highest rates—Miami is the extreme example—are usually urban.

Climate, too, has a striking connection with breaking the law. Police and criminals are busier in warmer regions of the country than in colder ones. Moreover, in the Sun Belt and in the Frost Belt, these adversaries are particularly active during July and August, when all crimes except robbery are more likely to occur. Why? Since people spend more time outdoors during these months, they are more vulnerable. Homes are vulnerable during this time of year, too, because they are more frequently left with open windows and unlocked doors. Robbery, the cold weather exception, is highest in December because pedestrians and stores doing brisk holiday business make tempting targets.

Time of day is another factor. After sundown is the time that most cars are stolen, most individuals and businesses are held up, most persons are assaulted, and most thefts are committed. Burglaries involving illegal entry or break-in, on the other hand, as well as purse-snatching and pocket-picking, happen more often during daylight hours.

Florida's Defense

When he was writing his famous piece "The Worst American State," H. L. Mencken found the best source of information for causes of death to be the nation's life insurance industry and that, when it came to murder, Florida had the highest rate.

The year was 1931. Not much has changed since then. Most of the Florida places profiled in this book rank near the bottom in personal safety. Of the 50 states, Florida has the highest rates for violent crime and for property crime. The state is the scene for Elmore Leonard's and John D. MacDonald's best-selling crime fiction, and its largest city, Miami, is the tropical backdrop for a bloody Friday evening television series.

Is this fair to the Sunshine State? Not entirely. Local crime rates per 100,000 people are computed on the number of full-time residents. But some resorts draw thousands of four-season visitors. A better way to measure crime rates in resorts, according to Florida's Department of Law Enforcement, is to add the average daily number of tourists to the number of year-round residents. Statewide, this would produce dramatically lower crime rates.

Violent vs. Property Crime: The Smaller the Place, the Better

If you look at the crime rates for the places detailed in the Place Profiles later in this chapter, one factor stands out. Whether you're considering property crimes or crimes of violence, the larger urban areas suffer far greater levels of crime than the smaller, more rural places.

Violent crimes, which make up only 10 percent of total crime in the United States, involve injury or the threat of injury. The FBI defines the following as violent crimes: murder, forcible rape (including attempted rape), robbery (which differs from burglary and larceny-theft because victims are threatened with harm if they don't turn over their property), and aggravated assault (an attack on a person with intent to injure or kill). Of the retirement areas with the highest violent crime rates, seven are larger urban areas.

The FBI classifies four offenses as property crimes: burglary (the illegal entry to a building to commit a felony or theft), larceny-theft (which can include anything from purse-snatching and shoplifting to bicycle theft and pocket-picking), motor-vehicle theft, and arson. Although arson was designated an Index Crime in 1979, data aren't yet available for all of the retirement places. For this reason, *Retirement Places Rated* doesn't include arson in its survey.

Violent Crime in the Retirement Places

SAFEST RETIREMENT PLACES	Violent Crime Rate
Clayton–Clarkesville, GA	29
Door County, WI	30
Mountain Home–Bull Shoals, AR	42
Eagle River, WI	43
Oak Harbor–Whidbey Island, WA	63
Fredericksburg, TX	75
Franklin County, TN	87
Rhinelander, WI	87
Bar Harbor–Frenchman Bay, ME	93
Camden–Penobscot Bay, ME	98

MOST DANGEROUS RETIREMENT PLACES	Violent Crime Rate
Miami–Hialeah, FL	1,639
Santa Fe, NM	1,043
West Palm Beach–Boca Raton– Delray Beach, FL	1,024
Charleston, SC	1,013
Hilton Head–Beaufort, SC	974
Brunswick–Golden Isles, GA	958
Las Vegas, NV	927
Orlando, FL	902
Albuquerque, NM	866
Clear Lake, CA	828

Source: FBI, unpublished "Crime by County" reports, 1981, 1982, 1983, 1984, and 1985.

The violent crime rate is the sum of rates for murder, forcible rape, robbery, and aggravated assault.

Property Crime in the Retirement Places

SAFEST RETIREMENT PLACES	Property Crime Rate
Clayton–Clarkesville, GA	591
Mountain Home–Bull Shoals, AR	1,095
Branson–Cassville–Table Rock Lake, MO	1,160
Southport, NC	1,475
Fredericksburg, TX	1,594
Franklin County, TN	1,834
Burnet–Marble Falls–Llano, TX	1,962
Paris–Big Sandy, TN	1,973
Hendersonville–Brevard, NC	2,005
Crossville, TN	2,108

MOST DANGEROUS RETIREMENT PLACES	Property Crime Rate
Miami–Hialeah, FL	8,718
Ocean City–Assateague Island, MD	8,344
Cape May, NJ	7,973
West Palm Beach–Boca Raton– Delray Beach, FL	7,926
Las Vegas, NV	7,631
Maui, HI	7,559
Santa Fe, NM	7,509
Houghton Lake, MI	7,351
Las Cruces, NM	7,210
Yuma, AZ	7,158

Source: FBI, unpublished "Crime by County" reports, 1981, 1982, 1983, 1984, and 1985.

The property crime rate is the sum of rates for burglary, larceny-theft, and motor-vehicle theft.

Age and sex figure into the equation, too. Some 40 million persons in this country have arrest records for offenses other than traffic tickets. The proportion of offenders who are male is much higher than their proportion in the general population. Half the persons picked up by the police for violent and property crimes are under 20 years of age and four fifths are male. None of this should be taken to mean that persons knock off grocery stores or become involved in bar fights *because* they are young and male, but these characteristics are associated with other factors in crime.

Economics also play a role. Every time the nation's unemployment rate goes up 10 percent, the police make a half million more arrests according to a Johns Hopkins University study on unemployment's hidden costs. But joblessness and loss of income don't automatically make a place dangerous. Many of the safer retirement places in America are poorer than average and suffer job losses during business slumps. Some more affluent communities, given similar sets of circumstances, aren't as safe as they appear: rich offenders tend to be arrested less frequently than poor ones, especially on suspicion. Once arrested, they are con-

Crime Trends

Are the *Retirement Places Rated* crime scores improving for certain retirement places and getting worse for others? The answer to both parts of the question is yes.

RETIREMENT PLACES BECOMING SAFER	Crime Score 5-Year Trend
Southport, NC	−48%
Franklin County, TN	−33
Friday Harbor–San Juan Islands, WA	−31
Bar Harbor–Frenchman Bay, ME	−23
Athens, GA	−22
Bend, OR	−22
Tucson, AZ	−21
Easton–Chesapeake Bay, MD	−20
Las Vegas, NV	−19
Portsmouth–Dover–Durham, NH	−18

RETIREMENT PLACES BECOMING MORE DANGEROUS	Crime Score 5-Year Trend
Clayton–Clarkesville, GA	+73%
Hamilton–Bitterroot Valley, MT	+50
Las Cruces, NM	+49
Kalispell, MT	+39
Carson City–Minden, NV	+37
Roswell, NM	+33
Burnet–Marble Falls–Llano, TX	+31
Chapel Hill, NC	+30
Santa Fe, NM	+30
Port Angeles–Strait of Juan de Fuca, WA	+23

Source: Retirement Places Rated average annual scores for the period 1981 through 1985 for each retirement place, compared with their 1981 scores.

victed with less frequency. This is especially true in juvenile cases involving thefts and break-ins.

Transience affects crime rates. A big deterrent to crime is a strong neighborhood where people know one another and look out for one another's safety and property, regardless of the number of police that patrol the area. This is the reason that high turnover, which results in strangers living next to each other, is associated with high crime rates. Moreover, resort areas that draw transients—Ocean City–Assateague Island, Maryland, and Myrtle Beach, South Carolina, for example—also have serious crime problems. When visitors are added to the year-round residents, the higher population improves the chances that victim and crook will eventually meet.

Police strength, too, is linked to crime rate. Among the retirement places profiled in this book, the employment of sworn uniformed police officers ranges from 1 for every 2,000 residents in Southport, North Carolina, all the way up to 1 for every 150 residents in Carson City–Minden, Nevada. In Manhattan, there are 1,300 police officers per square mile. It's natural to think the

safety of any community rises or falls in direct proportion to the size of the local police force, but it just isn't so. Police definitely fight crime, but most of what they do is after the fact. They respond to complaints; they follow up on tips; they catch criminals and bring them to trial. A large number of police per capita is usually an indication of a high-crime area rather than an area where crime is being prevented.

Other factors the FBI has found to be related to crime rates include the attitudes and practices of local prosecutors, judges, juries, and parole boards; the attitudes of the community toward crime; and the community's willingness to report crime.

KEEPING TRACK OF CRIME

Each year some 16,000 police departments send figures for the number of crimes reported in their jurisdictions to FBI headquarters in Washington. Eight categories of these crimes, because of their seriousness, frequency, and likelihood of being reported, serve as the FBI Crime Index for measuring criminal activity across the nation. Four are classified as violent crimes; the other four are classified as property crimes:

Violent Crimes	Property Crimes
murder	burglary
forcible rape	larceny-theft
robbery	motor-vehicle theft
aggravated assault	arson

Many of these crimes aren't always reported to the police, and this affects the accuracy of the FBI Crime Index. Moreover, in the past, some police departments either padded the figures to oust a judge considered soft on crime or to persuade the city council to increase the department's budget, or they fudged the number of crimes to create an image of effective law enforcement.

It's important to distinguish between the *incidence* of crime and the crime *rate*. Incidence is simply the number of crimes that are committed in a given place. The more people living in a place, the greater the crime incidence will be. In Lancaster, Pennsylvania, an average of 170 robberies are reported to the police each year. Therefore, Lancaster's incidence of robbery is 170. Las Cruces, New Mexico, averages 89 robberies. From these figures, you might think that Lancaster is far more dangerous than Las Cruces. However, 387,000 people live in Lancaster, while only 106,000 live in Las Cruces.

A truer measure of safety is the crime rate—the number of crimes per 100,000 people. Lancaster's robbery rate is 44.4. Las Cruces' rate is 87.5, or nearly twice that of Lancaster. But neither one of these retirement places experiences robbery rates near the national average—225.6.

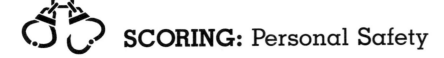

SCORING: Personal Safety

One flaw in the FBI Crime Index totals for places is that the numbers mask the seriousness of violent crime. The most common crime by far is larceny-theft (walking off with an unattended garden hose is one example; shoplifting a can of peas is another). Yet the FBI counts these heists as heavily as first-degree murder when it determines a place's crime rate. When it comes to comparing places, this method doesn't realistically show relative danger.

Austin, Texas, for instance, has a total crime rate of 7,103, roughly on par with Charleston, South Carolina, at 7,133. Are the two places equally dangerous? Hardly. Charleston's violent crime rate is two-and-one-half times as high as Austin's (1,013 versus 418). Although the Texas capital has a high property crime rate, it nevertheless is comparatively safe for its size.

The realistic way to rate the 131 retirement places for personal safety is simple: for each place, *Retirement Places Rated* averages the rates for violent and property crimes for the latest five-year period for which FBI data are available, but since we view property crimes to be much less serious than crimes against people, we give them one tenth the weight of violent crimes. (Although arson was designated a property crime in 1979, arson figures aren't included in the scoring because they are unavailable for many of the retirement places.) Each place starts with a base score of zero, and points are added according to these indicators:

1. *Violent crime rate.* The rates for all violent crimes—murder, rape, robbery, and aggravated assault—are totaled.
2. *Property crime rate.* The rates for burglary, larceny-theft, and motor-vehicle theft are added together, and the result is divided by 10.

The sum of a place's violent crime rate and one tenth its property crime rate, rounded off, represents the score (the higher the score, the more dangerous the place).

SCORING EXAMPLES

A small southern Appalachian retirement place, a Sun Belt capital, a New England college town, and a popular Florida resort illustrate the scoring method for personal safety.

Clayton–Clarkesville, Georgia (#1)

The mountainous area where Georgia, North Carolina, and Tennessee come together has steadily attracted retired people over the years. If sparse population and farming jobs make a place rural, then Clayton–Clarkesville, composed of adjacent Habersham and Rabun counties in northeastern Georgia, is about as rural as you can get.

Here the attraction is low-cost, quiet living near the spectacular Chattahoochee National Forest—yet within striking distance of Atlanta, Knoxville, and Asheville. The town names—Clayton, Clarkesville, Mount Airy, and Cornelia—evoke places in the mind where town dogs live out their lives without being kicked and where your neighbor helps you without being asked. Indeed, a look at Clayton–Clarkesville's crime figures makes you wonder whether anything "interesting" goes on here at all.

The area is cruised by the Georgia Highway Patrol and two county sheriff departments. Along with town police, these sworn officers have fewer murders, rapes, robberies, assaults, burglaries, and thefts reported to them each year than all the arrests they make for drunk driving. Adding its violent crime rate (29) to one tenth its property crime rate (59) results in a total score of 88, the lowest of 131 retirement areas.

Miami–Hialeah, Florida (#131)

In contrast to Clayton–Clarkesville, metropolitan Miami far to the south has a crime score of 2,511, the sum of its violent crime rate (1,639) and one tenth its property crime rate (872). The idea that this area is a crime capital, not just for Florida or the southeastern states, but for the entire country, isn't drawn from television drama—it's based on fact.

In Miami's favor, the crime rate has been edging downward since 1981. Of all the retirement places profiled here, the size of the local police force in Miami and surrounding Dade County is by far the largest. For all that, criminal activity is shockingly high. Last year nearly 200,000 violent and property crimes were reported to the police. Most of the arrests are for larceny, drunk driving, possession of drugs, sale of drugs, prostitution and commercial vice, and disorderly conduct.

Amherst–Northampton, Massachusetts (#25)

If crime rates tend to be higher where there are young populations, Amherst–Northampton is an exception to the rule. One quarter of the place's population are students at the Five Colleges—Amherst, Hampshire, Mount Holyoke, Smith, and the University of Massachusetts. Yet for each of the seven crimes on the FBI Crime Index, Amherst–Northampton and surrounding Hampshire County experience rates far below the national average. Moreover, these rates have been dropping since 1981.

Larceny-theft is the most common complaint

among the 3,200 crimes reported to the police in any year. Adding Amherst–Northampton's violent crime rate (162) to one tenth its property crime rate (287) results in a total score of 449.

Fort Lauderdale–Hollywood–Pompano Beach, Florida (#122)

If there are an estimated 1 million visitors in Florida on any given day, a hundred thousand of them are probably having fun in Fort Lauderdale–Hollywood–Pompano Beach in the middle of Florida's Gold Coast. Given New England's weather, it's likely that undergraduates from Amherst–Northampton's Five Colleges join the annual student migration here each spring break.

That's just the problem, according to Florida's Division of Tourism. Resorts here see a high level of disorderly conduct by young outsiders, *plus* scams by professional crooks from northern cities and not a little violence carried out by persons just passing through. But because the FBI doesn't take into account the thousands of visitors when per capita crime rates are calculated, resorts seem more dangerous places to live than they actually are.

Certainly Fort Lauderdale–Hollywood–Pompano Beach has lower crime statistics than neighboring Miami–Hialeah to the south and West Palm Beach–Boca Raton–Delray Beach immediately north. Lumping year-round residents and seasonal visitors together when calculating per capita crime may brighten the picture even more. Nevertheless, the violent crime rate (795) and one tenth the property crime rate (696) here are far above the national average, producing a crime score of 1,491.

 # RANKINGS: Personal Safety

In ranking 131 retirement places for relative personal safety, *Retirement Places Rated* uses two criteria: (1) the violent crime rate and (2) the property crime rate (because property crimes are generally less serious than violent crimes, the property crime rate is divided by 10). The sum of these rates is the retirement place's score. The higher the score, the more dangerous the place.

Places receiving tie scores are given the same rank and are listed in alphabetical order.

Retirement Places from Safest to Most Dangerous

Rank	Score	Rank	Score	Rank	Score
1. Clayton–Clarkesville, GA	88	22. Canandaigua, NY	428	41. Oscoda–Huron Shore, MI	584
2. Mountain Home–Bull Shoals, AR	152	23. Camden–Penobscot Bay, ME	432	44. Bend, OR	585
3. Branson–Cassville–Table Rock Lake, MO	227	24. Kerrville, TX	443	45. Prescott, AZ	593
4. Fredericksburg, TX	234	25. Amherst–Northampton, MA	449	46. Columbia County, NY	607
5. Franklin County, TN	270	26. St. George–Zion, UT	450	47. Port Angeles–Strait of Juan de Fuca, WA	608
6. Oak Harbor–Whidbey Island, WA	291	27. Portsmouth–Dover–Durham, NH	480	48. Asheville, NC	617
7. Southport, NC	293	28. State College, PA	482	49. Fairhope–Gulf Shores, AL	625
8. Door County, WI	308	29. Athens–Cedar Creek Lake, TX	486	50. Olympia, WA	632
9. Crossville, TN	335	30. Blacksburg, VA	500	51. Bloomington–Brown County, IN	635
10. Litchfield County, CT	346	31. Hamilton–Bitterroot Valley, MT	507	52. Petoskey–Straits of Mackinac, MI	639
11. Murray–Kentucky Lake, KY	347	32. Friday Harbor–San Juan Islands, WA	520	53. Grass Valley–Truckee, CA	660
12. Burnet–Marble Falls–Llano, TX	352	33. Bennington, VT	527	54. Gainesville–Lake Lanier, GA	671
13. Hanover, NH	362	34. Rhinelander, WI	529	55. Monticello–Liberty, NY	676
14. Hendersonville–Brevard, NC	377	35. Fayetteville, AR	545	56. Kalispell, MT	681
15. Canton–Lake Tawakoni, TX	378	36. Winchester, VA	546	57. Easton–Chesapeake Bay, MD	684
16. Grand Lake–Lake Tenkiller, OK	389	37. North Conway–White Mountains, NH	553	58. Carson City–Minden, NV	704
16. Paris–Big Sandy, TN	389	38. Burlington, VT	554	59. Laconia–Lake Winnipesaukee, NH	711
18. Keene, NH	390	39. Front Royal, VA	557	60. Medford–Ashland, OR	723
19. Eagle River, WI	392	40. Traverse City–Grand Traverse Bay, MI	580	61. Hot Springs–Lake Ouachita, AR	727
20. Lancaster, PA	393	41. Fort Walton Beach, FL	584	62. Ocean County, NJ	729
21. Bar Harbor–Frenchman Bay, ME	404	41. New Paltz–Ulster County, NY	584	63. San Luis Obispo, CA	731

Rank	Score		Rank	Score		Rank	Score
64. Missoula, MT	735		87. Deming, NM	969		110. Ann Arbor, MI	1,177
65. Chapel Hill, NC	736		88. Sarasota, FL	975			
			89. Naples, FL	1,013		111. Athens, GA	1,190
66. Grand Junction, CO	741		90. Virginia Beach–Norfolk, VA	1,014		112. San Antonio, TX	1,201
67. Kauai, HI	742					113. Phoenix, AZ	1,259
68. Fort Myers–Cape Coral, FL	782		91. Lexington, KY	1,021		114. Yuma, AZ	1,260
69. McAllen–Edinburg–			92. Maui, HI	1,022		115. Ocala, FL	1,295
Mission, TX	790		93. Brownsville–Harlingen, TX	1,026			
70. Charlottesville, VA	796		94. Cape Cod, MA	1,035		116. Bradenton, FL	1,324
			95. Houghton Lake, MI	1,042		117. Daytona Beach, FL	1,340
71. Bellingham, WA	797					118. Myrtle Beach, SC	1,366
72. Coeur d'Alene, ID	798		96. Flagstaff, AZ	1,043		119. Clear Lake, CA	1,383
73. Santa Rosa–Petaluma, CA	802		97. Colorado Springs, CO	1,063		120. Lakeland–Winter Haven, FL	1,400
74. Newport–Lincoln City, OR	808		98. Salinas–Seaside–				
75. Madison, WI	809		Monterey, CA	1,077		121. Ocean City–	
			99. St. Petersburg–			Assateague Island, MD	1,440
76. Iowa City, IA	823		Clearwater, FL	1,079		122. Fort Lauderdale–Hollywood–	
77. Red Bluff–			100. San Diego, CA	1,082		Pompano Beach, FL	1,491
Sacramento Valley, CA	831					123. Orlando, FL	1,567
78. Boise, ID	840		101. Roswell, NM	1,083		124. Albuquerque, NM	1,579
79. Fort Collins–Loveland, CO	848		102. Austin, TX	1,087		125. Hilton Head–Beaufort, SC	1,591
80. Springfield, MO	867		103. Melbourne–Titusville–				
			Palm Bay, FL	1,124		126. Charleston, SC	1,625
81. Rehoboth Bay–Indian River			104. Cape May, NJ	1,140		127. Brunswick–	
Bay, DE	880		105. Tucson, AZ	1,144		Golden Isles, GA	1,669
82. Eugene–Springfield, OR	881					128. Las Vegas, NV	1,690
83. Redding, CA	904		106. Lake Havasu City–			129. Santa Fe, NM	1,794
84. Biloxi–Gulfport, MS	921		Kingman, AZ	1,156		130. West Palm Beach–	
85. Chico–Paradise, CA	932		107. Reno, NV	1,161		Boca Raton–	
			108. Las Cruces, NM	1,170		Delray Beach, FL	1,817
86. Twain Harte–Yosemite, CA	934		109. Panama City, FL	1,173		131. Miami–Hialeah, FL	2,511

Retirement Places Listed Alphabetically

Retirement Place	Rank	Retirement Place	Rank	Retirement Place	Rank
Albuquerque, NM	124	Charlottesville, VA	70	Hamilton–Bitterroot Valley, MT	31
Amherst–Northampton, MA	25			Hanover, NH	13
Ann Arbor, MI	110	Chico–Paradise, CA	85		
Asheville, NC	48	Clayton–Clarkesville, GA	1	Hendersonville–Brevard, NC	14
Athens, GA	111	Clear Lake, CA	119	Hilton Head–Beaufort, SC	125
		Coeur d'Alene, ID	72	Hot Springs–Lake Ouachita, AR	61
Athens–Cedar Creek Lake, TX	29	Colorado Springs, CO	97	Houghton Lake, MI	95
Austin, TX	102			Iowa City, IA	76
Bar Harbor–Frenchman Bay, ME	21	Columbia County, NY	46		
Bellingham, WA	71	Crossville, TN	9	Kalispell, MT	56
Bend, OR	44	Daytona Beach, FL	117	Kauai, HI	67
		Deming, NM	87	Keene, NH	18
Bennington, VT	33	Door County, WI	8	Kerrville, TX	24
Biloxi–Gulfport, MS	84			Laconia–	
Blacksburg, VA	30	Eagle River, WI	19	Lake Winnipesaukee, NH	59
Bloomington–		Easton–Chesapeake Bay, MD	57		
Brown County, IN	51	Eugene–Springfield, OR	82	Lake Havasu City–Kingman, AZ	106
Boise, ID	78	Fairhope–Gulf Shores, AL	49	Lakeland–Winter Haven, FL	120
		Fayetteville, AR	35	Lancaster, PA	20
Bradenton, FL	116			Las Cruces, NM	108
Branson–Cassville–		Flagstaff, AZ	96	Las Vegas, NV	128
Table Rock Lake, MO	3	Fort Collins–Loveland, CO	79		
Brownsville–Harlingen, TX	93	Fort Lauderdale–Hollywood–		Lexington, KY	91
Brunswick–Golden Isles, GA	127	Pompano Beach, FL	122	Litchfield County, CT	10
Burlington, VT	38	Fort Myers–Cape Coral, FL	68	Madison, WI	75
		Fort Walton Beach, FL	41	Maui, HI	92
Burnet–Marble Falls–				McAllen–Edinburg–Mission, TX	69
Llano, TX	12	Franklin County, TN	5		
Camden–Penobscot Bay, ME	23	Fredericksburg, TX	4	Medford–Ashland, OR	60
Canandaigua, NY	22	Friday Harbor–San Juan		Melbourne–Titusville–	
Canton–Lake Tawakoni, TX	15	Islands, WA	32	Palm Bay, FL	103
Cape Cod, MA	94	Front Royal, VA	39	Miami–Hialeah, FL	131
		Gainesville–Lake Lanier, GA	54	Missoula, MT	64
Cape May, NJ	104			Monticello–Liberty, NY	55
Carson City–Minden, NV	58	Grand Junction, CO	66		
Chapel Hill, NC	65	Grand Lake–Lake Tenkiller, OK	16	Mountain Home–Bull Shoals, AR	2
Charleston, SC	126	Grass Valley–Truckee, CA	53	Murray–Kentucky Lake, KY	11

Retirement Place	Rank	Retirement Place	Rank	Retirement Place	Rank
Myrtle Beach, SC	118	Phoenix, AZ	113	San Luis Obispo, CA	63
Naples, FL	89	Port Angeles–Strait of		Santa Fe, NM	129
		Juan de Fuca, WA	47		
New Paltz–Ulster County, NY	41			Santa Rosa–	
Newport–Lincoln City, OR	74	Portsmouth–Dover–Durham, NH	27	Petaluma, CA	73
North Conway–		Prescott, AZ	45	Sarasota, FL	88
White Mountains, NH	37	Red Bluff–Sacramento Valley, CA	77	Southport, NC	7
Oak Harbor–Whidbey Island, WA	6	Redding, CA	83	Springfield, MO	80
Ocala, FL	115	Rehoboth Bay–Indian River		State College, PA	28
		Bay, DE	81		
Ocean City–				Traverse City–Grand Traverse	
Assateague Island, MD	121	Reno, NV	107	Bay, MI	40
Ocean County, NJ	62	Rhinelander, WI	34	Tucson, AZ	105
Olympia, WA	50	Roswell, NM	101	Twain Harte–Yosemite, CA	86
Orlando, FL	123	St. George–Zion, UT	26	Virginia Beach–Norfolk, VA	90
Oscoda–Huron Shore, MI	41	St. Petersburg–Clearwater, FL	99	West Palm Beach–Boca Raton–	
				Delray Beach, FL	130
Panama City, FL	109	Salinas–Seaside–Monterey, CA	98		
Paris–Big Sandy, TN	16	San Antonio, TX	112	Winchester, VA	36
Petoskey–Straits of Mackinac, MI	52	San Diego, CA	100	Yuma, AZ	114

 # PLACE PROFILES: Personal Safety

The Place Profiles show each retirement place's average annual rates for seven crimes: murder, forcible rape, robbery, aggravated assault, burglary, larceny-theft, and motor-vehicle theft for 1981 through 1985. These rates are divided into violent and property categories, and a total rate for each of these categories is given. A star preceding a retirement place's name highlights it as one of the top 15 places for personal safety.

The next-to-last column indicates the crime score trend over five years: 32 retirement places have an arrow pointing upward, meaning their *Retirement Places Rated* crime rates during this period have risen more than 5 percent; 48 places have an arrow pointing downward, meaning their rates have dropped more than 10 percent; a dash for the remaining 51 places means the rates have neither risen more than 5 percent nor dropped more than 10 percent.

All figures are from the FBI's unpublished "Crime by County" reports for 1982, 1983, 1984, 1985, and 1986.

	Violent Crime Rates					Property Crime Rates						
	Murder	Rape	Robbery	Assault	Total	Burglary	Larceny-Theft	Motor-Vehicle Theft	Total	SCORE	TREND	RANK
United States	**8.6**	**35.2**	**225.6**	**290.2**	**560**	**1,405.4**	**2,957.2**	**452.7**	**4,815**	**1,041**	▼	
Albuquerque, NM	9.5	59.0	264.4	533.0	866	2,273.4	4,437.1	415.5	7,126	**1,579**	—	124
Amherst–Northampton, MA	1.6	13.7	27.5	119.5	162	835.2	1,812.1	224.3	2,872	**449**	▼	25
Ann Arbor, MI	5.1	61.8	114.7	378.9	561	1,414.6	4,299.0	443.2	6,157	**1,177**	—	110
Asheville, NC	5.7	15.3	63.2	184.3	269	940.7	2,337.7	198.4	3,477	**617**	▲	48
Athens, GA	7.3	46.1	113.5	359.5	526	1,611.6	4,730.7	298.6	6,641	**1,190**	▼	111
Athens–Cedar Creek Lake, TX	11.5	9.3	17.6	162.1	201	1,062.4	1,681.4	102.8	2,847	**486**	▲	29
Austin, TX	11.8	60.7	144.3	201.3	418	1,907.7	4,430.9	346.7	6,685	**1,087**	—	102
Bar Harbor–Frenchman Bay, ME	2.8	7.0	8.0	74.8	93	952.6	2,034.8	120.9	3,108	**404**	▼	21
Bellingham, WA	2.4	32.1	33.3	178.8	247	1,425.7	3,813.6	260.0	5,499	**797**	▼	71
Bend, OR	4.4	23.1	26.1	83.7	137	1,057.8	3,207.4	218.9	4,484	**585**	▼	44
Bennington, VT	1.8	26.5	19.9	78.4	127	1,259.8	2,531.3	203.9	3,995	**527**	▲	33
Biloxi–Gulfport, MS	9.0	44.9	122.4	230.9	407	1,724.0	3,094.7	317.4	5,136	**921**	—	84

	Violent Crime Rates					Property Crime Rates						
	Murder	Rape	Robbery	Assault	Total	Burglary	Larceny-Theft	Motor-Vehicle Theft	Total	SCORE	TREND	RANK
United States	**8.6**	**35.2**	**225.6**	**290.2**	**560**	**1,405.4**	**2,957.2**	**452.7**	**4,815**	**1,041**	▼	
Blacksburg, VA	5.5	14.6	19.2	106.6	146	681.3	2,738.0	120.7	3,540	500	▲	30
Bloomington–Brown County, IN	2.2	17.3	21.0	173.9	214	940.6	3,069.6	197.5	4,208	635	—	51
Boise, ID	3.1	30.9	51.3	285.3	371	1,304.9	3,167.0	212.8	4,685	840	▼	78
Bradenton, FL	8.0	51.9	148.6	517.5	726	1,918.4	3,722.1	342.9	5,983	1,324	▲	116
★ Branson–Cassville–Table Rock Lake, MO	2.8	9.7	3.0	95.4	111	359.2	735.2	65.7	1,160	227	▲	3
Brownsville–Harlingen, TX	8.0	21.6	79.3	372.2	481	1,878.1	3,006.2	564.8	5,449	1,026	—	93
Brunswick–Golden Isles, GA	11.5	82.7	188.4	675.1	958	2,338.3	4,426.7	347.9	7,113	1,669	—	127
Burlington, VT	2.4	28.4	27.5	68.5	127	1,279.3	2,799.8	195.1	4,274	554	▲	38
★ Burnet–Marble Falls–Llano, TX	3.9	17.0	11.7	123.6	156	672.9	1,194.0	95.5	1,962	352	▲	12
Camden–Penobscot Bay, ME	1.2	14.9	16.2	65.2	98	780.3	2,400.1	156.0	3,336	432	▼	23
Canandaigua, NY	2.0	13.0	19.3	96.3	131	770.9	2,099.4	100.0	2,970	428	▲	22
★ Canton–Lake Tawakoni, TX	2.9	11.0	28.4	113.3	156	814.8	1,250.2	155.4	2,220	378	▲	15
Cape Cod, MA	2.1	25.6	40.1	394.3	462	2,234.7	3,169.1	321.9	5,726	1,035	—	94
Cape May, NJ	4.3	45.0	100.8	193.2	343	2,396.4	5,256.8	319.5	7,973	1,140	—	104
Carson City–Minden, NV	1.7	30.9	134.7	138.5	306	1,012.5	2,705.7	265.2	3,983	704	▲	58
Chapel Hill, NC	8.0	22.1	49.1	195.4	275	1,267.4	3,134.9	211.5	4,614	736	▲	65
Charleston, SC	10.1	64.2	291.0	647.7	1,013	1,821.9	3,869.3	429.2	6,120	1,625	—	126
Charlottesville, VA	11.2	25.1	66.4	181.5	284	863.0	4,065.0	194.7	5,123	796	—	70
Chico–Paradise, CA	3.5	44.2	68.2	277.6	394	1,772.2	3,357.9	253.9	5,384	932	▼	85
★ Clayton–Clarkesville, GA	1.6	3.0	4.9	19.9	29	258.4	292.1	40.5	591	88	▲	1
Clear Lake, CA	5.9	30.0	46.9	745.1	828	2,373.4	2,926.5	244.8	5,545	1,383	—	119
Coeur d'Alene, ID	2.6	24.9	34.2	284.4	346	1,304.1	3,021.6	196.9	4,523	798	▼	72
Colorado Springs, CO	5.3	61.5	143.5	235.8	446	1,803.5	4,047.2	323.4	6,174	1,063	—	97
Columbia County, NY	2.1	9.7	22.2	307.1	341	883.6	1,693.5	86.9	2,664	607	—	46
★ Crossville, TN	6.8	11.6	24.9	80.4	124	873.3	1,104.5	130.5	2,108	335	—	9
Daytona Beach, FL	9.4	56.1	178.7	425.1	669	2,207.4	4,175.8	321.8	6,705	1,340	▼	117
Deming, NM	3.6	32.5	52.2	298.4	387	1,791.3	3,769.6	259.4	5,820	969	—	87
★ Door County, WI	2.3	6.2	3.9	17.2	30	649.3	2,023.5	104.1	2,777	308	▼	8
Eagle River, WI	2.3	15.1	9.3	16.4	43	1,184.5	2,106.5	196.6	3,488	392	▲	19
Easton–Chesapeake Bay, MD	4.5	23.5	53.2	275.0	356	863.9	2,267.1	145.9	3,277	684	▼	57
Eugene–Springfield, OR	3.2	41.4	87.3	141.6	274	1,648.7	4,170.9	253.5	6,073	881	▼	82
Fairhope–Gulf Shores, AL	7.3	19.3	41.8	276.4	345	944.9	1,730.2	125.0	2,800	625	—	49
Fayetteville, AR	3.9	25.3	28.6	115.6	173	1,033.0	2,490.9	191.8	3,716	545	—	35
Flagstaff, AZ	5.7	38.0	92.0	317.9	454	1,285.0	4,389.4	216.0	5,890	1,043	▼	96
Fort Collins–Loveland, CO	3.7	30.9	25.5	267.9	328	1,140.3	3,849.0	209.7	5,199	848	▲	79
Fort Lauderdale–Hollywood–Pompano Beach, FL	12.6	46.3	352.0	383.7	795	2,128.4	4,251.3	583.1	6,963	1,491	▼	122
Fort Myers–Cape Coral, FL	9.3	36.3	149.9	204.7	400	1,221.2	2,381.1	219.7	3,822	782	▼	68
Fort Walton Beach, FL	4.9	29.0	65.3	155.5	255	969.2	2,105.4	219.2	3,294	584	▲	41

	Violent Crime Rates					Property Crime Rates						
	Murder	Rape	Robbery	Assault	Total	Burglary	Larceny-Theft	Motor-Vehicle Theft	Total	SCORE	TREND	RANK
United States	8.6	35.2	225.6	290.2	560	1,405.4	2,957.2	452.7	4,815	1,041	▼	
★ Franklin County, TN	4.4	9.5	13.0	59.8	87	520.3	1,166.3	147.5	1,834	270	▼	5
★ Fredericksburg, TX	1.3	9.6	9.5	54.9	75	456.4	1,050.3	87.1	1,594	234	▲	4
Friday Harbor–San Juan Islands, WA	14.2	7.1	2.5	138.9	163	871.8	2,507.1	195.1	3,574	520	▼	32
Front Royal, VA	8.2	33.5	30.2	121.1	193	968.4	2,501.4	165.0	3,635	557	—	39
Gainesville–Lake Lanier, GA	9.7	18.6	54.9	212.6	296	1,122.3	2,349.5	280.2	3,752	671	▼	54
Grand Junction, CO	3.4	27.6	50.0	151.8	233	1,233.9	3,600.4	244.4	5,079	741	—	66
Grand Lake–Lake Tenkiller, OK	6.5	9.2	17.7	94.7	128	945.3	1,469.8	195.4	2,611	389	▲	16
Grass Valley–Truckee, CA	8.5	21.5	30.1	247.4	308	1,114.0	2,196.1	208.6	3,519	660	▼	53
Hamilton–Bitterroot Valley, MT	3.3	11.6	6.0	243.1	264	363.1	1,937.1	124.9	2,425	507	▲	31
★ Hanover, NH	1.3	14.2	9.7	74.4	100	571.0	1,939.8	111.2	2,622	362	▼	13
★ Hendersonville–Brevard, NC	5.8	8.8	21.8	140.0	176	742.3	1,102.5	160.0	2,005	377	—	14
Hilton Head–Beaufort, SC	7.3	60.5	82.5	824.0	974	2,038.7	3,858.8	272.2	6,170	1,591	—	125
Hot Springs–Lake Ouachita, AR	10.0	25.1	92.3	249.5	377	1,200.1	2,088.4	206.9	3,495	727	—	61
Houghton Lake, MI	0.0	48.7	42.4	215.6	307	2,890.7	4,089.3	371.2	7,351	1,042	—	95
Iowa City, IA	2.9	31.0	23.6	250.8	308	1,007.8	3,940.5	203.8	5,152	823	▼	76
Kalispell, MT	2.6	24.8	10.9	240.2	279	817.2	2,987.0	213.7	4,018	681	▲	56
Kauai, HI	3.8	25.7	34.5	142.5	207	1,462.8	3,704.2	183.9	5,351	742	▼	67
Keene, NH	2.7	21.9	17.5	81.7	124	633.8	1,905.5	122.6	2,662	390	▼	18
Kerrville, TX	8.7	9.4	25.5	108.7	152	1,106.2	1,717.1	90.5	2,914	443	▲	24
Laconia–Lake Winnipesaukee, NH	1.8	33.1	22.5	140.3	198	1,544.7	3,344.5	240.3	5,130	711	—	59
Lake Havasu City–Kingman, AZ	7.2	19.0	61.2	527.7	615	1,488.3	3,529.1	396.5	5,414	1,156	—	106
Lakeland–Winter Haven, FL	10.6	49.7	150.7	589.9	801	1,745.6	3,947.0	297.4	5,990	1,400	—	120
Lancaster, PA	1.5	11.6	44.4	80.4	138	677.4	1,738.8	131.5	2,548	393	—	20
Las Cruces, NM	7.8	47.7	87.5	305.8	449	1,662.6	5,185.6	361.7	7,210	1,170	▲	108
Las Vegas, NV	17.3	67.5	486.3	356.3	927	2,726.6	4,239.4	664.7	7,631	1,690	▼	128
Lexington, KY	6.9	49.0	156.4	280.8	493	1,376.8	3,602.5	296.8	5,276	1,021	—	91
★ Litchfield County, CT	1.8	16.8	19.6	62.3	101	713.3	1,528.8	202.6	2,445	346	—	10
Madison, WI	2.2	31.3	71.0	115.1	220	1,273.2	4,396.6	215.0	5,885	809	▼	75
Maui, HI	4.1	35.5	58.3	168.0	266	2,170.1	5,073.2	315.9	7,559	1,022	—	92
McAllen–Edinburg–Mission, TX	6.8	15.0	39.0	261.9	323	1,684.5	2,675.3	304.8	4,665	790	—	69
Medford–Ashland, OR	3.3	30.3	45.0	152.2	231	1,235.7	3,467.5	217.2	4,920	723	—	60
Melbourne–Titusville–Palm Bay, FL	5.3	42.0	118.3	396.5	562	1,701.5	3,623.7	290.0	5,615	1,124	—	103
Miami–Hialeah, FL	26.4	55.8	741.2	815.8	1,639	2,494.1	5,219.8	1,004.1	8,718	2,511	—	131
Missoula, MT	5.5	32.6	32.7	144.2	215	883.0	4,040.3	275.1	5,198	735	—	64
Monticello–Liberty, NY	4.9	21.2	54.9	251.7	333	1,693.9	1,557.5	176.7	3,428	676	▼	55
★ Mountain Home–Bull Shoals, AR	3.5	3.5	4.5	30.2	42	333.9	712.9	47.8	1,095	152	—	2

	Violent Crime Rates					Property Crime Rates						
	Murder	Rape	Robbery	Assault	Total	Burglary	Larceny-Theft	Motor-Vehicle Theft	Total	SCORE	TREND	RANK
United States	**8.6**	**35.2**	**225.6**	**290.2**	**560**	**1,405.4**	**2,957.2**	**452.7**	**4,815**	**1,041**	▼	
★ Murray–Kentucky Lake, KY	4.3	7.5	10.7	109.0	132	691.9	1,340.0	132.5	2,164	347	—	11
Myrtle Beach, SC	11.4	38.9	110.0	491.5	652	2,133.6	4,520.9	483.4	7,138	1,366	▲	118
Naples, FL	17.6	40.0	122.4	285.6	466	1,706.1	3,456.6	308.8	5,472	1,013	▼	89
New Paltz–Ulster County, NY	4.1	19.9	38.9	214.0	277	1,161.9	1,746.8	157.7	3,066	584	—	41
Newport–Lincoln City, OR	3.3	33.1	51.4	240.7	329	1,505.3	3,059.4	221.8	4,787	808	▼	74
North Conway–White Mountains, NH	4.8	15.6	9.3	111.0	141	1,239.7	2,739.4	145.0	4,124	553	▲	37
★ Oak Harbor–Whidbey Island, WA	1.7	11.2	10.5	39.1	63	715.8	1,497.6	69.9	2,283	291	▼	6
Ocala, FL	9.5	47.8	138.3	493.4	689	2,159.7	3,628.4	276.3	6,064	1,295	—	115
Ocean City–Assateague Island, MD	10.8	65.8	85.3	443.8	606	2,343.9	5,637.0	363.3	8,344	1,440	—	121
Ocean County, NJ	2.7	22.8	69.3	171.9	267	1,227.3	3,142.0	245.4	4,615	729	▼	62
Olympia, WA	2.8	29.6	33.4	120.9	187	1,223.1	3,058.5	167.1	4,449	632	▲	50
Orlando, FL	8.7	56.9	259.3	577.4	902	2,229.7	4,045.0	374.3	6,649	1,567	▼	123
Oscoda–Huron Shore, MI	4.2	23.8	13.4	190.9	232	1,114.5	2,276.7	129.9	3,521	584	▼	41
Panama City, FL	7.3	61.7	72.7	476.6	618	1,379.7	3,905.5	263.5	5,549	1,173	—	109
Paris–Big Sandy, TN	4.9	12.2	21.2	153.7	192	668.2	1,218.7	86.0	1,973	389	▼	16
Petoskey–Straits of Mackinac, MI	0.0	41.6	30.5	140.7	213	998.7	3,118.0	139.0	4,256	639	—	52
Phoenix, AZ	8.4	43.9	180.4	335.2	568	1,985.0	4,495.6	432.6	6,913	1,259	▼	113
Port Angeles–Strait of Juan de Fuca, WA	3.6	21.7	21.5	125.8	173	1,107.9	3,072.2	168.6	4,349	608	▲	47
Portsmouth–Dover–Durham, NH	1.7	11.3	28.4	82.5	124	857.6	2,449.0	250.3	3,557	480	▼	27
Prescott, AZ	4.5	14.8	36.3	179.0	235	1,072.0	2,301.7	202.9	3,577	593	—	45
Red Bluff–Sacramento Valley, CA	8.5	28.2	44.5	269.3	351	1,262.3	3,333.3	206.0	4,802	831	▼	77
Redding, CA	6.9	41.6	68.6	305.6	423	1,507.4	3,057.2	247.5	4,812	904	▼	83
Rehoboth Bay–Indian River Bay, DE	6.8	41.2	46.0	354.5	449	1,293.0	2,862.3	154.5	4,310	880	—	81
Reno, NV	7.9	69.6	214.6	246.7	539	1,806.3	4,002.5	415.6	6,224	1,161	—	107
Rhinelander, WI	2.0	7.9	9.0	68.3	87	1,018.2	3,186.1	217.8	4,422	529	—	34
Roswell, NM	10.8	33.6	63.1	334.1	442	1,550.0	4,601.1	255.7	6,407	1,083	▲	101
St. George–Zion, UT	1.9	15.1	13.5	104.6	135	477.4	2,449.6	220.0	3,147	450	▲	26
St. Petersburg–Clearwater, FL	5.3	40.2	165.1	387.8	598	1,517.5	3,099.6	188.8	4,806	1,079	▼	99
Salinas–Seaside–Monterey, CA	8.1	41.1	159.3	338.2	547	1,433.4	3,635.0	229.8	5,298	1,077	—	98
San Antonio, TX	17.0	56.2	215.3	243.8	532	2,223.2	3,881.4	585.0	6,690	1,201	▲	112
San Diego, CA	7.4	40.3	228.5	269.5	546	1,609.7	3,081.3	665.4	5,356	1,082	▼	100
San Luis Obispo, CA	5.0	34.1	52.6	229.6	321	1,264.9	2,602.7	230.0	4,098	731	▼	63
Santa Fe, NM	7.3	47.4	104.5	883.5	1,043	2,098.2	4,948.7	462.5	7,509	1,794	▲	129
Santa Rosa–Petaluma, CA	5.1	35.1	79.2	207.6	327	1,561.3	2,967.8	216.4	4,746	802	▼	73
Sarasota, FL	5.9	48.4	113.2	261.2	429	1,614.3	3,623.3	218.9	5,457	975	—	88
★ Southport, NC	4.8	9.7	17.7	112.6	145	621.5	703.6	150.3	1,475	293	▼	7
Springfield, MO	4.7	27.7	73.9	136.4	243	1,711.0	4,291.7	241.2	6,244	867	▼	80

	Violent Crime Rates					Property Crime Rates						
	Murder	Rape	Robbery	Assault	Total	Burglary	Larceny-Theft	Motor-Vehicle Theft	Total	SCORE	TREND	RANK
United States	8.6	35.2	225.6	290.2	560	1,405.4	2,957.2	452.7	4,815	1,041	▼	
State College, PA	1.2	16.4	21.8	90.4	130	675.8	2,752.0	95.1	3,523	482	—	28
Traverse City–Grand Traverse Bay, MI	0.4	48.7	30.5	93.8	173	972.9	2,956.3	145.2	4,074	580	▼	40
Tucson, AZ	6.5	44.6	149.2	331.9	532	1,833.0	3,961.3	328.9	6,123	1,144	▼	105
Twain Harte–Yosemite, CA	3.3	29.5	25.1	512.4	570	1,233.9	2,258.7	150.4	3,643	934	▲	86
Virginia Beach–Norfolk, VA	9.7	44.6	210.9	222.0	487	1,287.2	3,728.6	251.2	5,267	1,014	—	90
West Palm Beach–Boca Raton–Delray Beach, FL	11.4	57.2	285.2	670.0	1,024	2,581.9	4,832.2	512.0	7,926	1,817	▼	130
Winchester, VA	4.6	15.7	41.7	119.7	182	823.3	2,656.3	158.5	3,638	546	▼	36
Yuma, AZ	10.2	46.7	119.1	367.8	544	1,651.0	5,117.3	389.4	7,158	1,260	▲	114

 ET CETERA: Personal Safety

CRIMES BY REGION

Although criminal activity varies from place to place and from year to year, regional patterns haven't changed much in decades. The murder rate in the West South Central states, where the frequency of people's killing one another has traditionally been the country's highest, is nearly three times that of the Plains states. Rape is highest in the West South Central and Pacific regions and lowest in New England and the Plains states. Armed robbery, a crime of big cities, is highest in the Mid-Atlantic states, lowest in the Plains states. The Plains states also have the lowest rates for assault, while the South Atlantic states experience the highest.

Criminologists recognize the geographic pattern of crime-ridden places immediately. Many of the country's more dangerous places are located on the East Coast from New Jersey southward. This area is rapidly growing. The resulting transience, which leads to strangers living close together, is strongly associated with crime. There are other reasons for high crime in this area. Professional crooks migrate to where the living is easy and the pickings bountiful; they don't stay in the industrial towns of the North but head South to warm weather and popular resorts. This is one reason Miami has been plagued by high crime for decades.

Finally, most of the dangerous places are hot much of the year. Knowing what we do about climate's influence on crime, it isn't surprising that large southern cities going through a steamy summer are America's most crime-ridden. Retired persons bidding farewell to Cedar Rapids, Milwaukee, Pittsburgh, or Syracuse to make their new homes in West Palm Beach, Orlando, Phoenix, or Las Vegas may need time not only for acclimatizing to warm weather, but also for getting used to crime's share in the local evening news.

RETIREMENT HOUSING DEVELOPMENTS: FOUR FACTORS FOR SECURITY

If you are considering life in a retirement development —whether a high-rise apartment or condominium, trailer park, townhouse complex, housing tract, or enclosed dwelling with adjoining courtyards and interior patios—check for these basic security factors.

Opportunity for Surveillance. The ease with which both residents and police patrols can watch what is going on is determined almost totally by the design of the building complex. The ability to survey, supervise, and question strangers will depend on how each residence is designed and on its relationship to neighboring dwellings. The proximity of elevator doors to apartment entrances, the number of apartments opening onto each landing, the location and nearness of parking lots and open spaces, the layout of streets and walkways, the evenness and intensity of both exterior and interior lighting—all of these factors affect ease of surveillance.

All entryways and walkways should be clearly visible to residents and police at any time of day or night. This means that the landscaping surrounding them should be low and free from obstacles and heavy foliage. Walkways should be evenly illuminated at

Regional Crime Rates

Region	Violent Crime Rates				Property Crime Rates		
	Murder	Rape	Robbery	Assault	Burglary	Larceny-Theft	Motor-Vehicle Theft
U.S. National Average	**7.9**	**36.6**	**208.5**	**302.9**	**1,287.3**	**2,901.2**	**462.0**
New England: Maine, New Hampshire, Vermont, Massachusetts, Rhode Island, Connecticut	6.1	28.5	291.2	270.5	1,050.2	2,436.9	543.8
Mid-Atlantic: New York, New Jersey, Pennsylvania	7.1	29.6	339.8	284.2	1,040.3	2,448.0	526.0
Great Lakes: Ohio, Indiana, Illinois, Michigan, Wisconsin	7.1	37.2	197.9	275.8	1,111.9	2,781.2	504.1
Plains: Minnesota, Iowa, Missouri, North Dakota, South Dakota, Nebraska, Kansas	4.2	25.0	85.9	203.9	960.0	2,521.2	245.4
South Atlantic: District of Columbia, Delaware, Maryland, Virginia, West Virginia, North Carolina, South Carolina, Georgia, Florida	9.3	39.0	196.6	387.2	1,367.3	3,018.2	357.6
East South Central: Kentucky, Tennessee, Alabama, Mississippi	9.0	30.5	114.4	239.2	1,009.2	1,952.4	296.1
West South Central: Arkansas, Louisiana, Oklahoma, Texas	11.5	45.6	171.1	312.2	1,601.6	3,322.7	526.5
Mountain: Montana, Idaho, Wyoming, Colorado, New Mexico, Arizona, Utah, Nevada	6.6	38.4	115.0	314.3	1,513.7	3,844.2	350.4
Pacific: Washington, Oregon, California, Alaska, Hawaii	9.2	45.4	281.8	350.5	1,705.1	3,507.1	587.2

Source: FBI, *Crime in the United States*, 1986.

Personal Safety: The States Ranked from Safest to Most Dangerous

State	Violent Crime Rate (Rank)	Property Crime Rate (Rank)	Score	State	Violent Crime Rate (Rank)	Property Crime Rate (Rank)	Score
1. North Dakota	47 (1)	2,632 (3)	310	26. Alabama	458 (30)	3,485 (11)	807
2. West Virginia	166 (5)	2,087 (1)	375	27. Connecticut	402 (25)	4,303 (27)	832
3. South Dakota	137 (2)	2,504 (2)	387	28. Tennessee	474 (32)	3,692 (15)	843
4. New Hampshire	141 (3)	3,111 (7)	452	29. Delaware	433 (29)	4,528 (30)	886
5. Maine	168 (6)	3,504 (12)	518	30. Missouri	504 (33)	3,863 (22)	890
6. Vermont	148 (4)	3,740 (18)	522	31. Oklahoma	422 (27)	5,003 (38)	922
7. Kentucky	306 (18)	2,642 (4)	570	32. Massachusetts	538 (35)	4,220 (26)	960
8. Mississippi	271 (16)	2,995 (6)	571	33. Georgia	507 (34)	4,603 (34)	967
9. Nebraska	238 (12)	3,457 (9)	584	34. New Jersey	545 (36)	4,550 (32)	1,000
10. Iowa	212 (9)	3,731 (17)	585	35. Washington	425 (28)	6,103 (46)	1,035
11. Wisconsin	207 (7)	3,810 (21)	588	36. South Carolina	631 (41)	4,210 (25)	1,052
12. Pennsylvania	331 (20)	2,706 (5)	602	37. Alaska	582 (39)	5,295 (40)	1,112
12. Idaho	235 (11)	3,673 (14)	602	38. Colorado	471 (31)	6,448 (48)	1,116
14. Wyoming	257 (14)	3,758 (19)	633	39. Texas	550 (37)	6,019 (45)	1,152
15. Montana	209 (8)	4,341 (28)	643	40. Illinois	703 (44)	4,597 (33)	1,163
15. Virginia	295 (17)	3,484 (10)	643	41. Oregon	551 (38)	6,179 (47)	1,169
17. Minnesota	256 (13)	3,878 (23)	644	42. Louisiana	694 (43)	4,869 (36)	1,181
18. Indiana	309 (19)	3,605 (13)	670	43. Arizona	603 (40)	6,514 (49)	1,254
19. Arkansas	348 (22)	3,237 (8)	672	44. Nevada	667 (42)	5,908 (44)	1,258
20. Hawaii	219 (10)	4,981 (37)	717	45. New Mexico	704 (45)	5,782 (43)	1,282
21. Kansas	356 (23)	4,019 (24)	758	46. Maryland	835 (48)	4,538 (31)	1,289
22. Ohio	382 (24)	3,806 (20)	763	47. Michigan	734 (46)	5,632 (41)	1,297
23. Utah	267 (15)	5,050 (39)	772	48. California	765 (47)	5,753 (42)	1,340
24. Rhode Island	347 (21)	4,377 (29)	785	49. New York	930 (49)	4,659 (35)	1,396
25. North Carolina	421 (26)	3,701 (16)	791	50. Florida	941 (50)	6,633 (50)	1,604

Source: FBI, *Crime in the United States*, 1986.

The score is the sum of the violent crime rate and one tenth the property crime rate.

Crime Compared with Other Events in Life

The rates of some violent crimes are higher than those of other harmful life events. For example, the risk of being the victim of violent crime is higher than the risk of being affected by divorce, death from cancer, or injury or death from a fire. Anyone over 15 years old runs a greater risk of being a violent crime victim, with or without injury, than being hurt in a traffic accident. Still, a person is much more likely to die from natural causes than from being a victim of crime.

Event	Annual Rate per 1,000 Adults
Accidental injury, all circumstances	290.000
Accidental injury at home	105.000
Personal theft	**82.000**
Accidental injury at work	68.000
Divorce	23.000
Injury in motor-vehicle accident	23.000
Death, all causes	11.000
Aggravated assault	**9.000**
Death of spouse	9.000
Robbery	**7.000**
Heart disease death	4.000
Cancer death	2.000
Accidental death, all circumstances	0.500
Motor-vehicle accident death	0.300
Pneumonia/influenza death	0.300
Suicide	0.200
Injury from fire	0.100
Murder	**0.100**
Death from fire	0.003

Source: Bureau of Justice Statistics, *Report to the Nation on Crime and Justice*, 1983.

night with lamps that are not so bright as to cause light "tunnels."

Clustered housing units in which residents know their neighbors generally are conducive to watchfulness. In large buildings, if only a few apartments open onto a common landing or hallway, the same sort of neighborly concern is promoted.

Differentiation of Space and Territory. The most dangerous places within large buildings are interior public areas with no definite territorial boundaries. Areas seemingly belonging to no one are, in effect, open to everyone. When places are definitely marked off, an intruder will be more obvious, and owners and neighbors will be alerted to potential danger more quickly.

Access Control. Obviously, the quality of locks, doors, door frames, and windows affects the ease with which your residence can be entered. Yet many builders give little attention to these details. Still less may be given to entrances, a surprising fact when you consider that the design and layout of entrances are crucial elements in security, since they define territory and boundaries to residents, visitors, and intruders.

Entrances and exits to a complex should be limited in number, and entrance routes should pass near activity areas so that those who come and go can be observed by many people. An increasingly popular type of retirement community designed for metropolitan areas high in crime (like many found in Florida, for example) consists of an enclosed complex of either condominium townhouses or cluster homes surrounded by a wall or secure fence and connected by courtyards and terraces. The entrance in these developments is usually a single gate guarded by a watchman who probably has closed-circuit television and elaborate communications systems.

Siting and Clustering. The placement of buildings on the grounds and their relationship to one another affect the ease of access. In complexes where the design allows anyone to wander at will between dwellings or through courtyards, the opportunity for crime increases. When residences are clustered so that entrances face each other and access is limited, strangers are less likely to wander through and are more apt to be questioned if they do. The practice of clustering units together, then, limits access naturally and unobtrusively, while at the same time providing a setting for the casual social contacts between neighbors that promote security.

Despite the obvious feeling of security that walls, fences, guard posts, and television scanners provide for retired persons in a community setting, too heavy a concentration of these precautions should be a warning flag to the potential resident. Security measures piled on top of one another, like excessive numbers of police with attack dogs, are an indicator of unacceptably high crime in the area. If, upon inspecting your "model community," you sense an inordinate preoccupation with security, it's wise to make local inquiries about crime or simply eliminate the community from consideration altogether.

JUST HOW VULNERABLE ARE YOU?

Most older adults' dread of violent crime is out of proportion to the odds of their being victimized. But the consequences of burglary, robbery, and fraud are certainly real enough. It is difficult enough for anyone to return to a ransacked home or bounce back after being robbed on the street, or defrauded of savings. Why shouldn't older adults living on fixed incomes be more fearful when the impact of these crimes is deeper and longer lasting?

Besides common sense defenses that include staying away from dark streets, locking your doors and windows, not talking to strangers, and being alert, aware, and accompanied when going out, here are a few more defenses drawn from various sources, including the Dade County (Miami) Department of Public Safety and the U.S. Department of Justice.

Burglary Defenses

For most households, minimum security (defined by police as preventing entry into a home through any door or window *except* by destructive force) is enough to frustrate intruders. It's usually *after* they've been burglarized, experts note, that people learn additional ways to make their homes secure.

If your home is going to be hit, the chances are greater that it will happen during the day while you are out (even if you're gardening in the backyard) than at night when you're asleep, and that the burglar will be an unemployed young person who lives in or knows the neighborhood, and that the job will be done on the spur of the moment because the home looks empty and easy to enter.

From the viewpoint of the crook, the job's quick rewards also entail the risk of doing time in jail. He may turn back at any of three points:

1. Casing the house. If doors and windows are in plain sight and the sounds are unmistakable that someone is inside, most intruders will turn down the risk and search instead for an easier target.

TACTICS FOR DEFENSE:
- Trim or remove shrubbery near doors and windows to limit an intruder's potential hiding places.
- Leave your air conditioner's fan on when you are away; most burglaries occur in August, and an idle air conditioner is the crook's tip to an empty house.
- If you leave the house during the day, walk out to the sidewalk and turn and wave at the front door.
- Turn on a radio or a television, porch light and yard light, and one or two interior lights (the bathroom is one of the best rooms in which to leave a light on) if you are going out for the evening.

2. Entering the house. Even if the front door is unlocked, an intruder commits a crime once he is inside the house— whether or not anything is stolen. If doors and windows are locked and it looks as if it will take time and energy to break in, he will often go elsewhere.

3. Prowling the house. A burglar inside a target house is a very dangerous person to confront; however, he might still be discouraged if he could not quickly find loot or if he thought the police were on their way.

TACTICS FOR DEFENSE:
- Maintain a secure closet (not a safe) with an outward-opening door for storing furs, cameras, guns, silverware, and jewelry; on the door, install a one-inch deadbolt lock. Place an annunciator alarm on the inside. If the door is paneled or of hollow-core construction, strengthen it with ¾-inch plywood or galvanized sheet steel backing.
- Install a telephone extension in your bedroom

and add a rim lock with a 1-inch deadbolt to the interior side of the bedroom door (ideally, a "thumb turn" with *no* exterior key); then if you hear an intruder, you can retreat to the bedroom, lock the door, and call the police.

In addition, you should avoid:

- Displaying guns on interior walls that can be seen from the street. Guns are big drawing cards for burglars.
- Hiding door keys in the mailbox, under the doormat, atop the door casing, in a flowerpot, or any "secret" place seasoned burglars search first.
- Keeping a safe in your house. If an intruder finds a safe, he will assume you have something of great value and may come back later and force you to open it.
- Leaving window fans and air conditioners in unlocked windows when you are away from home.
- Entering your home or calling out if you find a window or door forced when you return home. Go to a neighbor and call the police. Wait there until the police come.
- Attaching tags on your key ring that identify you, your car, or your address.

Personal Larceny Defenses

Personal larceny with contact, a police blotter term for purse-snatching and pocket-picking, is the only crime

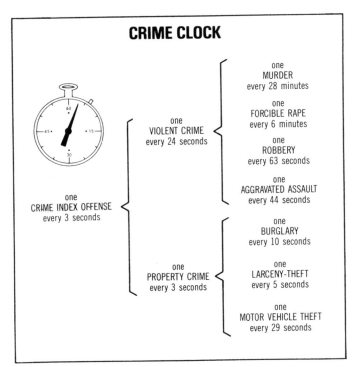

CRIME CLOCK

one
CRIME INDEX OFFENSE
every 3 seconds

one
VIOLENT CRIME
every 24 seconds

one
MURDER
every 28 minutes

one
FORCIBLE RAPE
every 6 minutes

one
ROBBERY
every 63 seconds

one
AGGRAVATED ASSAULT
every 44 seconds

one
PROPERTY CRIME
every 3 seconds

one
BURGLARY
every 10 seconds

one
LARCENY-THEFT
every 5 seconds

one
MOTOR VEHICLE THEFT
every 29 seconds

Source: FBI, *Crime in the United States,* 1986.
Figures are for 1985.

Neighborhood Crime Watches

It is not uncommon to see a crime in progress without recognizing it as such. Here are some situations, drawn from the Justice Department's *Crime Prevention Handbook for* *Senior Citizens*, that might be observed in any neighborhood. These are situations a trained police officer would investigate if he or she were making the observation.

Situations Involving Vehicles

Situations	Possible Significance
Moving vehicles, especially if moving slowly without lights, following an aimless or repetitive course	Casing for a place to rob or burglarize; drug pusher, sex offender, or vandal
Parked, occupied vehicle, especially at an unusual hour	Lookout for burglary in progress (sometimes two people masquerading as lovers)
Vehicle parked in neighbor's drive being loaded with valuables, even if the vehicle looks legitimate, i.e., moving van or commercial van	Burglary or larceny in progress
Abandoned vehicle with or without license plate	Stolen or abandoned after being used in a crime
Persons loitering around parked cars	Burglary of vehicle contents, theft of accessories, vandalism
Persons detaching accessories and mechanical parts	Theft or vandalism
Apparent business transactions from a vehicle near school, park, or quiet residential neighborhood	Drug sales
Persons being forced into vehicle	Kidnapping, rape, robbery
Objects thrown from a moving vehicle	Disposal of contraband

Situations Involving Property

Situations	Possible Significance
Property in homes, garages, or storage areas, especially if several items of the same kind such as TVs and bicycles	Storage of stolen property

Situations Involving Property

Situations	Possible Significance
Property in vehicles, especially meaningful at night or if property is household goods, appliances, unmounted tape decks, stereo equipment	Stolen property, burglary in progress
Property being removed from a house or building; meaningful if residents are at work, on vacation, or are known to be absent	Burglary or larceny in progress
Open doors, broken doors or windows, or other signs of a forced entry	Burglary in progress or the scene of a recent burglary

Situations Involving Persons

Situations	Possible Significance
Door-to-door solicitors— especially significant if one goes to the back of the house and one stays in front. Can be men or women, clean-cut and well dressed	Casing for burglary, burglary in progress, soliciting violation
Waiting in front of a house	Lookout for burglary in progress
Forced entry or entry through window	Burglary, vandalism, theft
Persons short-cutting through yards	Fleeing the scene of a crime
Persons running, especially if carrying items of value	Fleeing the scene of a crime
Person carrying property, especially if property isn't boxed or wrapped	Offender leaving the scene of a burglary, robbery, or larceny
High volume of human traffic in and out of residence	Drug sales, vice activities, "fence" operation

If you see any of these suspicious activities, call the police. Don't hesitate to call because you think the incident is insignificant or that the police will be bothered in responding to your call. Many occurrences could be completely innocent, but this is something for the police to determine. Your name and the information you provide them will be kept confidential.

---

that strikes older adults more frequently than the rest of the population. It is a common way a street crook gets cash in a hurry. The target is the person who looks the easiest to attack, has the most money or valuables to lose, and appears the least likely to give chase.

Purses. If you can do without a purse, do without it. Instead, tuck money and credit cards in an inside pocket. If you must carry a purse, carry it under your arm with its opening facing down; if you're attacked, let the purse's contents fall to the ground, then sit down on the sidewalk before you are knocked down.

Wallets. Never carry a wallet in your back pocket; even an amateur can lift it and escape before you realize what's happening. Carry it in the front pocket of your trousers; pin this pocket closed above the wallet with a safety pin, or wrap a large rubber band around the wallet so that it can't be withdrawn smoothly and can't fall through if your pocket is cut by a razor blade.

In addition, you should avoid:

- Letting strangers stop you for conversation.
- Approaching cars parked on the street with motors running.

- Flashing your jewelry or cash. This is a signal to street thugs, especially if you seem neither strong nor quick. They may follow you to a more convenient spot for a holdup.
- Walking close to building entrances or shrubbery.
- Getting separated from your purse or wallet in a crowded rest room or other public place, or leaving your purse or wallet unattended in a shopping cart, or on a counter.
- Mingling with adolescents leaving school or groups of adolescents anywhere.
- Using shortcuts, alleys, or dark ways, and walking through sparsely traveled areas or near thick trees and shrubs.

TYPICAL FRAUDS

P. T. Barnum is credited with the wise but cynical comment that there is "a sucker born every minute and two [con men] to take advantage of him." He spoke from bitter experience; twice in his lifetime he was the victim of swindlers.

Why do people continue to fall for con games? The answer is that the proposals sound too good to pass up and are presented with urgency by persons who appear to be sincere and honest. The favorite targets of these crooks are older adults who are likely to have liquid assets in their savings accounts.

It's hard to believe that people can still be taken in by the "pigeon drop," a thousand-year-old scam in which the "mark" is expected to ante up some of his or her own money in order to be cut in on an imaginary find of a small fortune. A similar game involves persuading a victim to help bank examiners and the FBI catch an embezzler by withdrawing some of his or her funds and turning them over to the supposed law enforcement officer.

Both of these scams have been exposed time after time, yet victims continue to be bilked out of millions of dollars every year. Consumer and business frauds, too, net billions for their perpetrators. Here are some common examples.

Building Inspector and Contractor Scams

Code violation frauds are perpetrated by crooks working in tandem. One poses as a building inspector who "discovers" serious violations and the need for immediate repairs, for example, to a homeowner's furnace. Shortly afterward the accomplice arrives, pretending to be a repairman who can perform the needed work at low cost. Typically, little or nothing is done to the furnace, but the victim gets a bill for several hundred dollars.

Home improvement swindles are played by con men who usually show up late in the day offering to perform some service such as installing insulation at half price. They claim they have just finished a job in the neighborhood and have material left over, which accounts for the good deal they can pass on to you. You have to make up your mind on the spot and shell out the money immediately. The job probably never gets finished, and the materials used are worth even less than the bargain price you paid.

Work-at-Home Schemes

IDEAS, INVENTIONS, new products needed by innovative manufacturers. Marketing assistance available to individuals, tinkerers, universities, companies. Call free: 1-800-528-6050. Arizona residents: 1-800-352-0458, extension 831.

EARN $200 weekly, part-time taking short phone messages at home. Call 1-615-779-3235 extension 267.

Assemble electronic devices in your home spare time. $300.00–$600.00/week possible. Experience, knowledge, not necessary. No investment. Write for free information. Electronic Development Lab, Drawer 1560-L, Pinellas Park, FL 33565.

Work-at-home schemes are almost exclusively targeted toward older adults who respond to newspaper and magazine advertisements such as the above examples noted in a recent U.S. House of Representatives hearing on mail fraud. The ads promise extra income each month, all yours for addressing envelopes, making wreaths or plaques in your living room, knitting baby bootees, assembling fishing tackle in your basement,

---

RELOCATION RESOURCES

Concerned about personal safety in your prospective retirement haven? The following may help in your relocation decision making.

Finding crime rates in smaller places. This book uses counties to define retirement places. One caveat: just as crime rates are variable from one county to another, so do crime rates vary among towns within a *single* county. Though a retirement place may end up with a crime score that makes it look as dangerous as the rough-cut 19th-century frontier, certain towns within its county boundaries are havens of rectitude and serenity.

Two examples are Phoenix (Maricopa County), Arizona, and Daytona Beach (Volusia County), Florida. With respective rankings of 113 and 117 out of 131 retirement places, these two are among the most crime-ridden in this book. Yet despite these poor rankings, both counties contain suburban towns that contrast sharply with their more dangerous surroundings. Within metropolitan Phoenix, the towns of Avondale, Buckeye, El Mirage, and Paradise Valley are extremely safe. So are Edgewater, Lake Helen, Ponce Inlet, and Port Orange within metropolitan Daytona Beach.

How safe are Phoenix and Daytona Beach? There, as elsewhere, it all depends on where you live within the county. One source that helps you determine the relative safety of hundreds of places is the FBI's annual *Crime in the United States.* It is available in libraries, or for $13 you can order it postpaid from:

Superintendent of Documents
U.S. Government Printing Office
Washington, DC 20402–9325
(202) 783-3238

Sometimes It's Better If Your Check *Isn't* in the Mail

Do you recall the public service TV spot showing the neighborhood thug lamenting how tough it is to make a buck, now that folks don't get their Social Security checks in the mail anymore? Actually, two out of three older adults still do. They may want to reconsider the advantages of direct deposit.

There's one big disadvantage to receiving your benefits in the mail, according to the Treasury Department: because of checks being lost, stolen, or otherwise uncashable, you are seven times more likely to encounter a "nonreceipt" problem than persons who have their money directly deposited in a bank.

Direct deposit gives you quicker access to funds and faster posting to interest-bearing accounts. It certainly saves time, especially if you don't drive. It also saves you money; some banks offer older adults who sign up for direct deposit free 5.25 percent NOW accounts that otherwise would entail a $5 monthly service charge and require a minimum balance of $1,500.

To sign up for direct deposit, all you have to do is fill out a form from the Treasury Department's Financial Management Service and take it to your bank. Better yet, your bank has copies of the form; ask them to send you one.

Commodities Sales

Commodities swindles have become one of the biggest consumer frauds in years. Government investigators estimate these schemes are defrauding the public of as much as $1 billion a year.

The term *commodities* refers to a wide range of investments, from metals and gems to wholesale food products and foreign currencies. Although most investment firms are reputable, there are a growing number of illegitimate firms who illegally sell off-exchange investments to the unwary. Because commodities issues are complex, even highly educated persons are taken in. Indeed, convicted swindlers have testified in recent congressional hearings that the preferred customer is a retired physician, engineer, college professor, or military officer. Moreover, according to these crooks, the best parts of the country to "mine" are the Midwest and Far West because, they allege, people there are less cynical.

Commodities investments are perfect vehicles for swindlers, since the payment of profits to investors can often be deferred for six months to a year, leaving plenty of time for the operators to skip town before the investors suspect a scam. Moreover, since commodities are by nature very complicated and risky investments, many investors are never sure whether they've been had or not.

There are two basic ways to invest in commodities. The first is to pay the full price and take immediate possession of the items. The second is to buy on margin, which involves putting up a percentage of the total purchase price with the balance being due on a future date.

A commodities scheme typically involves a "boiler room" operation, which is a room full of telephones in which 10 to 100 salespeople make calls to persons who responded to newspaper advertising. The salespersons are paid by commission, and high-pressure sales are the name of the game. In many cases, a sale is consummated on the telephone. If the person called doesn't agree to purchase anything in the initial call, he or she will be inundated with literature and harassed until a sale is made. The salesperson usually requires the deposit to be wired from the investor's bank, leaving no time for second thoughts.

growing earthworms, watching television, or raising house plants at home. U.S. Postal Service investigators, who have been looking into these scams for years, say that they haven't encountered one legitimate work-at-home offer that requires payment from the person who responds to the advertisement.

That's the key to work-at-home scams. A fee is required in order for the person to get in on the opportunity. The promoter claims that the money is for a start-up kit or for other expenses. The promise is that the promoter will buy back the finished product or that he will arrange for it to be purchased by others in the marketplace. Unfortunately, the promoter seldom if ever buys back the products, and the consumer is not only robbed of his or her initial cash outlay but is also stuck with a large quantity of products for which there is no market.

Services:

Health Care, Public Transportation, and Continuing Education

INTRODUCTION: Services

"Why do people move to rural parts?" a government specialist wondered in the late 1970s when rapid population growth was dramatically changing the countryside. "Do they do it because they're unaware some of these places don't provide much in the way of services, or because there aren't any services that they will have to pay taxes for?"

The level of services, that aspect of urban living most taken for granted until one relocates, is one thing that improves with population size. (Up to a point, experts will argue; above one-half million residents, some say, local services start crumbling.) It certainly takes in a lot of line items on local budgets: public health, schools, parks, public transit, roads, safety, water and sewerage, trash pickup, energy, and even telecommunications.

From the many possible services that you might expect of any retirement destination, let's look at three: health care, public transportation, and continuing education.

HEALTH CARE

For many older adults, health care quality plays the biggest part in their decision whether to stay in familiar territory or move to a distant place. And why shouldn't it? In later life, visits to the doctor become more frequent; short-term hospital stays are a distinct possibility; and as each year passes, doctor fees and prescriptions take a bigger chunk from the household budget.

Retirement Places Rated doesn't attempt to judge the relative quality of health care in 131 retirement places. From Albuquerque to Yuma, this book simply looks at their local supply of physicians and hospitals. True enough, these two parts of the health care system are found in greater abundance in larger retirement places. This doesn't mean that quality health care in a small Ozark clinic is a contradiction. Nor does it mean that poor health care won't be encountered in a huge university medical center in the big city. The quality of medical care most people receive depends on many things, including their own ability to pay for it, the luck of the draw, professional incompetence, and human error.

Physicians and Their Specialties

Not every physician is listed in the Yellow Pages. Some are hospital administrators, medical school professors, journalists, lawyers, or researchers for pharmaceutical companies. Others work for the federal government's Public Health Service, Veteran's Administration, or Department of Defense service branches. Still others

are in residency training or are full-time members of hospital staffs. When it comes to the number of physicians per capita, what really counts are the number of doctors who maintain offices and see patients.

Where doctors end up practicing is partly determined by sentiment, their perceptions of local quality of life, or both. But mainly it's a matter of economics. The physician has invested three to seven years in graduate medical education and frequently has to start out with a monstrous loan to repay.

Some begin work on a hospital staff, develop a practice, get loose from the hospital, and open an office. Others are taken into someone else's practice as a partner or as one of a group of physicians. Still others buy practices from doctors who are preparing to retire. By whatever means they launch themselves professionally, for new M.D.s who wish to specialize, the primary concern is a place's population size.

Depending on how they spend their professional hours, the American Medical Association classifies office-based physicians into four groups.

General practitioners use all accepted methods of medical care. They treat diseases and injuries, provide preventive care, do routine checkups, prescribe drugs, and do some surgery. They also refer patients to medical specialists.

General Practitioners in the Retirement Places

	General Practitioners
Clear Lake, CA	20
Deming, NM	7
Fredericksburg, TX	9
Grass Valley–Truckee, CA	29
Hanover, NH	31
Kalispell, MT	28
North Conway–White Mountains, NH	13
Oscoda–Huron Shore, MI	12
Port Angeles–Strait of Juan de Fuca, WA	29

Source: American Medical Association, *Physician Characteristics and Distribution*, 1985, and Woods & Poole Economics, Inc., population forecasts.

Medical Specialists in the Retirement Places

	Medical Specialists
Ann Arbor, MI	219
Chapel Hill, NC	95
Charlottesville, VA	101
Easton–Chesapeake Bay, MD	23
Hanover, NH	66
Iowa City, IA	94
Lexington, KY	232
Madison, WI	238
Missoula, MT	52
Petoskey–Straits of Mackinac, MI	25

Source: American Medical Association, *Physician Characteristics and Distribution*, 1985, and Woods & Poole Economics, Inc., population forecasts.

The AMA's Physician Classifications

The American Medical Association classifies a physician as a general practitioner, medical specialist, surgeon, or other specialist by 35 specialties in which the physician reports spending the largest number of his or her professional hours.

General Practitioners
General Practice
Family Practice

Medical Specialists
Allergy
Cardiovascular Diseases
Dermatology
Gastroenterology
Internal Medicine
Pediatrics
Pediatric Allergy
Pediatric Cardiology
Pulmonary Diseases

Surgical Specialists
General Surgery
Neurological Surgery
Obstetrics and Gynecology
Ophthalmology
Orthopedic Surgery
Otolaryngology
Plastic Surgery
Colon and Rectal Surgery
Thoracic Surgery
Urology

Other Specialists
Aerospace Medicine
Anesthesiology
Child Psychiatry
Diagnostic Radiology
Forensic Pathology
Neurology
Occupational Medicine
Psychiatry
Pathology
Physical Medicine and Rehabilitation
General Preventive Medicine
Public Health
Radiology
Therapeutic Radiology

Source: American Medical Association, *Physician Characteristics and Distribution,* 1986.

Medical specialists focus on specific medical disciplines such as cardiology, allergy, gastroenterology, or dermatology. Medical specialists (and general practitioners) are likely to give attention to surgical and nonsurgical approaches to treatment. If it is decided that surgery is the method of treatment, they refer patients to surgeons.

Surgical specialists operate on a regular basis several times a week. The letters F.A.C.S. (Fellow of the American College of Surgeons) after the surgeon's name indicate that he or she has passed an evaluation of surgical training and skills as well as ethical fitness.

Other specialists concentrate on disciplines as familiar as psychiatry or as exotic as aerospace medicine and forensic medicine.

Accredited Hospitals

The word *health* can also mean its opposite, *illness.* A hospital is not really a health care institution; its business is to take care of sick people. The truly healthy need little health care except for an occasional shot or checkup; the unhealthy need a lot more.

Just as not all M.D.s see patients, not all hospitals handle typical illnesses and emergencies. Many of the 7,150 U.S. hospitals exclusively treat chronic diseases or alcohol and drug addiction, or they may be burn centers, psychiatric hospitals or rehabilitation hospitals. *Retirement Places Rated* counts only general hospitals certified for Medicare participation by the U.S. Department of Health and Human Services and accredited for acute care by the Joint Commission on Accreditation of Hospitals (JCAH).

The number of Medicare-certified and JCAH-accredited acute-care hospitals and their inpatient beds varies among retirement places. Although the number of hospital beds isn't as valuable an indicator as it once was before advances in medicine and pharmacology shortened a hospital stay, it is still valid for gauging relative health care supply. Places with large numbers of beds per capita, for example, are regional medical

Veterans Administration (VA) Hospitals

In addition to hospitals that are both JCAH-accredited and Medicare-certified, 22 retirement places also have a VA hospital.

Albuquerque, NM
Amherst–Northampton, MA
Ann Arbor, MI
Asheville, NC
Biloxi–Gulfport, MS
Boise, ID
Canandaigua, NY
Charleston, SC
Fayetteville, AR
Grand Junction, CO
Iowa City, IA
Kerrville, TX
Lexington, KY
Madison, WI
Miami–Hialeah, FL
Phoenix, AZ
Prescott, AZ
Reno, NV
St. Petersburg–Clearwater, FL
San Antonio, TX
San Diego, CA
Tucson, AZ

Source: Veterans Administration, *Annual Report,* 1986.

centers; other places have just one general hospital.

If an area appeals to you, don't be discouraged by its apparent lack of hospitals. There are usually good facilities a short drive away. Residents of Ocean City–Assateague Island, for example, may have to drive to Washington or Baltimore for specialized care, but there are many good small hospitals on the Eastern Shore that are more than adequate for routine care.

PUBLIC TRANSPORTATION

If it's a toss-up between Cape Cod and Cape May in your mind, in which place can you do without a car? Probably neither one, unless you're very deliberate in finding a neighborhood with a nearby bus stop.

Public transportation is a costly urban service. In spite of rising fares, it operates at a loss nearly everywhere. Moreover, transit routes are mapped so that a limited number of buses can serve the largest number of persons who don't own an automobile (or want the convenience of doing without one) and need a reliable, cheap way to get to work or into town for shopping. Nevertheless, in places where the tab for parking in a downtown lot or garage costs $10, where rush-hour traffic jams approach grid-lock, where distances are long and time always seems short, the options for public transportation in retirement places really count.

Fixed-route systems pick up passengers at predetermined stops on a regular schedule and provide rides within town or commuter rides from outside of town. Except for San Diego's and Miami's rapid rail systems, fixed-route public transit and "the bus" are synonymous in 80 retirement places.

Demand-response systems operate like a taxi service in low-density markets not served by fixed-route transit. Unlike taxis, demand-response minibuses are run by the local government and the waiting times may be excessive.

Special-service carriers are found in larger places (San Diego, for example, has 26; Phoenix has 19, and

---

Rising Hospital Costs

It's bad enough that consumer prices tripled from 1965 to 1984. But the average hospital stay jumped more than *ninefold* (from $316 to $2,995) during the same period.

Last year, the typical bill for a semiprivate hospital room was $226 for one day; prices were generally highest in the West, Midwest, and East, and lowest in the South.

Daily Hospital Room Rates: The States Ranked

State	Daily Room Charge	State	Daily Room Charge
1. Alaska	$345	26. Maryland	$200
2. California	299	26. New Jersey	200
3. Pennsylvania	276	28. Kansas	198
4. Michigan	274	29. Missouri	195
5. Delaware	264	30. Florida	194
6. Illinois	258	31. Indiana	193
7. Hawaii	253	32. Kentucky	188
8. Washington	245	33. Iowa	187
9. New York	241	34. West Virginia	175
10. Massachusetts	240	35. North Dakota	172
11. Ohio	239	36. Virginia	171
12. Oregon	236	37. Texas	170
13. Vermont	234	37. Wisconsin	170
14. Nevada	230	39. Alabama	169
15. Colorado	225	39. South Dakota	169
16. Rhode Island	221	41. Oklahoma	167
17. Connecticut	218	42. Louisiana	166
18. New Mexico	212	43. Nebraska	164
19. Minnesota	211	44. Wyoming	159
20. Maine	210	45. Georgia	155
21. Arizona	209	46. Arkansas	150
22. Montana	208	47. Tennessee	148
22. New Hampshire	208	48. South Carolina	146
24. Idaho	204	49. North Carolina	145
25. Utah	203	50. Mississippi	116

Source: Health Insurance Association of America, *Source Book of Health Insurance Data*, 1986.

Figures are for 1986 cost to a patient for a semiprivate room.

Hospital Inpatient Bed Supply

	Number of Hospitals/Beds
Charlottesville, VA	2/941
Hanover, NH	5/559
Iowa City, IA	2/1,122
Petoskey–Straits of Mackinac, MI	1/260
Rhinelander, WI	2/296
Springfield, MO	3/1,692

For every 100,000 residents, the above retirement places have more than 750 inpatient hospital beds. The retirement places below have fewer than 150.

	Number of Hospitals/Beds
Athens–Cedar Creek Lake, TX	1/77
Branson–Cassville–Table Rock Lake, MO	1/78
Brownsville–Harlingen, TX	3/328
Burnet–Marble Falls–Llano, TX	1/50
Franklin County, TN	1/34
Oak Harbor–Whidbey Island, WA	1/51
Salinas–Seaside–Monterey, CA	4/457

Source: American Hospital Association, *Guide to the Health Care Field,* 1986, and Woods & Poole Economics, Inc., population forecasts.

Hospitals in Deming, New Mexico; Eagle River, Wisconsin; Hamilton–Bitterroot Valley, Montana; and Southport, North Carolina, are Medicare-certified, but not accredited for acute care by the JCAH. There are no hospitals in Canton–Lake Tawakoni, Texas; Friday Harbor–San Juan Islands, Washington; Houghton Lake, Michigan; and Ocean City–Assateague Island, Maryland.

Tucson has 17), but for many small retirement places, special-service carriers are the only kind of public transit rolling. This isn't truly *public* transit, though—like fixed-route and demand-response systems—special-service carriers get some of their money from the federal government. Operated by nonprofit organizations like the Red Cross, the American Cancer Society, or the American Association of Retired Persons, their market is a specific group such as older adults or the handicapped.

CONTINUING EDUCATION

When most of us look back over our lives, we see a passage from school in youth, through work during the middle years, to retirement.

Education–work–leisure are commonly called the "linear life plan," and many persons question whether it is the best plan for the future, given people's lengthening life spans. Retirement, frankly, can be a period of boredom and anxiety for some persons who miss the world of work. For others, it would be an empty time indeed if there weren't opportunities for learning new things.

A generation ago, few educational opportunities were available for older adults because the classroom was perceived as the exclusive province of the young. Today, many public and private colleges and universities reduce tuition fees or waive them entirely for older

adults who wish to finish their college degree, or earn a college degree, or just study for the sheer joy of learning.

Of the 131 retirement places featured in this book, 106 have at least one college. The U.S. Department of Education classifies higher education institutions into one of four basic types.

Two-year colleges include junior colleges, community colleges, and technical institutes that offer at least one year of college-level courses leading to an associate degree or are creditable toward a bachelor's degree at a four-year college.

Four-year colleges offer undergraduate courses leading to a bachelor of arts or bachelor of science degree and either award fewer than 30 masters degrees a year or aren't engaged in graduate education at all.

Comprehensive colleges and universities have diverse undergraduate and graduate courses (including professional programs in dentistry, law, medicine, and theology) but either award fewer than 30 doctoral degrees a year or aren't engaged in doctoral-level education at all.

Doctoral-level universities offer undergraduate and graduate courses, but they also grant at least 30 Ph.Ds a year in at least 3 program areas.

Medical Schools: A Major Health Care Asset

Medical schools are associated with local teaching hospitals where state-of-the-art techniques, equipment, and therapy are used, and where one can receive care supervised by medical school faculty. Of the 127 medical schools in the United States, just 15 are in the retirement places profiled in this book.

Albuquerque, NM—University of New Mexico School of Medicine
Ann Arbor, MI—University of Michigan Medical School
Burlington, VT—University of Vermont College of Medicine
Chapel Hill, NC—University of North Carolina School of Medicine
Charleston, SC—Medical University of South Carolina
Charlottesville, VA—University of Virginia School of Medicine
Hanover, NH—Dartmouth Medical School
Iowa City, IA—University of Iowa College of Medicine
Lexington, KY—University of Kentucky College of Medicine
Madison, WI—University of Wisconsin Medical School
Miami–Hialeah, FL—University of Miami School of Medicine
Reno, NV—University of Nevada School of Medicine
San Antonio, TX—University of Texas Medical School
San Diego, CA—University of California School of Medicine
Tucson, AZ—University of Arizona College of Medicine

Source: Association of American Medical Colleges, 1987.

SCORING: Services

That services are in greater supply in bigger places than they are in smaller ones is simply common sense. This doesn't mean health care needs, public transit options, and continuing-education opportunities will be satisfied only in places the scale of a Miami–Hialeah, a Phoenix, or a San Diego.

Ultimately, ranking retirement places by available services can't be done to everyone's satisfaction. "Services" fills a laundry list of everything from trash pickup and street repair to fire protection and gypsy moth spraying. If you agree that health care, public transit, and the chance to take a college course or finish a degree is as good a set of services as any other, then you won't always be disappointed by smaller places, particularly college areas with a medical school.

In spotlighting these selected services, *Retirement Places Rated* doesn't criticize the quality of local hospitals, the credentials of local physicians, the breadth of local college course offerings, or the current state of repair of the local bus fleet. We simply indicate the presence or absence of certain services that many older adults agree enhance retirement living.

Each place starts with a base score of zero; points are added according to the following criteria.

Health Care

Points are awarded on the basis of how accessible physicians and hospitals are to residents within each place. Per capita access to these items is rated AA, A, B, or C (AA indicating the best access and C the least), and the retirement place is awarded points accordingly: 400 points for an AA rating, 300 points for A, 200 points for B, and 100 points for C.

1. *General practitioners.*

A retirement place gets a rating of:	If there is one general practitioner for every:
AA	3,200 or fewer people
A	4,500 to 3,201 people
B	5,700 to 4,501 people
C	5,701 or more people

2. *Medical specialists.*

A retirement place gets a rating of:	If there is one medical specialist for every:
AA	2,500 or fewer people
A	3,600 to 2,501 people
B	6,000 to 3,601 people
C	6,001 or more people

3. *Surgical specialists.*

A retirement place gets a rating of:	If there is one surgeon for every:
AA	2,200 or fewer people
A	2,900 to 2,201 people
B	4,000 to 2,901 people
C	4,001 or more people

4. *Other specialists.*

A retirement place gets a rating of:	If there is one specialist for every:
AA	2,900 or fewer people
A	3,800 to 2,901 people
B	7,000 to 3,801 people
C	7,001 or more people

5. *Accredited hospital beds.* Accredited hospitals are defined here as institutions certified for acute care by the Joint Committee on Accreditation of Hospitals and for Medicare participation by the U.S. Department of Human Services.

A retirement place gets a rating of:	If for every 100,000 persons, there are:
AA	430 or more beds
A	300 to 429 beds
B	230 to 299 beds
C	229 or fewer beds in local accredited hospitals.

Public Transportation: Buses, Rapid Rail Cars, and Demand-Response Vehicles

Based on federal Urban Mass Transportation Administration averages for the annual distance a typical bus travels over a fixed route (41,161 miles), a minibus travels in demand-response service (28,738 miles), and a rapid rail car travels over its track (55,328 miles), the total annual fleet mileage in each retirement place is divided by the population and then multiplied by 100.

For example, the Pioneer Valley Transportation Authority's 12 buses in Amherst–Northampton log a total of 493,932 miles in scheduled service in a year's time. This works out to 3.53 miles for each person, good for 353 points.

Continuing Education

While local colleges and universities with open admissions policies and tuition waivers for older adults are special assets, all nonprofit, privately run or public-run institutions that have undergraduate programs contribute points. The percent of the retirement place's population enrolled in these colleges and universities is multiplied by 100 and added to the score.

The enrollment at San Antonio's seven colleges and universities, for example, is 3.88 percent of the three-county area's population, good for 388 points. Tucson's two colleges enroll 51,189 students, or 8.12 percent of its population, good for 812 points.

SCORING EXAMPLES

A college area in Big Ten Country and a small Texas

Interior retirement place illustrate the scoring method for services.

Iowa City, Iowa (#1)

This retirement place on the eastern Iowa prairie is a regional medical center in every sense of the term. A large medical school, two large hospitals, and an abundance of office-based physicians earn Iowa City the maximum 2,000 points in health care facilities. Iowa City also has an established system of public transit, including buses and demand-response mini-buses in town and buses in suburban Coralville. By *Retirement Places Rated*'s measurement for supply, this service is good for 1,568 points. And finally, with a student population of 30,798, Iowa City is a preeminent college area. The total score for Iowa City is 7,124, which places it comfortably in the leading slot, over 700 points ahead of runner-up Chapel Hill.

Canton–Lake Tawakoni, Texas (#131)

This small East Texas retirement place has no public transportation, no local colleges, and no hospital. Its resident physicians include four general practitioners and one medical specialist, good for 200 points. This marks the extent of the services for which Canton–Lake Tawakoni can receive points.

This doesn't mean that Canton and surrounding Van Zandt County aren't good places to live. It does mean that residents will need a car for getting around, and that most health care and continuing-education services must be obtained elsewhere. Fortunately, this retirement place is within commuting distance of Dallas on the west and Tyler on the east via Interstate 20. People who opt for Canton–Lake Tawakoni are attracted for other reasons, mainly its extremely low cost of living and its high degree of personal safety.

RANKINGS: Services

Four criteria are used to derive the score for a retirement place's supply of selected services: (1) physicians, (2) accredited Medicare hospitals, (3) public transportation, and (4) colleges and universities. Places that receive tie scores are given the same rank and listed alphabetically.

Retirement Places from First to Last

Rank	Score	Rank	Score	Rank	Score
1. Iowa City, IA	7,124	27. Flagstaff, AZ	2,954	52. Keene, NH	2,180
2. Chapel Hill, NC	6,371	28. Bellingham, WA	2,887	53. Coeur d'Alene, ID	2,161
3. Athens, GA	5,775	29. Albuquerque, NM	2,862	54. Daytona Beach, FL	2,153
4. Blacksburg, VA	5,682	30. Charleston, SC	2,838	55. Melbourne–Titusville–	
5. Madison, WI	5,204			Palm Bay, FL	2,127
		31. Murray–Kentucky Lake, KY	2,776		
6. State College, PA	4,749	32. San Luis Obispo, CA	2,761	56. Bennington, VT	2,099
7. Ann Arbor, MI	4,606	33. Phoenix, AZ	2,707	56. Salinas–Seaside–Monterey,	
8. Hanover, NH	4,292	34. Fort Collins–Loveland, CO	2,669	CA	2,099
9. Charlottesville, VA	4,275	35. Asheville, NC	2,642	58. Rhinelander, WI	2,058
10. Bloomington–		36. Hot Springs–Lake Ouachita,		59. Sarasota, FL	2,054
Brown County, IN	4,130	AR	2,607	60. Camden–Penobscot Bay, ME	2,052
11. Amherst–Northampton, MA	4,117	37. Medford–Ashland, OR	2,555	61. Carson City–Minden, NV	2,048
12. Missoula, MT	4,056	38. Santa Rosa–Petaluma, CA	2,502	62. Gainesville–Lake Lanier, GA	2,013
13. Miami–Hialeah, FL	3,915	39. Olympia, WA	2,477	63. Brunswick–Golden Isles, GA	2,008
14. San Diego, CA	3,747	40. Las Cruces, NM	2,464	64. New Paltz–Ulster County, NY	2,004
15. Reno, NV	3,744			65. Virginia Beach–Norfolk, VA	2,000
		41. Redding, CA	2,426		
16. Port Angeles–Strait of		42. Boise, ID	2,411	66. Santa Fe, NM	1,972
Juan de Fuca, WA	3,743	43. Petoskey–Straits of		67. Orlando, FL	1,934
17. Burlington, VT	3,486	Mackinac, MI	2,396	68. Colorado Springs, CO	1,931
18. Tucson, AZ	3,413	44. Grand Junction, CO	2,376	69. Kauai, HI	1,853
19. Austin, TX	3,350	45. Cape Cod, MA	2,374	70. Bar Harbor–Frenchman Bay,	
20. Springfield, MO	3,347			ME	1,838
		46. Bradenton, FL	2,370		
21. Chico–Paradise, CA	3,249	47. Twain Harte–Yosemite, CA	2,308	71. West Palm Beach–	
22. Fayetteville, AR	3,245	48. Bend, OR	2,284	Boca Raton–	
23. Lexington, KY	3,215	49. St. Petersburg–Clearwater,		Delray Beach, FL	1,836
24. Eugene–Springfield, OR	3,103	FL	2,267	72. Lancaster, PA	1,822
25. San Antonio, TX	3,038	50. Fort Lauderdale–Hollywood–		73. Lakeland–Winter Haven, FL	1,820
		Pompano Beach, FL	2,257	74. Canandaigua, NY	1,803
26. Traverse City–Grand Traverse				75. Grand Lake–Lake Tenkiller,	
Bay, MI	3,037	51. Cape May, NJ	2,198	OK	1,748

Rank	Score		Rank	Score		Rank	Score
76. Laconia–			96. Newport–Lincoln City, OR	1,412		115. Yuma, AZ	1,055
Lake Winnipesaukee, NH	1,747		97. Houghton Lake, MI	1,411			
77. Fort Myers–Cape Coral, FL	1,729		98. Hendersonville–Brevard, NC	1,391		116. Franklin County, TN	1,051
78. Las Vegas, NV	1,721		99. Portsmouth–Dover–Durham,			117. Clayton–Clarkesville, GA	1,001
79. Winchester, VA	1,708		NH	1,382		118. Door County, WI	1,000
80. Easton–Chesapeake Bay,			100. Mountain Home–Bull Shoals,			119. Fairhope–	
MD	1,700		AR	1,373		Gulf Shores, AL	985
						120. Ocala, FL	964
81. Myrtle Beach, SC	1,667		101. Panama City, FL	1,359			
82. Grass Valley–Truckee, CA	1,644		102. Litchfield County, CT	1,342		121. Burnet–Marble Falls–	
83. Kalispell, MT	1,635		103. Crossville, TN	1,300		Llano, TX	800
84. Kerrville, TX	1,626		103. Naples, FL	1,300		121. Paris–Big Sandy, TN	800
85. Columbia County, NY	1,598		105. Monticello–Liberty, NY	1,257		121. Red Bluff–Sacramento	
						Valley, CA	800
86. Hilton Head–Beaufort, SC	1,597		106. Lake Havasu City–Kingman,			124. Branson–Cassville–	
87. Biloxi–Gulfport, MS	1,584		AZ	1,223		Table Rock Lake, MO	772
88. St. George–Zion, UT	1,513		107. McAllen–Edinburg–Mission,			125. Friday Harbor–San Juan	
89. Roswell, NM	1,478		TX	1,208		Islands, WA	700
90. Rehoboth Bay–Indian River			108. Oscoda–Huron Shore, MI	1,194			
Bay, DE	1,465		109. Ocean County, NJ	1,189		125. Oak Harbor–Whidbey Island,	
			110. Clear Lake, CA	1,156		WA	700
91. Brownsville–Harlingen, TX	1,433					127. Eagle River, WI	600
91. Ocean City–			111. Fredericksburg, TX	1,100		128. Southport, NC	598
Assateague Island, MD	1,433		111. Front Royal, VA	1,100		129. Deming, NM	500
93. Maui, HI	1,422		111. North Conway–			130. Hamilton–Bitterroot Valley,	
93. Prescott, AZ	1,422		White Mountains, NH	1,100		MT	400
95. Athens–Cedar Creek Lake, TX	1,417		114. Fort Walton Beach, FL	1,067		131. Canton–Lake Tawakoni, TX	200

Retirement Places Listed Alphabetically

Retirement Place	Rank		Retirement Place	Rank		Retirement Place	Rank
Albuquerque, NM	29		Coeur d'Alene, ID	53		Kauai, HI	69
Amherst–Northampton, MA	11		Colorado Springs, CO	68		Keene, NH	52
Ann Arbor, MI	7					Kerrville, TX	84
Asheville, NC	35		Columbia County, NY	85		Laconia–	
Athens, GA	3		Crossville, TN	103		Lake Winnipesaukee, NH	76
			Daytona Beach, FL	54			
Athens–Cedar Creek Lake, TX	95		Deming, NM	129		Lake Havasu City–Kingman, AZ	106
Austin, TX	19		Door County, WI	118		Lakeland–Winter Haven, FL	73
Bar Harbor–Frenchman Bay, ME	70					Lancaster, PA	72
Bellingham, WA	28		Eagle River, WI	127		Las Cruces, NM	40
Bend, OR	48		Easton–Chesapeake Bay, MD	80		Las Vegas, NV	78
			Eugene–Springfield, OR	24			
Bennington, VT	56		Fairhope–Gulf Shores, AL	119		Lexington, KY	23
Biloxi–Gulfport, MS	87		Fayetteville, AR	22		Litchfield County, CT	102
Blacksburg, VA	4					Madison, WI	5
Bloomington–			Flagstaff, AZ	27		Maui, HI	93
Brown County, IN	10		Fort Collins–Loveland, CO	34		McAllen–Edinburg–Mission, TX	107
Boise, ID	42		Fort Lauderdale–Hollywood–				
			Pompano Beach, FL	50		Medford–Ashland, OR	37
Bradenton, FL	46		Fort Myers–Cape Coral, Fl	77		Melbourne–Titusville–	
Branson–Cassville–			Fort Walton Beach, FL	114		Palm Bay, FL	55
Table Rock Lake, MO	124					Miami–Hialeah, FL	13
Brownsville–Harlingen, TX	91		Franklin County, TN	116		Missoula, MT	12
Brunswick–Golden Isles, GA	63		Fredericksburg, TX	111		Monticello–Liberty, NY	105
Burlington, VT	17		Friday Harbor–San Juan				
			Islands, WA	125		Mountain Home–Bull Shoals, AR	100
Burnet–Marble Falls–			Front Royal, VA	111		Murray–Kentucky Lake, KY	31
Llano, TX	121		Gainesville–Lake Lanier, GA	62		Myrtle Beach, SC	81
Camden–Penobscot Bay, ME	60					Naples, FL	103
Canandaigua, NY	74		Grand Junction, CO	44		New Paltz–Ulster County, NY	64
Canton–Lake Tawakoni, TX	131		Grand Lake–Lake Tenkiller, OK	75			
Cape Cod, MA	45		Grass Valley–Truckee, CA	82		Newport–Lincoln City, OR	96
			Hamilton–Bitterroot Valley, MT	130		North Conway–	
Cape May, NJ	51		Hanover, NH	8		White Mountains, NH	111
Carson City–Minden, NV	61					Oak Harbor–Whidbey Island, WA	125
Chapel Hill, NC	2		Hendersonville–Brevard, NC	98		Ocala, FL	120
Charleston, SC	30		Hilton Head–Beaufort, SC	86		Ocean City–	
Charlottesville, VA	9		Hot Springs–Lake Ouachita, AR	36		Assateague Island, MD	91
			Houghton Lake, MI	97			
Chico–Paradise, CA	21		Iowa City, IA	1		Ocean County, NJ	109
Clayton–Clarkesville, GA	117					Olympia, WA	39
Clear Lake, CA	110		Kalispell, MT	83		Orlando, FL	67

Retirement Place	Rank	Retirement Place	Rank	Retirement Place	Rank
Oscoda–Huron Shore, MI	108	Reno, NV	15	Southport, NC	128
Panama City, FL	101	Rhinelander, WI	58	Springfield, MO	20
Paris–Big Sandy, TN	121	Roswell, NM	89	State College, PA	6
Petoskey–Straits of Mackinac, MI	43	St. George–Zion, UT	88		
Phoenix, AZ	33	St. Petersburg–Clearwater, FL	49	Traverse City–Grand Traverse Bay, MI	26
Port Angeles–Strait of Juan de Fuca, WA	16			Tucson, AZ	18
		Salinas–Seaside–Monterey, CA	56	Twain Harte–Yosemite, CA	47
Portsmouth–Dover–Durham, NH	99	San Antonio, TX	25	Virginia Beach–Norfolk, VA	65
Prescott, AZ	93	San Diego, CA	14		
Red Bluff–Sacramento Valley, CA	121	San Luis Obispo, CA	32	West Palm Beach–Boca Raton–Delray Beach, FL	71
Redding, CA	41	Santa Fe, NM	66		
Rehoboth Bay–Indian River Bay, DE	90	Santa Rosa–Petaluma, CA	38	Winchester, VA	79
		Sarasota, FL	59	Yuma, AZ	115

PLACE PROFILES: Services

The following pages show the supply of health care, public transportation, and college-level continuing-education facilities in each of the 131 retirement places.

Health Care, the first heading in each profile, details how many office-based physicians practice there according to the American Medical Association's basic classifications of general practice, surgery, medical specialties, and other specialties. The number of local hospitals accredited by the Joint Commission on Accreditation of Hospitals (JCAH) and certified for Medicare participation by the U.S. Department of Human Services is also included, as are their total number of inpatient beds. Each item's access rating is shown in the right-hand column. (AA indicates the best access and C the worst.) Because VA hospitals do not participate in the Medicare system, and because only military veterans may be patients, they aren't counted when determining a place's access rating.

The second heading, Public Transportation, gives the name of the transit agency that regularly operates over a fixed route or has a fleet of vehicles in demand-response service. Also included is the number of nonprofit special-service carriers, such as a county Senior Center or the American Red Cross, which operate vans and minibuses irregularly.

Continuing Education, the last category, shows the types and enrollment size of local private and public colleges and universities.

The sources for the information are the American Association of Retired Persons, *Tuition Policies in Higher Education for Older Adults*, 1985, and *State Legislative and Administrative Tuition Policies Affecting Older Adults in Higher Education*, 1985; American Hospital Association, *Guide to the Health Care Field*, 1986; American Medical Association, *Physician Characteristics and Distribution in the U.S.*, 1985; U.S. Department of Education, *Education Directory, Colleges and Universities, 1985–86*, 1986; U.S. Department of Transportation, *A Directory of Rural and Specialized Transit Operators*, 1986, and *A Directory of Urban Public Transportation Service*, 1986.

A star preceding a retirement place's name highlights it as one of the top 15 places for services.

Albuquerque, NM

Rating

Health Care (1,500 points)
Office-based physicians
General practitioners: 70	C
Medical specialists: 238	AA
Surgical specialists: 252	AA
Other specialists: 238	AA
Accredited hospitals: 6 (1,411 beds)	B
VA Medical Center	

Public Transportation (801 points)
Fixed route: Suntran (89 buses)
Demand response: Suntran (8 minibuses)
Special service: 7
Continuing Education (561 points)
4 year: University of Albuquerque (1,181, private)
Doctoral: University of New Mexico (26,079, public)

Score: 2,862
Rank: 29

★ Amherst–Northampton, MA

Rating

Health Care (1,300 points)
Office-based physicians
General practitioners: 43	A
Medical specialists: 52	A
Surgical specialists: 34	C
Other specialists: 75	AA
Accredited hospitals: 3 (339 beds)	B
VA Medical Center	

Public Transportation (353 points)
Fixed route: Pioneer Valley TA (12 buses)
Special service: 6
Continuing Education (2,464 points)
4 year:
    Amherst College (1,543, private)
    Hampshire College (1,049, private)
    Mount Holyoke College (1,966, private)
    Smith College (2,752, private)

Rating

Doctoral: University of Massachusetts (27,162, public)
Score: 4,117
Rank: 11

★ Ann Arbor, MI
Health Care (1,700 points)
Office-based physicians
General practitioners: 58 — B
Medical specialists: 219 — AA
Surgical specialists: 192 — AA
Other specialists: 273 — AA
Accredited hospitals: 4 (924 beds) — A
VA Medical Center
Public Transportation (605 points)
Fixed route: Ann Arbor TA (40 buses)
Special service: 5
Continuing Education (2,301 points)
2 year: Washtenaw Community College (7,858, public)
4 year:
Cleary College (969, private)
Concordia College (487, private)
Comprehensive: Eastern Michigan University (18,802, public)
Doctoral: University of Michigan (34,467, public)
Score: 4,606
Rank: 7

Asheville, NC
Health Care (1,900 points)
Office-based physicians
General practitioners: 48 — A
Medical specialists: 86 — AA
Surgical specialists: 101 — AA
Other specialists: 71 — AA
Accredited hospitals: 4 (889 beds) — AA
VA Medical Center
Public Transportation (392 points)
Fixed route: Asheville TA (16 buses)
Special service: 4
Continuing Education (350 points)
2 year:
Asheville-Buncombe Technical College (2,406, public)
Montreat-Anderson College (366, private)
4 year:
University of North Carolina (2,651, public)
Warren Wilson College (463, private)
Score: 2,642
Rank: 35

★ Athens, GA
Health Care (1,900 points)
Office-based physicians
General practitioners: 18 — A
Medical specialists: 37 — AA
Surgical specialists: 56 — AA
Other specialists: 33 — AA
Accredited hospitals: 2 (477 beds) — AA
Public Transportation (590 points)
Fixed route: Athens Transit (11 buses)
Special service: 1
Continuing Education (3,285 points)
Doctoral: University of Georgia (25,230, public)
Score: 5,775
Rank: 3

Athens–Cedar Creek Lake, TX
Health Care (700 points)
Office-based physicians
General practitioners: 14 — A
Medical specialists: 1 — C
Surgical specialists: 3 — C
Other specialists: 2 — C

Rating

Accredited hospitals: 1 (77 beds) — C
Continuing Education (717 points)
2 year: Henderson County Junior College (3,795, public)
Score: 1,417
Rank: 95

Austin, TX
Health Care (1,400 points)
Office-based physicians
General practitioners: 133 — B
Medical specialists: 220 — A
Surgical specialists: 261 — A
Other specialists: 196 — A
Accredited hospitals: 9 (2,576 beds) — A
Public Transportation (700 points)
Fixed route: Capital Metro TA (112 buses)
Demand response: Capital Metro TA (13 minibuses)
Special service: 8
Continuing Education (1,250 points)
2 year: Austin Community College (17,807, public)
4 year:
Huston-Tillotson College (587, private)
St. Edward's University (2,356, private)
Southwestern University (1,001, private)
Comprehensive: SW Texas State University (19,222, public)
Doctoral: University of Texas (47,973, public)
Score: 3,350
Rank: 19

Bar Harbor–Frenchman Bay, ME
Health Care (1,400 points)
Office-based physicians
General practitioners: 14 — A
Medical specialists: 8 — B
Surgical specialists: 16 — A
Other specialists: 12 — A
Accredited hospitals: 3 (156 beds) — A
Public Transportation (274 points)
Fixed route: Downeast Transportation (3 buses)
Special service: 1
Continuing Education (164 points)
4 year:
College of the Atlantic (117, private)
Maine Maritime Academy (621, public)
Score: 1,838
Rank: 70

Bellingham, WA
Health Care (1,300 points)
Office-based physicians
General practitioners: 36 — A
Medical specialists: 35 — A
Surgical specialists: 46 — A
Other specialists: 38 — A
Accredited hospitals: 2 (225 beds) — C
Public Transportation (635 points)
Fixed route: Whatcom TA (18 buses)
Special service: 2
Continuing Education (952 points)
2 year: Whatcom Community College (1,963, public)
Comprehensive: Western Washington University (9,144, public)
Score: 2,887
Rank: 28

Bend, OR
Health Care (1,800 points)
Office-based physicians
General practitioners: 25 — AA
Medical specialists: 20 — A
Surgical specialists: 36 — AA

Other specialists: 25   AA
Accredited hospitals: 2 (231 beds)   A
Public Transportation (233 points)
Fixed route: City of Bend Transit (4 buses)
Special service: 3
Continuing Education (251 points)
2 year: Central Oregon Community College (1,769, public)

Score: 2,284
Rank: 48

Bennington, VT
Health Care (1,800 points)
Office-based physicians
General practitioners: 14   AA
Medical specialists: 15   AA
Surgical specialists: 16   A
Other specialists: 11   A
Accredited hospitals: 1 (160 beds)   AA
Public Transportation
Special service: 2
Continuing Education (299 points)
4 year:
    Bennington College (584, private)
    Southern Vermont College (482, private)

Score: 2,099
Rank: 56

Biloxi–Gulfport, MS
Health Care (1,300 points)
Office-based physicians
General practitioners: 36   B
Medical specialists: 48   B
Surgical specialists: 72   A
Other specialists: 47   B
Accredited hospitals: 6 (879 beds)   AA
    VA Medical Center
Public Transportation (284 points)
Fixed route: Mississippi Coast TA (12 buses)
Demand response: Mississippi Coast TA (3 minibuses)
Special service: 2

Score: 1,584
Rank: 87

★ Blacksburg, VA
Health Care (900 points)
Office-based physicians
General practitioners: 23   AA
Medical specialists: 12   B
Surgical specialists: 15   C
Other specialists: 6   C
Accredited hospitals: 1 (146 beds)   C
Public Transportation (1,505 points)
Fixed route: Blacksburg Transit (26 buses)
Continuing Education (3,277 points)
Doctoral: Virginia Polytechnic Institute (23,303, public)

Score: 5,682
Rank: 4

★ Bloomington–Brown County, IN
Health Care (1,100 points)
Office-based physicians
General practitioners: 28   A
Medical specialists: 29   B
Surgical specialists: 31   B
Other specialists: 38   A
Accredited hospitals: 1 (257 beds)   C
Public Transportation (308 points)
Fixed route: Bloomington Transit (9 buses)
Special service: 1

Continuing Education (2,722 points)
Doctoral: Indiana University (32,715, public)

Score: 4,130
Rank: 10

Boise, ID
Health Care (1,400 points)
Office-based physicians
General practitioners: 39   B
Medical specialists: 57   A
Surgical specialists: 93   AA
Other specialists: 50   B
Accredited hospitals: 3 (615 beds)   A
    VA Medical Center
Public Transportation (423 points)
Fixed route: Boise Urban Stages (19 buses)
Demand response: Boise Urban Stages (2 minibuses)
Special service: 4
Continuing Education (588 points)
4 year: Boise Bible College (80, private)
Comprehensive: Boise State University (11,584, public)

Score: 2,411
Rank: 42

Bradenton, FL
Health Care (1,600 points)
Office-based physicians
General practitioners: 46   A
Medical specialists: 59   A
Surgical specialists: 70   A
Other specialists: 50   A
Accredited hospitals: 2 (895 beds)   AA
Public Transportation (432 points)
Fixed route: Manatee County Transit (11 buses)
Demand response: Manatee County Transit (11 minibuses)
Continuing Education (338 points)
2 year: Manatee Junior College (6,025, public)

Score: 2,370
Rank: 46

Branson–Cassville–Table Rock Lake, MO
Health Care (600 points)
Office-based physicians
General practitioners: 13   B
Medical specialists: 5   C
Surgical specialists: 8   C
Other specialists: 2   C
Accredited hospitals: 1 (78 beds)   C
Public Transportation
Special service: 1
Continuing Education (172 points)
4 year: School of the Ozarks (1,222, private)

Score: 772
Rank: 124

Brownsville–Harlingen, TX
Health Care (600 points)
Office-based physicians
General practitioners: 35   C
Medical specialists: 55   B
Surgical specialists: 62   C
Other specialists: 33   C
Accredited hospitals: 3 (328 beds)   C
Public Transportation (554 points)
Fixed route:
    Brownsville Urban System (15 buses)
    Valley Transit (20 buses)
Special service: 1

Continuing Education (279 points)
2 year:
   Texas Southmost College (4,886, public)
   Texas State Technical Institute (2,359, public)
Score: 1,433
Rank: 91

Brunswick–Golden Isles, GA

Health Care (1,800 points)
Office-based physicians

	Rating
General practitioners: 13	B
Medical specialists: 24	AA
Surgical specialists: 32	AA
Other specialists: 31	AA
Accredited hospitals: 1 (340 beds)	AA

Public Transportation
Special service: 1
Continuing Education (208 points)
2 year: Brunswick Junior College (1,243, public)
Score: 2,008
Rank: 63

Burlington, VT

Health Care (1,600 points)
Office-based physicians

	Rating
General practitioners: 21	C
Medical specialists: 83	AA
Surgical specialists: 73	AA
Other specialists: 85	AA
Accredited hospitals: 2 (553 beds)	A

Public Transportation (725 points)
Fixed route: Chittenden County TA (24 buses)
Special service: 3
Continuing Education (1,161 points)
2 year: Champlain College (1,801, private)
4 year:
   Burlington College (167, private)
   Trinity College (945, private)
Comprehensive: St. Michael's College (2,009, private)
Doctoral: University of Vermont (10,908, public)
Score: 3,486
Rank: 17

Burnet–Marble Falls–Llano, TX

Health Care (800 points)
Office-based physicians

	Rating
General practitioners: 14	AA
Medical specialists: 5	C
Surgical specialists: 4	C
Other specialists: 2	C
Accredited hospitals: 1 (50 beds)	C

Public Transportation
Special service: 1
Score: 800
Rank: 121

Camden–Penobscot Bay, ME

Health Care (1,700 points)
Office-based physicians

	Rating
General practitioners: 8	A
Medical specialists: 14	A
Surgical specialists: 19	AA
Other specialists: 15	AA
Accredited hospitals: 1 (106 beds)	A

Public Transportation (352 points)
Fixed route: Coastal Transportation (3 buses)
Special service: 1
Score: 2,052
Rank: 60

Canandaigua, NY

Health Care (1,300 points)
Office-based physicians

	Rating
General practitioners: 14	C
Medical specialists: 39	AA
Surgical specialists: 38	A
Other specialists: 19	B
Accredited hospitals: 3 (391 beds)	A
VA Medical Center	

Public Transportation
Special service: 1
Continuing Education (503 points)
2 year: Community College of the Finger Lakes (2,952, public)
4 year: Hobart–William Smith Colleges (1,829, private)
Score: 1,803
Rank: 74

Canton–Lake Tawakoni, TX

Health Care (200 points)
Office-based physicians

	Rating
General practitioners: 4	C
Medical specialists: 1	C

Score: 200
Rank: 131

Cape Cod, MA

Health Care (1,500 points)
Office-based physicians

	Rating
General practitioners: 38	A
Medical specialists: 68	A
Surgical specialists: 67	A
Other specialists: 59	AA
Accredited hospitals: 3 (414 beds)	B

Public Transportation (578 points)
Fixed route: Cape Cod RTA (24 buses)
Special service: 1
Continuing Education (296 points)
2 year: Cape Cod Community College (4,251, public)
4 year: Massachusetts Maritime Academy (803, public)
Score: 2,374
Rank: 45

Cape May, NJ

Health Care (800 points)
Office-based physicians

	Rating
General practitioners: 17	B
Medical specialists: 11	C
Surgical specialists: 21	C
Other specialists: 22	B
Accredited hospitals: 1 (239 beds)	B

Public Transportation (1,398 points)
Fixed route: Cape May County Transit (30 buses)
Special service: 3
Score: 2,198
Rank: 51

Carson City–Minden, NV

Health Care (1,000 points)
Office-based physicians

	Rating
General practitioners: 23	AA
Medical specialists: 10	C
Surgical specialists: 19	B
Other specialists: 15	B
Accredited hospitals: 1 (97 beds)	C

Public Transportation (527 points)
Fixed route: Tahoe Transit District (8 buses)
Special service: 3
Continuing Education (521 points)
2 year: Western Nevada Community College (3,256, public)
Score: 2,048
Rank: 61

Rating

★ Chapel Hill, NC
Health Care (1,900 points)
Office-based physicians
General practitioners: 26 — A
Medical specialists: 95 — AA
Surgical specialists: 66 — AA
Other specialists: 128 — AA
Accredited hospitals: 1 (576 beds) — AA
Public Transportation (1,945 points)
Fixed route: Chapel Hill Transit (37 buses)
Demand Response: Town of Chapel Hill (5 minibuses)
Continuing Education (2,526 points)
Doctoral: University of North Carolina (21,652, public)

Score: 6,371
Rank: 2

Charleston, SC
Health Care (1,900 points)
Office-based physicians
General practitioners: 70 — A
Medical specialists: 174 — AA
Surgical specialists: 188 — AA
Other specialists: 148 — AA
Accredited hospitals: 6 (1,713 beds) — AA
  VA Medical Center
Public Transportation (449 points)
Fixed route: South Carolina Electric (33 buses)
Special service: 6
Continuing Education (489 points)
2 year: Trident Technical College (4,685, public)
4 year: Baptist College at Charleston (1,649, private)
Comprehensive:
  Citadel Military College (3,048, public)
  College of Charleston (5,395, public)

Score: 2,838
Rank: 30

★ Charlottesville, VA
Health Care (1,800 points)
Office-based physicians
General practitioners: 25 — B
Medical specialists: 101 — AA
Surgical specialists: 90 — AA
Other specialists: 124 — AA
Accredited hospitals: 2 (941 beds) — AA
Public Transportation (812 points)
Fixed route: Charlottesville Transit (10 buses)
Demand response: JAUNT (21 minibuses)
Special service: 1
Continuing Education (1,663 points)
2 year: Piedmont Community College (3,644, public)
Doctoral: University of Virginia (17,143, public)

Score: 4,275
Rank: 9

Chico–Paradise, CA
Health Care (1,700 points)
Office-based physicians
General practitioners: 48 — A
Medical specialists: 58 — A
Surgical specialists: 78 — AA
Other specialists: 65 — AA
Accredited hospitals: 6 (701 beds) — A
Public Transportation (296 points)
Fixed route: Chico Area Transit (5 buses)
Demand response: Chico Clipper (10 minibuses)
Special service: 4
Continuing Education (1,253 points)
2 year: Butte College (6,697, public)
Comprehensive: California State University (14,196,
  public)

Score: 3,249
Rank: 21

Clayton–Clarkesville, GA
Health Care (900 points)
Office-based physicians
General practitioners: 13 — AA
Medical specialists: 8 — B
Surgical specialists: 3 — C
Accredited hospitals: 2 (104 beds) — B
Public Transportation
Special service: 1
Continuing Education (101 points)
4 year: Piedmont College (387, private)

Score: 1,001
Rank: 117

Clear Lake, CA
Health Care (800 points)
Office-based physicians
General practitioners: 20 — AA
Medical specialists: 7 — C
Surgical specialists: 5 — C
Other specialists: 6 — C
Accredited hospitals: 2 (73 beds) — C
Public Transportation (356 points)
Demand response: Clearlake Dial-A-Ride (6 minibuses)
Special service: 2

Score: 1,156
Rank: 110

Coeur d'Alene, ID
Health Care (1,200 points)
Office-based physicians
General practitioners: 21 — A
Medical specialists: 12 — B
Surgical specialists: 26 — A
Other specialists: 11 — B
Accredited hospitals: 1 (168 beds) — B
Public Transportation (640 points)
Fixed route: Panhandle Area Transit (11 buses)
Special service: 3
Continuing Education (321 points)
2 year: North Idaho College (2,274, public)

Score: 2,161
Rank: 53

Colorado Springs, CO
Health Care (1,100 points)
Office-based physicians
General practitioners: 49 — C
Medical specialists: 114 — A
Surgical specialists: 126 — B
Other specialists: 99 — A
Accredited hospitals: 4 (1,086 beds) — B
Public Transportation (469 points)
Fixed route: Colorado Springs Transit (42 buses)
Special service: 4
Continuing Education (362 points)
2 year:
  Nazarene Bible College (433, private)
  Pikes Peak Community College (5,545, public)
4 year: Colorado College (1,923, private)
Comprehensive: University of Colorado (5,445, public)

Score: 1,931
Rank: 68

Columbia County, NY
Health Care (1,100 points)
Office-based physicians
General practitioners: 14 — A
Medical specialists: 20 — A
Surgical specialists: 14 — C
Other specialists: 13 — B
Accredited hospitals: 1 (170 beds) — B

Rating

Public Transportation (273 points)
Fixed route: Hudson Bus System (4 buses)
Continuing Education (225 points)
2 year: Columbia-Greene Community College (1,356,
    public)

Score: 1,598
Rank: 85

Crossville, TN
Health Care (1,300 points)
Office-based physicians
General practitioners: 11   AA
Medical specialists: 5   C
Surgical specialists: 11   A
Other specialists: 3   C
Accredited hospitals: 1 (172 beds)   AA
Public Transportation
Special service: 2

Score: 1,300
Rank: 103

Daytona Beach, FL
Health Care (1,400 points)
Office-based physicians
General practitioners: 70   A
Medical specialists: 65   B
Surgical specialists: 98   B
Other specialists: 80   A
Accredited hospitals: 7 (1,388 beds)   AA
Public Transportation (367 points)
Fixed route: Volusia County TA (25 buses)
Demand response: Volusia County TA (3 minibuses)
Special service: 2
Continuing Education (386 points)
2 year: Daytona Beach Community College (7,271, public)
4 year: Bethune Cookman College (1,708, private)
Comprehensive: Stetson University (2,739, private)

Score: 2,153
Rank: 54

Deming, NM
Health Care (500 points)
Office-based physicians
General practitioners: 7   AA
Medical specialists: 1   C
Public Transportation
Special service: 1

Score: 500
Rank: 129

Door County, WI
Health Care (1,000 points)
Office-based physicians
General practitioners: 11   AA
Medical specialists: 4   C
Surgical specialists: 6   C
Other specialists: 4   B
Accredited hospitals: 1 (71 beds)   B
Public Transportation
Special service: 2

Score: 1,000
Rank: 118

Eagle River, WI
Health Care (600 points)
Office-based physicians
General practitioners: 3   B
Medical specialists: 3   B
Surgical specialists: 4   C
Other specialists: 2   C

Rating

Public Transportation
Special service: 3

Score: 600
Rank: 127

Easton–Chesapeake Bay, MD
Health Care (1,700 points)
Office-based physicians
General practitioners: 5   C
Medical specialists: 23   AA
Surgical specialists: 30   AA
Other specialists: 17   AA
Accredited hospitals: 1 (186 beds)   AA
Public Transportation
Special service: 2

Score: 1,700
Rank: 80

Eugene–Springfield, OR
Health Care (1,300 points)
Office-based physicians
General practitioners: 77   A
Medical specialists: 105   A
Surgical specialists: 107   A
Other specialists: 86   A
Accredited hospitals: 4 (603 beds)   C
Public Transportation (949 points)
Fixed route: Lane County MTD (57 buses)
Demand response: Mobility, Inc. (8 minibuses)
Special service: 1
Continuing Education (854 points)
2 year: Lane Community College (6,944, public)
4 year:
    Eugene Bible College (162, private)
    Northwest Christian College (236, private)
Doctoral: University of Oregon (15,840, public)

Score: 3,103
Rank: 24

Fairhope–Gulf Shores, AL
Health Care (800 points)
Office-based physicians
General practitioners: 17   B
Medical specialists: 11   C
Surgical specialists: 16   C
Other specialists: 17   B
Accredited hospitals: 3 (217 beds)   B
Public Transportation
Special service: 1
Continuing Education (185 points)
2 year: Faulkner State Junior College (1,710, public)

Score: 985
Rank: 119

Fayetteville, AR
Health Care (1,700 points)
Office-based physicians
General practitioners: 38   AA
Medical specialists: 34   A
Surgical specialists: 40   A
Other specialists: 30   A
Accredited hospitals: 3 (508 beds)   AA
    VA Medical Center
Public Transportation (154 points)
Fixed route: Ozark Transit (4 buses)
Special service: 3
Continuing Education (1,391 points)
Doctoral: University of Arkansas (14,882, public)

Score: 3,245
Rank: 22

Rating

Flagstaff, AZ
Health Care (1,000 points)
Office-based physicians
General practitioners: 28 — AA
Medical specialists: 15 — B
Surgical specialists: 19 — C
Other specialists: 21 — B
Accredited hospitals: 2 (135 beds) — C
Public Transportation (609 points)
Fixed route: Coconino Community Services (13 buses)
Special service: 4
Continuing Education (1,345 points)
Comprehensive: Northern Arizona University (11,824, public)

Score: 2,954
Rank: 27

Fort Collins–Loveland, CO
Health Care (1,000 points)
Office-based physicians
General practitioners: 54 — A
Medical specialists: 44 — B
Surgical specialists: 61 — B
Other specialists: 37 — B
Accredited hospitals: 3 (318 beds) — C
Public Transportation (678 points)
Fixed route: Fort Collins Transport (14 buses)
Demand response: Caravan (23 minibuses)
Continuing Education (991 points)
Doctoral: Colorado State University (18,094, public)

Score: 2,669
Rank: 34

Fort Lauderdale–Hollywood–Pompano Beach, FL
Health Care (1,400 points)
Office-based physicians
General practitioners: 209 — C
Medical specialists: 595 — AA
Surgical specialists: 528 — A
Other specialists: 380 — A
Accredited hospitals: 15 (4,639 beds) — A
Public Transportation (639 points)
Fixed route: Broward County MTA (151 buses)
Demand response: Broward Special Services (50 minibuses)
Special service: 8
Continuing Education (218 points)
2 year: Broward Community College (19,500, public)
Comprehensive: Nova University (6,641, private)

Score: 2,257
Rank: 50

Fort Myers–Cape Coral, FL
Health Care (1,300 points)
Office-based physicians
General practitioners: 55 — B
Medical specialists: 85 — A
Surgical specialists: 97 — B
Other specialists: 77 — A
Accredited hospitals: 3 (945 beds) — A
Public Transportation (217 points)
Fixed route: Lee County Transit (15 buses)
Special service: 3
Continuing Education (212 points)
2 year: Edison Community College (6,022, public)

Score: 1,729
Rank: 77

Rating

Fort Walton Beach, FL
Health Care (800 points)
Office-based physicians
General practitioners: 21 — C
Medical specialists: 26 — B
Surgical specialists: 26 — C
Other specialists: 23 — B
Accredited hospitals: 2 (311 beds) — B
Continuing Education (267 points)
2 year: Okaloosa-Walton Junior College (3,592, public)

Score: 1,067
Rank: 114

Franklin County, TN
Health Care (700 points)
Office-based physicians
General practitioners: 7 — B
Medical specialists: 7 — B
Surgical specialists: 8 — C
Other specialists: 4 — C
Accredited hospitals: 1 (34 beds) — C
Public Transportation
Special service: 2
Continuing Education (351 points)
4 year: University of the South (1,158, private)

Score: 1,051
Rank: 116

Fredericksburg, TX
Health Care (1,100 points)
Office-based physicians
General practitioners: 9 — AA
Medical specialists: 3 — B
Surgical specialists: 1 — C
Other specialists: 2 — C
Accredited hospitals: 1 (61 beds) — A
Public Transportation
Special service: 1

Score: 1,100
Rank: 111

Friday Harbor–San Juan Islands, WA
Health Care (700 points)
Office-based physicians
General practitioners: 3 — A
Surgical specialists: 1 — C
Other specialists: 3 — A
Public Transportation
Special service: 1

Score: 700
Rank: 125

Front Royal, VA
Health Care (1,100 points)
Office-based physicians
General practitioners: 5 — B
Medical specialists: 5 — B
Surgical specialists: 7 — B
Other specialists: 3 — C
Accredited hospitals: 1 (111 beds) — AA

Score: 1,100
Rank: 111

Gainesville–Lake Lanier, GA
Health Care (1,600 points)
Office-based physicians
General practitioners: 8 — C
Medical specialists: 33 — AA
Surgical specialists: 44 — AA
Other specialists: 25 — A
Accredited hospitals: 2 (476 beds) — AA

Rating

Public Transportation
Special service: 2
Continuing Education (413 points)
2 year: Gainesville Junior College (1,744, public)
4 year: Brenau College (1,602, private)

Score: 2,013
Rank: 62

Grand Junction, CO

Health Care (1,400 points)
Office-based physicians
General practitioners: 33   AA
Medical specialists: 29   A
Surgical specialists: 38   A
Other specialists: 27   B
Accredited hospitals: 1 (264 beds)   B
  VA Medical Center
Public Transportation (635 points)
Demand response: Mesa County Human Resources (23
  minibuses)
Continuing Education (341 points)
4 year: Mesa College (3,552, public)

Score: 2,376
Rank: 44

Grand Lake–Lake Tenkiller, OK

Health Care (600 points)
Office-based physicians
General practitioners: 13   B
Medical specialists: 7   C
Surgical specialists: 4   C
Other specialists: 5   C
Accredited hospitals: 3 (120 beds)   C
Public Transportation
Special service: 4
Continuing Education (1,148 points)
Comprehensive: Northeastern State University (7,266,
  public)

Score: 1,748
Rank: 75

Grass Valley–Truckee, CA

Health Care (1,300 points)
Office-based physicians
General practitioners: 29   AA
Medical specialists: 16   B
Surgical specialists: 23   B
Other specialists: 23   A
Accredited hospitals: 2 (166 beds)   B
Public Transportation (344 points)
Fixed route: Nevada County TA (6 buses)
Special service: 2

Score: 1,644
Rank: 82

Hamilton–Bitterroot Valley, MT

Health Care (400 points)
Office-based physicians
General practitioners: 5   B
Medical specialists: 4   C
Surgical specialists: 3   C
Public Transportation
Special service: 1

Score: 400
Rank: 130

★ Hanover, NH

Health Care (2,000 points)
Office-based physicians
General practitioners: 31   AA
Medical specialists: 66   AA

Rating

Surgical specialists: 58   AA
Other specialists: 60   AA
Accredited hospitals: 5 (559 beds)   AA
Public Transportation (1,277 points)
Fixed route: Advance Transit (22 buses)
Special service: 4
Continuing Education (1,015 points)
4 year: University of New Hampshire (2,577, public)
Doctoral: Dartmouth College (4,622, private)

Score: 4,292
Rank: 8

Hendersonville–Brevard, NC

Health Care (1,200 points)
Office-based physicians
General practitioners: 23   A
Medical specialists: 24   B
Surgical specialists: 30   B
Other specialists: 17   B
Accredited hospitals: 3 (400 beds)   A
Public Transportation
Special service: 2
Continuing Education (191 points)
2 year:
  Blue Ridge Technical College (1,134, public)
  Brevard College (658, private)

Score: 1,391
Rank: 98

Hilton Head–Beaufort, SC

Health Care (700 points)
Office-based physicians
General practitioners: 12   C
Medical specialists: 18   B
Surgical specialists: 27   B
Other specialists: 11   C
Accredited hospitals: 2 (163 beds)   C
Public Transportation (658 points)
Fixed route: Lowcountry RTA (13 buses)
Special service: 2
Continuing Education (239 points)
2 year:
  Beaufort Technical College (1,187, public)
  University of South Carolina (753, public)

Score: 1,597
Rank: 86

Hot Springs–Lake Ouachita, AR

Health Care (1,800 points)
Office-based physicians
General practitioners: 18   A
Medical specialists: 30   A
Surgical specialists: 39   AA
Other specialists: 27   AA
Accredited hospitals: 3 (484 beds)   AA
Public Transportation (633 points)
Fixed Route: Hot Springs Transit (12 buses)
Special service: 1
Continuing Education (174 points)
2 year: Garland County Community College (1,356,
  public)

Score: 2,607
Rank: 36

Houghton Lake, MI

Health Care (200 points)
Office-based physicians
General practitioners: 3   C
Other specialists: 2   C
Public Transportation (561 points)
Demand response: Roscommon Mini-Bus (4 minibuses)

Rating

Continuing Education (650 points)
2 year: Kirtland Community College (1,333, public)
Score: 1,411
Rank: 97

★ Iowa City, IA

Health Care (2,000 points)
Office-based physicians
General practitioners: 33 — AA
Medical specialists: 94 — AA
Surgical specialists: 116 — AA
Other specialists: 117 — AA
Accredited hospitals: 2 (1,122 beds) — AA
   VA Medical Center
Public Transportation (1,568 points)
Fixed route:
   Coralville Transit (7 buses)
   Iowa City Transit (19 buses)
Demand response: Johnson County SEATS (10
   minibuses)
Continuing Education (3,556 points)
Doctoral: University of Iowa (30,798, public)
Score: 7,124
Rank: 1

Kalispell, MT

Health Care (1,300 points)
Office-based physicians
General practitioners: 28 — AA
Medical specialists: 12 — B
Surgical specialists: 23 — A
Other specialists: 19 — A
Accredited hospitals: 1 (107 beds) — C
Public Transportation
Special service: 3
Continuing Education (335 points)
2 year: Flathead Valley Community College (1,874, public)
Score: 1,635
Rank: 83

Kauai, HI

Health Care (1,600 points)
Office-based physicians
General practitioners: 15 — AA
Medical specialists: 14 — A
Surgical specialists: 17 — A
Other specialists: 18 — AA
Accredited hospitals: 2 (113 beds) — B
Public Transportation
Special service: 3
Continuing Education (253 points)
2 year: Kauai Community College (1,159, public)
Score: 1,853
Rank: 69

Keene, NH

Health Care (1,300 points)
Office-based physicians
General practitioners: 17 — A
Medical specialists: 21 — A
Surgical specialists: 18 — B
Other specialists: 18 — A
Accredited hospitals: 1 (173 beds) — B
Public Transportation
Special service: 2
Continuing Education (880 points)
4 year:
   Franklin Pierce College (2,293, private)
   University of New Hampshire Keene State College
   (3,512, public)
Score: 2,180
Rank: 52

Rating

Kerrville, TX

Health Care (1,500 points)
Office-based physicians
General practitioners: 12 — A
Medical specialists: 14 — A
Surgical specialists: 16 — A
Other specialists: 9 — B
Accredited hospitals: 2 (171 beds) — AA
   VA Medical Center
Public Transportation
Special service: 2
Continuing Education (126 points)
2 year: Schreiner College (489, private)
Score: 1,626
Rank: 84

Laconia–Lake Winnipesaukee, NH

Health Care (1,700 points)
Office-based physicians
General practitioners: 10 — B
Medical specialists: 22 — AA
Surgical specialists: 21 — AA
Other specialists: 17 — AA
Accredited hospitals: 1 (157 beds) — A
Public Transportation
Special service: 3
Continuing Education (47 points)
2 year: New Hampshire Vocational Technical College
   (214, public)
Score: 1,747
Rank: 76

Lake Havasu City–Kingman, AZ

Health Care (700 points)
Office-based physicians
General practitioners: 15 — B
Medical specialists: 7 — C
Surgical specialists: 17 — C
Other specialists: 16 — B
Accredited hospitals: 2 (171 beds) — C
Public Transportation (109 points)
Fixed route: Colorado River Transit (2 buses)
Special service: 7
Continuing Education (414 points)
2 year: Mohave Community College (3,121, public)
Score: 1,223
Rank: 106

Lakeland–Winter Haven, FL

Health Care (1,400 points)
Office-based physicians
General practitioners: 65 — B
Medical specialists: 115 — A
Surgical specialists: 130 — A
Other specialists: 98 — A
Accredited hospitals: 5 (1,275 beds) — A
Public Transportation (159 points)
Fixed route: Lakeland Area Mass Transit (11 buses)
Demand response: Lakeland Area Mass Transit (4
   minibuses)
Special service: 4
Continuing Education (261 points)
2 year:
   Polk Community College (4,488, public)
   Webber College (353, private)
4 year:
   Florida Southern College (3,096, private)
   Southeastern College (1,021, private)
   Spurgeon Baptist Bible College (65, private)
   Warner Southern College (335, private)
Score: 1,820
Rank: 73

Rating

Lancaster, PA
Health Care (1,200 points)
Office-based physicians
General practitioners: 143   AA
Medical specialists: 72   B
Surgical specialists: 97   B
Other specialists: 76   B
Accredited hospitals: 4 (1,138 beds)   B
Public Transportation (319 points)
Fixed route: Red Rose TA (30 buses)
Special service: 1
Continuing Education (303 points)
4 year:
   Elizabethtown College (1,788, private)
   Franklin and Marshall College (2,783, private)
   Lancaster Bible College (389, private)
Comprehensive: Millersville University (6,770, public)
Score: 1,822
Rank: 72

Las Cruces, NM
Health Care (1,000 points)
Office-based physicians
General practitioners: 19   B
Medical specialists: 24   B
Surgical specialists: 33   B
Other specialists: 20   B
Accredited hospitals: 1 (286 beds)   B
Public Transportation (189 points)
Demand response: Las Cruces Metro Planning (7 buses)
Special service: 5
Continuing Education (1,275 points)
Doctoral: New Mexico State University (13,540, public)
Score: 2,464
Rank: 40

Las Vegas, NV
Health Care (1,100 points)
Office-based physicians
General practitioners: 104   C
Medical specialists: 146   B
Surgical specialists: 177   B
Other specialists: 158   A
Accredited hospitals: 7 (1,901 beds)   A
Public Transportation (270 points)
Fixed route: Las Vegas Transit System (39 buses)
Special service: 4
Continuing Education (351 points)
2 year: Clark County Community College (9,824, public)
Comprehensive: University of Nevada (10,989, public)
Score: 1,721
Rank: 78

Lexington, KY
Health Care (1,900 points)
Office-based physicians
General practitioners: 81   A
Medical specialists: 232   AA
Surgical specialists: 214   AA
Other specialists: 212   AA
Accredited hospitals: 8 (2,037 beds)   AA
   VA Medical Center
Public Transportation (610 points)
Fixed route: LEXTRAN (43 buses)
Demand response: Red Cross WHEELS (11 minibuses)
Special service: 5
Continuing Education (705 points)
2 year: Midway College (352, private)
4 year:
   Asbury College (1,067, private)
   Georgetown College (1,290, private)
   Transylvania University (787, private)

Rating

Doctoral: University of Kentucky (20,637, public)
Score: 3,215
Rank: 23

Litchfield County, CT
Health Care (1,200 points)
Office-based physicians
General practitioners: 29   B
Medical specialists: 88   AA
Surgical specialists: 54   B
Other specialists: 40   B
Accredited hospitals: 4 (414 beds)   B
Public Transportation
Special service: 5
Continuing Education (142 points)
2 year: NW Connecticut Community College (2,343, public)
Score: 1,342
Rank: 102

★ Madison, WI
Health Care (1,900 points)
Office-based physicians
General practitioners: 92   A
Medical specialists: 238   AA
Surgical specialists: 205   AA
Other specialists: 242   AA
Accredited hospitals: 5 (1,557 beds)   AA
   VA Medical Center
Public Transportation (1,867 points)
Fixed route: Madison Metro (145 buses)
Demand response:
   Independent Living (16 minibuses)
   Metro Plus (6 minibuses)
Special service: 2
Continuing Education (1,437 points)
2 year: Madison Area Technical College (5,930, public)
4 year: Edgewood College (681, private)
Doctoral: University of Wisconsin (44,218, public)
Score: 5,204
Rank: 5

Maui, HI
Health Care (1,200 points)
Office-based physicians
General practitioners: 29   A
Medical specialists: 25   B
Surgical specialists: 37   A
Other specialists: 26   A
Accredited hospitals: 2 (172 beds)   C
Public Transportation
Special service: 2
Continuing Education (222 points)
2 year: Maui Community College (2,087, public)
Score: 1,422
Rank: 93

McAllen–Edinburg–Mission, TX
Health Care (700 points)
Office-based physicians
General practitioners: 66   B
Medical specialists: 35   C
Surgical specialists: 58   C
Other specialists: 48   C
Accredited hospitals: 5 (1,061 beds)   B
Public Transportation (229 points)
Fixed route: Valley Transit (20 buses)
Continuing Education (279 points)
Comprehensive: Pan American University (10,042, public)
Score: 1,208
Rank: 107

Rating

Medford–Ashland, OR
Health Care (1,600 points)
Office-based physicians
General practitioners: 37 — A
Medical specialists: 49 — A
Surgical specialists: 71 — AA
Other specialists: 40 — A
Accredited hospitals: 4 (559 beds) — A
Public Transportation (641 points)
Fixed route: Rogue Valley TD (22 buses)
Special service: 1
Continuing Education (314 points)
Comprehensive: Southern Oregon State College (4,432, public)
Score: 2,555
Rank: 37

Melbourne–Titusville–Palm Bay, FL
Health Care (1,200 points)
Office-based physicians
General practitioners: 59 — B
Medical specialists: 82 — B
Surgical specialists: 101 — B
Other specialists: 90 — A
Accredited hospitals: 4 (1,064 beds) — A
Public Transportation (373 points)
Fixed route: Space Coast Transit (15 buses)
Demand response: Space Coast Transit (20 minibuses)
Special service: 4
Continuing Education (554 points)
2 year: Brevard Community College (10,709, public)
Comprehensive: Florida Institute of Technology (6,997, private)
Score: 2,127
Rank: 55

★ Miami–Hialeah, FL
Health Care (2,000 points)
Office-based physicians
General practitioners: 622 — AA
Medical specialists: 1,101 — AA
Surgical specialists: 1,025 — AA
Other specialists: 898 — AA
Accredited hospitals: 26 (8,516 beds) — AA
    VA Medical Center
Public Transportation (1,499 points)
Fixed route:
    Metro Dade County TA (56 rapid rail)
    Metro Dade County TA (600 buses)
Special service: 20
Continuing Education (416 points)
2 year: Miami-Dade Community College (37,675, public)
4 year:
    Florida Memorial College (1,760, private)
    Miami Christian College (353, private)
Comprehensive:
    Barry University (3,931, private)
    Florida International University (16,116, public)
    St. Thomas University (3,595, private)
Doctoral: University of Miami (13,708, private)
Score: 3,915
Rank: 13

★ Missoula, MT
Health Care (1,900 points)
Office-based physicians
General practitioners: 18 — A
Medical specialists: 52 — AA
Surgical specialists: 53 — AA
Other specialists: 40 — AA
Accredited hospitals: 3 (366 beds) — AA

Rating

Public Transportation (964 points)
Fixed route: Missoula Urban TD (16 buses)
Demand response: Missoula Urban TD (3 minibuses)
Special service: 2
Continuing Education (1,192 points)
Comprehensive: University of Montana (9,213, public)
Score: 4,056
Rank: 12

Monticello–Liberty, NY
Health Care (1,000 points)
Office-based physicians
General practitioners: 9 — C
Medical specialists: 18 — A
Surgical specialists: 13 — C
Other specialists: 12 — B
Accredited hospitals: 1 (275 beds) — A
Public Transportation
Special service: 1
Continuing Education (257 points)
2 year: Sullivan County Community College (1,656, public)
Score: 1,257
Rank: 105

Mountain Home–Bull Shoals, AR
Health Care (1,100 points)
Office-based physicians
General practitioners: 13 — A
Medical specialists: 10 — B
Surgical specialists: 10 — C
Other specialists: 12 — A
Accredited hospitals: 1 (133 beds) — B
Public Transportation (273 points)
Fixed route: NATS (3 buses)
Special service: 2
Score: 1,373
Rank: 100

Murray–Kentucky Lake, KY
Health Care (1,200 points)
Office-based physicians
General practitioners: 11 — B
Medical specialists: 10 — B
Surgical specialists: 15 — B
Other specialists: 9 — B
Accredited hospitals: 2 (258 beds) — AA
Public Transportation (289 points)
Fixed route: Murray-Calloway Transit System (4 buses)
Special service: 3
Continuing Education (1,287 points)
Comprehensive: Murray State University (7,335, public)
Score: 2,776
Rank: 31

Myrtle Beach, SC
Health Care (800 points)
Office-based physicians
General practitioners: 22 — C
Medical specialists: 21 — C
Surgical specialists: 39 — B
Other specialists: 22 — B
Accredited hospitals: 3 (357 beds) — B
Public Transportation (555 points)
Fixed route: Coastal RTA (17 buses)
Special service: 2
Continuing Education (312 points)
2 year: Horry-Georgetown Technical College (1,304, public)
4 year: University of South Carolina (2,627, public)
Score: 1,667
Rank: 81

Rating

Naples, FL
Health Care (1,300 points)
Office-based physicians
General practitioners: 26   B
Medical specialists: 37   A
Surgical specialists: 48   A
Other specialists: 26   B
Accredited hospitals: 1 (400 beds)   A

Score: 1,300
Rank: 103

New Paltz–Ulster County, NY
Health Care (1,300 points)
Office-based physicians
General practitioners: 40   A
Medical specialists: 50   A
Surgical specialists: 49   B
Other specialists: 40   B
Accredited hospitals: 3 (514 beds)   A
Public Transportation (74 points)
Fixed route: Kingston Citibus (3 buses)
Special service: 2
Continuing Education (630 points)
2 year: Ulster County Community College (3,197, public)
Comprehensive: State University of New York (7,344, public)

Score: 2,004
Rank: 64

Newport–Lincoln City, OR
Health Care (1,100 points)
Office-based physicians
General practitioners: 14   AA
Medical specialists: 10   B
Surgical specialists: 7   C
Other specialists: 7   B
Accredited hospitals: 2 (98 beds)   B
Public Transportation (312 points)
Fixed route: Newport Area Transit (3 buses)
Special service: 2

Score: 1,412
Rank: 96

North Conway–White Mountains, NH
Health Care (1,100 points)
Office-based physicians
General practitioners: 13   AA
Medical specialists: 3   C
Surgical specialists: 11   B
Other specialists: 8   B
Accredited hospitals: 2 (96 beds)   B

Score: 1,100
Rank: 111

Oak Harbor–Whidbey Island, WA
Health Care (700 points)
Office-based physicians
General practitioners: 12   A
Medical specialists: 4   C
Surgical specialists: 8   C
Other specialists: 4   C
Accredited hospitals: 1 (51 beds)   C

Score: 700
Rank: 125

Ocala, FL
Health Care (700 points)
Office-based physicians
General practitioners: 22   C
Medical specialists: 33   B
Surgical specialists: 40   C

Rating

Other specialists: 28   B
Accredited hospitals: 2 (414 beds)   C
Public Transportation (126 points)
Demand Response: Marion County Senior Services (8 minibuses)
Special service: 5
Continuing Education (138 points)
2 year: Central Florida Community College (2,522, public)

Score: 964
Rank: 120

Ocean City–Assateague Island, MD
Health Care (600 points)
Office-based physicians
General practitioners: 11   AA
Medical specialists: 1   C
Other specialists: 2   C
Public Transportation (833 points)
Fixed route: Ocean City Bus System (7 buses)
Special service: 3

Score: 1,433
Rank: 91

Ocean County, NJ
Health Care (1,000 points)
Office-based physicians
General practitioners: 36   C
Medical specialists: 108   A
Surgical specialists: 113   B
Other specialists: 53   C
Accredited hospitals: 4 (1,262 beds)   A
Public Transportation
Special service: 7
Continuing Education (189 points)
2 year: Ocean County College (5,612, public)
4 year: Georgian Court College (1,572, private)
Score: 1,189
Rank: 109

Olympia, WA
Health Care (1,100 points)
Office-based physicians
General practitioners: 39   A
Medical specialists: 45   A
Surgical specialists: 45   B
Other specialists: 31   B
Accredited hospitals: 1 (331 beds)   C
Public Transportation (968 points)
Fixed route: Intercity Transit (32 buses)
Demand response: Mobility Services (6 minibuses)
Continuing Education (409 points)
2 year: South Puget Sound Community College (2,959, public)
4 year:
    Evergreen State College (2,826, public)
    St. Martin's College (508, private)

Score: 2,477
Rank: 39

Orlando, FL
Health Care (1,200 points)
Office-based physicians
General practitioners: 140   C
Medical specialists: 260   A
Surgical specialists: 357   A
Other specialists: 229   B
Accredited hospitals: 8 (2,979 beds)   A
Public Transportation (331 points)
Fixed route: Tri-County Transit (69 buses)
Demand response: Orange County Community Affairs (7 minibuses)
Special service: 1

Rating

Continuing Education (403 points)
2 year:
Seminole Community College (5,092, public)
Valencia Community College (11,432, public)
4 year:
Central Florida Bible College (127, private)
Orlando College (906, private)
Comprehensive:
Rollins College (3,648, private)
University of Central Florida (15,822, public)
Score: 1,934
Rank: 67

Oscoda–Huron Shore, MI
Health Care (900 points)
Office-based physicians
General practitioners: 12 — AA
Medical specialists: 3 — C
Surgical specialists: 6 — C
Other specialists: 1 — C
Accredited hospitals: 1 (65 beds) — B
Public Transportation (294 points)
Fixed route: Iosco Transit Corporation (2 buses)
Special service: 1
Score: 1,194
Rank: 108

Panama City, FL
Health Care (1,000 points)
Office-based physicians
General practitioners: 13 — C
Medical specialists: 27 — B
Surgical specialists: 34 — B
Other specialists: 24 — B
Accredited hospitals: 2 (460 beds) — A
Continuing Education (359 points)
2 year: Gulf Coast Community College (3,976, public)
Score: 1,359
Rank: 101

Paris–Big Sandy, TN
Health Care (800 points)
Office-based physicians
General practitioners: 7 — C
Medical specialists: 8 — B
Surgical specialists: 9 — C
Other specialists: 4 — C
Accredited hospitals: 1 (140 beds) — A
Score: 800
Rank: 121

Petoskey–Straits of Mackinac, MI
Health Care (1,700 points)
Office-based physicians
General practitioners: 2 — C
Medical specialists: 25 — AA
Surgical specialists: 29 — AA
Other specialists: 25 — AA
Accredited hospitals: 1 (260 beds) — AA
Continuing Education (696 points)
2 year: North Central Michigan College (1,692, public)
Score: 2,396
Rank: 43

Phoenix, AZ
Health Care (1,300 points)
Office-based physicians
General practitioners: 416 — B
Medical specialists: 654 — A
Surgical specialists: 743 — A
Other specialists: 610 — A

Rating

Accredited hospitals: 21 (5,098 beds) — B
VA Medical Center
Public Transportation (840 points)
Fixed route: Phoenix Transit System (337 buses)
Demand response:
City of Phoenix Aging Services (34 minibuses)
Glendale Dial-A-Ride (12 buses)
Mesa Dial-A-Ride (20 buses)
Special service: 19
Continuing Education (567 points)
2 year:
Glendale Community College (13,002, public)
Maricopa Community College (3,466, public)
Mesa Community College (14,907, public)
Phoenix College (11,836, public)
Rio Salado Community College (12,497, public)
Scottsdale Community College (7,313, public)
South Mountain Community College (1,154, public)
4 year:
American Indian Bible College (75, private)
Arizona College of the Bible (161, private)
Grand Canyon College (1,379, private)
Southwestern Baptist Bible College (147, private)
Doctoral: Arizona State University (40,538, public)
Score: 2,707
Rank: 33

Port Angeles–Strait of Juan de Fuca, WA
Health Care (1,200 points)
Office-based physicians
General practitioners: 29 — AA
Medical specialists: 10 — B
Surgical specialists: 18 — B
Other specialists: 10 — B
Accredited hospitals: 1 (126 beds) — B
Public Transportation (2,085 points)
Fixed route: Clallam Transit (27 buses)
Special service: 1
Continuing Education (458 points)
2 year: Peninsula College (2,441, public)
Score: 3,743
Rank: 16

Portsmouth–Dover–Durham, NH
Health Care (800 points)
Office-based physicians
General practitioners: 42 — C
Medical specialists: 79 — B
Surgical specialists: 86 — B
Other specialists: 79 — B
Accredited hospitals: 5 (541 beds) — C
Public Transportation (177 points)
Fixed route: COAST (14 buses)
Special service: 8
Continuing Education (405 points)
2 year:
Castle Junior College (149, private)
New Hampshire Vocational Technical College (673, public)
White Pines College (63, private)
Doctoral: University of New Hampshire (12,314, public)
Score: 1,382
Rank: 99

Prescott, AZ
Health Care (700 points)
Office-based physicians
General practitioners: 16 — C
Medical specialists: 11 — C
Surgical specialists: 31 — B
Other specialists: 12 — C
Accredited hospitals: 2 (217 beds) — B
VA Medical Center

Rating

Public Transportation (135 points)
Fixed route:
  Prescott-Whipple Stage (1 bus)
  Verde Valley TA (2 buses)
Special service: 4
Continuing Education (587 points)
2 year: Yavapai College (5,203, public)
4 year: Prescott College (187, private)
Score: 1,422
Rank: 93

Red Bluff–Sacramento Valley, CA
Health Care (800 points)
Office-based physicians
General practitioners: 14   A
Medical specialists: 5   C
Surgical specialists: 6   C
Other specialists: 6   C
Accredited hospitals: 2 (108 beds)   B
Public Transportation
Special service: 3
Score: 800
Rank: 121

Redding, CA
Health Care (1,500 points)
Office-based physicians
General practitioners: 45   AA
Medical specialists: 29   B
Surgical specialists: 52   A
Other specialists: 46   A
Accredited hospitals: 4 (454 beds)   A
Public Transportation (301 points)
Fixed route: NorCal Transit (8 buses)
Demand response: R & M Mini-Trans (3 minibuses)
Special service: 3
Continuing Education (625 points)
2 year: Shasta College (8,622, public)
Score: 2,426
Rank: 41

Rehoboth Bay–Indian River Bay, DE
Health Care (1,300 points)
Office-based physicians
General practitioners: 24   B
Medical specialists: 31   A
Surgical specialists: 35   B
Other specialists: 30   A
Accredited hospitals: 3 (430 beds)   A
Public Transportation
Special service: 7
Continuing Education (165 points)
2 year: Delaware Technical and Community (1,808,
  public)
Score: 1,465
Rank: 90

★ Reno, NV
Health Care (1,900 points)
Office-based physicians
General practitioners: 60   A
Medical specialists: 110   AA
Surgical specialists: 139   AA
Other specialists: 113   AA
Accredited hospitals: 5 (1,102 beds)   AA
  VA Medical Center
Public Transportation (1,104 points)
Fixed route: Citifare (31 buses)
Demand response: Elderport Services (46 minibuses)
Special service: 4

Rating

Continuing Education (740 points)
2 year: Truckee Meadows Community College (7,430,
  public)
4 year:
  Old College (155, private)
  Sierra Nevada College (152, private)
Doctoral: University of Nevada (9,681, public)
Score: 3,744
Rank: 15

Rhinelander, WI
Health Care (1,700 points)
Office-based physicians
General practitioners: 7   B
Medical specialists: 17   AA
Surgical specialists: 22   AA
Other specialists: 11   A
Accredited hospitals: 2 (296 beds)   AA
Public Transportation
Special service: 3
Continuing Education (358 points)
2 year: Nicolet College (1,168, public)
Score: 2,058
Rank: 58

Roswell, NM
Health Care (1,200 points)
Office-based physicians
General practitioners: 11   B
Medical specialists: 18   A
Surgical specialists: 19   B
Other specialists: 12   B
Accredited hospitals: 3 (238 beds)   A
Public Transportation
Special service: 1
Continuing Education (278 points)
2 year:
  Eastern New Mexico University (1,285, public)
  New Mexico Military Institute (424, private)
Score: 1,478
Rank: 89

St. George–Zion, UT
Health Care (1,000 points)
Office-based physicians
General practitioners: 12   AA
Medical specialists: 5   C
Surgical specialists: 6   C
Other specialists: 9   B
Accredited hospitals: 1 (106 beds)   B
Public Transportation
Special service: 1
Continuing Education (513 points)
2 year: Dixie College (1,904, public)
Score: 1,513
Rank: 88

St. Petersburg–Clearwater, FL
Health Care (1,500 points)
Office-based physicians
General practitioners: 159   B
Medical specialists: 312   A
Surgical specialists: 335   A
Other specialists: 288   A
Accredited hospitals: 17 (3,980 beds)   AA
  VA Medical Center
Public Transportation (568 points)
Fixed route: Suncoast TA (104 buses)
Demand response: Suncoast TA (21 minibuses)
Special service: 8
Continuing Education (199 points)
2 year: St. Petersburg Junior College (15,865, public)

Rating

4 year:
    Clearwater Christian College (199, private)
    Eckerd College (1,073, private)
Score: 2,267
Rank: 49

Salinas–Seaside–Monterey, CA

Health Care (1,200 points)
Office-based physicians

	Rating
General practitioners: 69	B
Medical specialists: 96	A
Surgical specialists: 122	A
Other specialists: 94	A
Accredited hospitals: 4 (457 beds)	C

Public Transportation (528 points)
Fixed route:
    King City Transit (2 buses)
    Monterey-Salinas Transit (39 buses)
Special service: 2
Continuing Education (371 points)
2 year:
    Hartnell College (6,210, public)
    Monterey Peninsula College (5,656, public)

Score: 2,099
Rank: 56

San Antonio, TX

Health Care (1,400 points)
Office-based physicians

	Rating
General practitioners: 241	B
Medical specialists: 409	A
Surgical specialists: 480	A
Other specialists: 435	A
Accredited hospitals: 15 (4,788 beds)	A
VA Medical Center	

Public Transportation (1,250 points)
Fixed route: VIA Metropolitan Transit (385 buses)
Demand response: VIA Metropolitan Transit (14 minibuses)
Special service: 19
Continuing Education (388 points)
2 year:
    St. Philip's College (6,313, public)
    San Antonio College (22,274, public)
Comprehensive:
    Incarnate Word College (1,350, private)
    Our Lady of the Lake University (1,685, private)
    St. Mary's University (3,305, private)
    Trinity University (2,850, private)
    University of Texas (12,612, public)

Score: 3,038
Rank: 25

★ San Diego, CA

Health Care (1,600 points)
Office-based physicians

	Rating
General practitioners: 565	A
Medical specialists: 922	AA
Surgical specialists: 947	A
Other specialists: 1,001	AA
Accredited hospitals: 30 (5,677 beds)	B
VA Medical Center	

Public Transportation (1,480 points)
Fixed route:
    Chula Vista Transit (9 buses)
    National City Transit (7 buses)
    San Diego County Transit System (537 buses)
    San Diego County Transit System (36 rapid rail)
Demand response:
    Chula Vista Transit (5 minibuses)
    City of El Cajon (15 minibuses)
    City of La Mesa (12 minibuses)
    North County Transit (10 minibuses)

    San Diego County Transit System (225 minibuses)
Special service: 26
Continuing Education (667 points)
2 year:
    Cuyamaca College (2,299, public)
    Grossmont College (13,472, public)
    Mira Costa College (5,274, public)
    Palomar College (15,261, public)
    San Diego City College (11,034, public)
    San Diego Mesa College (17,137, public)
    San Diego Miramar College (3,707, public)
    Southwestern College (10,146, public)
4 year:
    Christian Heritage College (434, private)
    Coleman College (771, private)
    National University (8,735, private)
    Point Loma Nazarene College (1,917, private)
Comprehensive:
    San Diego State University (33,898, public)
    University of San Diego (5,264, private)
Doctoral:
    United States International University (2,539, private)
    University of California (14,295, public)

Score: 3,747
Rank: 14

San Luis Obispo, CA

Health Care (1,400 points)
Office-based physicians

	Rating
General practitioners: 47	A
Medical specialists: 60	A
Surgical specialists: 71	A
Other specialists: 65	A
Accredited hospitals: 5 (565 beds)	B

Public Transportation (272 points)
Fixed route:
    North Coastal Transit (3 buses)
    South County Transit (3 buses)
Demand response:
    City of Atascadero (5 minibuses)
    City of Morro Bay (5 minibuses)
Special service: 1
Continuing Education (1,089 points)
2 year: Cuesta College (5,440, public)
Comprehensive: California Polytechnic University (15,968, public)

Score: 2,761
Rank: 32

Santa Fe, NM

Health Care (1,400 points)
Office-based physicians

	Rating
General practitioners: 21	B
Medical specialists: 43	AA
Surgical specialists: 41	A
Other specialists: 47	AA
Accredited hospitals: 1 (208 beds)	C

Public Transportation (447 points)
Demand response: Santa Fe Human Needs (15 minibuses)
Special service: 1
Continuing Education (125 points)
4 year:
    College of Santa Fe (854, private)
    St. John's College (353, private)

Score: 1,972
Rank: 66

Santa Rosa–Petaluma, CA

Health Care (1,400 points)
Office-based physicians

	Rating
General practitioners: 134	AA
Medical specialists: 124	A

Surgical specialists: 144   Rating **A**
Other specialists: 111   **A**
Accredited hospitals: 7 (724 beds)   **C**
Public Transportation (485 points)
Fixed route:
  Santa Rosa Municipal Transit (13 buses)
  Sonoma County Transit (21 buses)
Demand response:
  Sonoma Care-A-Van (2 minibuses)
  Volunteer Wheels (10 minibuses)
Special service: 6
Continuing Education (617 points)
2 year: Santa Rosa Junior College (16,804, public)
Comprehensive: Sonoma State University (5,364, public)

Score: 2,502
Rank: 38

Sarasota, FL
Health Care (1,800 points)
Office-based physicians
General practitioners: 60   **A**
Medical specialists: 127   **AA**
Surgical specialists: 134   **AA**
Other specialists: 94   **AA**
Accredited hospitals: 3 (1,104 beds)   **A**
Public Transportation (239 points)
Fixed route: Sarasota County Area Transit (15 buses)
Special service: 1
Continuing Education (15 points)
4 year: Ringling School of Art and Design (399, private)

Score: 2,054
Rank: 59

Southport, NC
Health Care (500 points)
Office-based physicians
General practitioners: 10   **B**
Medical specialists: 1   **C**
Surgical specialists: 4   **C**
Other specialists: 3   **C**
Public Transportation
Special service: 1
Continuing Education (98 points)
2 year: Brunswick Technical College (463, public)

Score: 598
Rank: 128

Springfield, MO
Health Care (1,700 points)
Office-based physicians
General practitioners: 31   **C**
Medical specialists: 114   **AA**
Surgical specialists: 128   **AA**
Other specialists: 85   **AA**
Accredited hospitals: 3 (1,692 beds)   **AA**
Public Transportation (576 points)
Fixed route: Springfield City Utilities (24 buses)
Demand response: Springfield City Utilities (6 minibuses)
Special service: 3
Continuing Education (1,071 points)
4 year:
  Baptist Bible College (1,227, private)
  Central Bible College (1,038, private)
  Drury College (2,400, private)
  Evangel College (1,777, private)
Comprehensive: SW Missouri State University (15,121, public)

Score: 3,347
Rank: 20

★ State College, PA
Health Care (1,200 points)
Office-based physicians
General practitioners: 33   **A**
Medical specialists: 26   **B**
Surgical specialists: 32   **B**
Other specialists: 18   **B**
Accredited hospitals: 3 (397 beds)   **A**
Public Transportation (685 points)
Fixed route: Centre Area TA (20 buses)
Continuing Education (2,864 points)
Doctoral: Pennsylvania State University (34,401, public)

Score: 4,749
Rank: 6

Traverse City–Grand Traverse Bay, MI
Health Care (1,800 points)
Office-based physicians
General practitioners: 12   **B**
Medical specialists: 27   **AA**
Surgical specialists: 33   **AA**
Other specialists: 33   **AA**
Accredited hospitals: 1 (286 beds)   **AA**
Public Transportation (694 points)
Fixed route: Bay Area TA (10 buses)
Continuing Education (543 points)
2 year: Northwestern Michigan College (3,222, public)

Score: 3,037
Rank: 26

Tucson, AZ
Health Care (1,600 points)
Office-based physicians
General practitioners: 104   **C**
Medical specialists: 309   **AA**
Surgical specialists: 293   **AA**
Other specialists: 270   **AA**
Accredited hospitals: 9 (1,935 beds)   **A**
  VA Medical Center
Public Transportation (1,001 points)
Fixed route: Tucson MTS (124 buses)
Demand response: Handicar (42 minibuses)
Special service: 17
Continuing Education (812 points)
2 year: Pima Community College (20,882, public)
Doctoral: University of Arizona (30,307, public)

Score: 3,413
Rank: 18

Twain Harte–Yosemite, CA
Health Care (1,500 points)
Office-based physicians
General practitioners: 16   **AA**
Medical specialists: 11   **B**
Surgical specialists: 15   **A**
Other specialists: 13   **A**
Accredited hospitals: 2 (152 beds)   **A**
Public Transportation (193 points)
Fixed route: Tuolumne County Transit (2 buses)
Continuing Education (615 points)
2 year: Columbia College (2,619, public)

Score: 2,308
Rank: 47

Virginia Beach–Norfolk, VA
Health Care (900 points)
Office-based physicians
General practitioners: 115   **C**
Medical specialists: 218   **B**
Surgical specialists: 256   **B**
Other specialists: 225   **B**
Accredited hospitals: 8 (2,296 beds)   **B**

Public Transportation (661 points)
Fixed route: Tidewater TDC (142 buses)
Continuing Education (439 points)
2 year: Tidewater Community College (14,976, public)
4 year: Virginia Wesleyan College (976, private)
Comprehensive:
    Norfolk State University (7,233, public)
    Old Dominion University (15,626, public)

Score: 2,000
Rank: 65

West Palm Beach–Boca Raton–Delray Beach, FL

Health Care (1,300 points)
Office-based physicians

	Rating
General practitioners: 131	C
Medical specialists: 341	AA
Surgical specialists: 349	A
Other specialists: 213	A
Accredited hospitals: 11 (2,350 beds)	B

Public Transportation (238 points)
Fixed route: COTRANS (46 buses)
Special service: 8
Continuing Education (298 points)
2 year:
    College of Boca Raton (823, private)
    Palm Beach Junior College (11,637, public)
4 year: Palm Beach Atlantic College (977, private)
Comprehensive: Florida Atlantic University (10,228, public)

Score: 1,836
Rank: 71

Winchester, VA

Health Care (800 points)
Office-based physicians

	Rating
General practitioners: 6	C
Medical specialists: 10	C
Surgical specialists: 10	C
Other Specialists: 8	C
Accredited hospitals: 1 (415 beds)	AA

Public Transportation (753 points)
Fixed route: Winchester TA (11 buses)
Continuing Education (155 points)
4 year: Shenandoah College (932, private)

Score: 1,708
Rank: 79

Yuma, AZ

Health Care (700 points)
Office-based physicians

	Rating
General practitioners: 23	B
Medical specialists: 16	C
Surgical specialists: 27	B
Other specialists: 13	C
Accredited hospitals: 1 (227 beds)	C

Public Transportation
Special service: 3
Continuing Education (355 points)
2 year: Arizona Western College (3,718, public)

Score: 1,055
Rank: 115

ET CETERA: Services

DRIVER LICENSING

When you settle in a new state, you have to surrender your out-of-state driver's license and get a new one. The time permitted to do this ranges from "immediately" in 13 states, up to 30 days in 14 states, and up to 90 days in 9 other states. New Hampshire and Vermont allow you as much time as your former state gives newcomers. Hawaii lets you keep your license until it expires.

Required Tests

For a new resident with a valid driver's license from a former state, the requirement for getting a license from the new state varies considerably. In Arkansas, all you do is apply and pay the fee. In Connecticut, Massachusetts, and New Hampshire, a vision test is required, but all other tests may be waived. West Virginia requires only a test of the state's rules of the road. Six states require you to get behind the wheel with a license examiner for a road test; in 20 other states, a road test may be waived or required at the discretion of the examiner.

"Problem" Drivers

If your license has been revoked, you won't get a new one simply by moving to another state. Every license application is checked with the National Driver Register, a federal data file of persons whose license to drive has been denied or withdrawn. Moreover, 30 states belong to the National Driver License Compact, an agreement among states to share information on drivers who accumulate tickets in one jurisdiction and try to escape control in another.

Driver Age Discrimination?

Once you start feeling your age, will insurance companies and state highway safety committees consider you dangerous when you get behind the wheel of your automobile?

On the face of it, older drivers have a better accident record than younger drivers; people over 65 represent one in nine persons in this country yet are involved in only 1 in 17 of the automobile accidents. According to the National Safety Council, however, people over 65 drive much less than younger people and actually have a poorer accident record in terms of the miles they drive.

At the 1974 Conference on the Aging Driver, the American Medical Association and the American Association of Motor Vehicle Administrators recommended that no driver's license should be placed in jeopardy just because the licensee is older, but added that "it does make sense for the licensing agency to conduct more frequent reexamination of the senior citizen." Accordingly, six states and Washington, D.C., now require special examinations or reexaminations based solely on age.

ILLINOIS	Complete reexamination every three years for drivers over 69.
INDIANA	Complete reexamination every three years for drivers over 75.
LOUISIANA	Physical examination every four years for drivers over 60.
MAINE	Vision reexamination at age 40, age 52, and 65 and over.
NEW HAMPSHIRE	Complete reexamination for drivers over 75.
OREGON	Vision reexamination at age 50 and over.
WASHINGTON, D.C.	Vision and reaction examination for drivers over 70; complete reexamination at age 75 and over.

DRIVING DANGER SIGNALS

Researching the records of insurance companies and state police agencies, Dr. Leon Pastalan of the University of Michigan found that older drivers receive a high number of tickets for the following five different traffic violations:

- Rear-end collisions
- Dangerously slow driving
- Failure to yield the right-of-way
- Driving the wrong way on one-way streets
- Illegal turns

Even though people age at different rates, normal changes that affect eyesight, muscle reflexes, and hearing are the reasons older adults are ticketed for these moving violations more often than the rest of the population. Simply recognizing your limitations will help you become a better driver.

Eyesight. Ninety percent of all sensory input needed to drive a car comes through the eyes. As vision loses its sharpness, the typical rectangular black-and-white road signs become hard to read. Night driving is especially risky, because the older we get, the more illumination we need. For example, an 80-year-old needs three times the light that a 20-year-old needs to read. Other problems include loss of depth perception (a major cause of rear-end collisions) and limited peripheral vision (dangerous when making turns at intersections).

You can adjust to these dangers by not driving at night, having regular eye checkups, wearing gray or green-tinted sunglasses on days with high sun glare, and replacing your car's standard rearview mirror with a wide-angle one to aid peripheral vision.

Muscle Reflexes. Many people slow down as they get older. Strength may dwindle, neck and shoulder joints may stiffen, and you may tire sooner. Most important to driving, your reflex reactions may slow. All of these symptoms can affect how safely you enter a busy freeway, change lanes to pass a plodding 18-wheel truck, or avoid a rear-end fender bender.

Ask your physician if any of the medication you're taking might decrease your alertness and ability to drive defensively. On long road trips, take along a companion to share the driving and break the day's distance into short stretches to reduce fatigue. Don't get caught on freeways and major arterial streets during morning and evening rush hours.

Hearing. One in every five persons over 55 and one of every three persons over 65 has impaired hearing. It is a gradual condition and can go unnoticed for a long time. When you can't hear the ambulance siren, a ticket for failing to yield the right-of-way to an emergency vehicle is the likely consequence.

You can compensate for hearing loss by having periodic checkups. When you drive, open a window, turn off the radio, keep the air conditioner fan on low speed, and cut unnecessary conversation.

---

55 Alive Driving

There is more to driving than just knowing the rules of the road. Knowing at what temperature an icy road is most slippery, for example, or what the danger spots are in a parking lot and which medications could cause problems for you behind the wheel are nuggets of information for driving defensively.

You can take an eight-hour course to refine your existing skills and review the rules of the road for safer driving. The classroom course is produced by the American Association of Retired Persons (AARP) and conducted throughout the country in two four-hour sessions.

The fee to take the class is $7 in every state except New York. AARP provides the program and materials; thousands of volunteers throughout the country provide the instruction.

If you are 50 or older and want to take the course, write

AARP 55/Mature Driving
1909 K St., NW
Washington, DC 20049

Obtaining a Driver's License After Relocating:
A Guide for Persons with a Current License from Their Former State

State	Time Limit for Obtaining License After Establishing Residence	Rules of the Road	Signs and Signals	Vision	Vehicle Operation	Member of National Driver License Compact
Alabama	30 days	•	•	•		•
Alaska	90 days	•	•	•		
Arizona	Immediately	•	•	•	•	•
Arkansas	Immediately					
California	10 days	•	•	•		•
Colorado	30 days	•	•	•	X	
Connecticut	60 days	X	X	•	X	
Delaware	60 days	•	•	•	X	•
Florida	30 days	•	•	•	•	
Georgia	30 days	•	•	•		
Hawaii	*	•	•	•	•	•
Idaho	90 days	•	•	•		•
Illinois	90 days	•	•	•		•
Indiana	60 days	•	•	•		•
Iowa	Immediately	•	•	•		
Kansas	90 days	•	•	•		•
Kentucky	Immediately	•	•	•		
Louisiana	90 days	•	•	•		•
Maine	30 days	•	•	•	X	
Maryland	30 days	•	•	•	X	
Massachusetts	Immediately	X	X	•		
Michigan	Immediately	•	•	•		
Minnesota	60 days	•	•	•	X	
Mississippi	60 days	•	•	•		•
Missouri	Immediately	•	•	•		•
Montana	90 days	•	•	•	•	•
Nebraska	30 days	•	•	•	X	•
Nevada	45 days	•	•	•	X	•
New Hampshire	Reciprocity	X	X	•	X	•
New Jersey	60 days	•		•	X	•
New Mexico	30 days	•		•		•
New York	30 days	•	•	•		
North Carolina	30 days	•	•	•	X	
North Dakota	60 days	•	•	•	X	•
Ohio	30 days	•	•	•	X	
Oklahoma	Immediately	•	•	•	•	•
Oregon	Immediately	•	•	•	X	•
Pennsylvania	60 days	•	•	•	X	
Rhode Island	30 days	•	•	•		
South Carolina	90 days	•	•	•	X	
South Dakota	90 days	•	•	•		•
Tennessee	90 days	•	•	•	X	•
Texas	30 days	•	•	•	X	
Utah	60 days	•	•	•		•
Vermont	Reciprocity	•	•	•	X	
Virginia	30 days	•	•	•		•
Washington	Immediately	•	•	•	•	•
West Virginia	Immediately	•				•
Wisconsin	Immediately	•	•	•	X	
Wyoming	Immediately	•	•	•	X	

Source: Federal Highway Administration, *Driver's License Administration Requirements and Fees*, 1986.

*In Hawaii, a drivers license from any state is valid until its expiration, if the driver is older than 18 years of age.

• Required

X May be waived at the discretion of the examiner

COLLEGE TUITION BREAKS FOR OLDER ADULTS

Thirty-six states waive or reduce tuition in their public colleges for persons who've reached a specific age. It's the law in 24 of these states; in the other 12, it's a policy adopted by the state's Board of Regents or its Board of Higher Education.

College Tuition Breaks: Waivers for Older Adults

State	Law	Policy	Minimum Age	All State-Supported Institutions
Alabama		•	60	
Arkansas	•		60	•
California		•	60	
Connecticut	•		62	•
Delaware	•		60	•
Florida	•		62	•
Georgia	•		62	•
Hawaii	•		60	•
Idaho		•	60	•
Illinois	•		65	•
Kansas		•	60	•
Kentucky	•		65	•
Louisiana	•		65	•
Maine		•	65	•
Maryland	•		60	•
Massachusetts	•		65	•
Minnesota	•		62	•
Nevada		•	62	•
New Hampshire		•	65	•
New Jersey	•		65	•
New Mexico	•		65	•
New York	•		60	•
North Carolina	•		65	•
North Dakota		•	65	•
Ohio	•		60	•
Oklahoma		•	65	•
Oregon		•	65	•
Rhode Island	•		65	•
South Carolina	•		60	•
South Dakota		•	65	•
Tennessee	•		60, 65	•
Texas	•		65	•
Utah	•		62	•
Virginia	•		60	•
Washington	•		60	•
Wisconsin		•	62	•

Source: American Association of Retired Persons, *State Legislative and Administrative Tuition Policies Affecting Older Adults in Higher Education,* 1985, and Places Rated Partnership survey, 1987.

The limitations on this benefit vary among the states. All of them grant it on a *space-available basis,* which simply means that older students who want to take advantage of the tuition break are admitted to courses only after tuition-paying students have enrolled. Eight states grant the benefit only for *auditing* courses, that is, enrolling for no credit. Four states—

Illinois, Maryland, South Carolina, and Virginia—look at the applicant's income to determine eligibility.

College Tuition Breaks: Waiver Limitations

ALABAMA
Tuition and general student fees are waived for courses in all state-supported 2-year colleges.

ARKANSAS
Tuition and general student fees are waived only for credit courses on a space-available basis.

CALIFORNIA
Tuition and general student fees waived only at participating campuses of the California State University system for credit courses on a space-available basis.

CONNECTICUT
Unless the student has been accepted into a degree-granting program, tuition fees are waived for courses only on a space-available basis.

DELAWARE
Tuition and general student fees are waived for auditing courses, or for taking courses for credit, on a space-available basis; students must be formal degree candidates.

FLORIDA
Tuition fees are waived for courses on a space-available basis.

GEORGIA
Tuition fees are waived only for credit courses on a space-available basis; dental, medical, veterinary, and law school courses are excluded. Regular admission procedures are required.

HAWAII
Tuition and general student fees are waived only for regularly scheduled credit courses on a space-available basis.

IDAHO
A $5 fee per registration is charged for courses on a space-available basis.

ILLINOIS
Tuition fees are waived for regularly scheduled credit courses on a space-available basis for older students whose income is less than the current threshold for property tax relief.

KANSAS
Tuition and general student fees are waived only for auditing courses on a space-available basis.

KENTUCKY
Tuition and general student fees are waived only for regularly scheduled credit courses on a space-available basis.

LOUISIANA
Tuition and other registration fees are waived for courses on a space-available basis.

MAINE

Tuition fees are waived for undergraduate courses on a space-available basis.

MARYLAND

Tuition fees are waived for 2-year college courses on a space-available basis, and up to three university or 4-year college courses per term on a space-available basis for students whose income is derived from retirement benefits and who aren't employed full time.

MASSACHUSETTS

Tuition fees are waived for courses on a space-available basis.

MINNESOTA

Except for an administration fee of $6 a credit hour, collected only when a course is taken for credit, tuition and activity fees are waived to attend courses for credit, to audit any course offered for credit, or enroll in any noncredit adult vocational education courses on a space-available basis.

NEVADA

Tuition fees are waived only for regularly scheduled courses; consent of the instructor may be required.

Establishing Residency for Tuition Benefits

Legal residency is not only important for tax purposes, it's a necessary step to qualify for in-state tuition fees or tuition waivers at local public colleges.

Of the states that offer some form of tuition reduction or waiver, most require proof of at least one year of residency. Here are several steps to take to satisfy that requirement:

- Ask the local county clerk for a certificate of domicile.
- Get a driver's license, and register your car in the new state.
- If you don't drive, ask the driver's license authority for a nondriver identification card. All states now issue them; some are similar to the driver's license format. Delaware, Illinois, and Minnesota will issue an ID card to all persons, not just nondrivers.
- File your final state income tax in your former state; file state and federal income taxes in the new state.
- At first opportunity, register and vote in an election in your new state.

NEW HAMPSHIRE

Tuition fees are waived for auditing Continuing Education Division courses up to a maximum of 8 academic credits per semester, university and college extension courses on a space-available basis, and vocational-technical courses on a space-available basis.

NEW JERSEY

Tuition fees are waived for courses on a space-available basis; students must be formal degree candidates and successfully complete at least 6 academic credits per semester.

NEW MEXICO

Tuition reduced to $5.00 per credit hour up to a maximum of 6 credit hours per semester on a space-available basis.

NEW YORK

Tuition fees are waived only for auditing courses on a space-available basis.

NORTH CAROLINA

Tuition fees are waived for auditing courses or for taking courses for credit on a space-available basis. Regular admission procedures are required.

NORTH DAKOTA

Tuition fees are waived only for auditing courses on a space-available basis.

OHIO

Tuition and matriculation fees are waived only for auditing courses on a space-available basis; approval of course instructor may be required.

OKLAHOMA

Tuition fees are waived only for auditing courses on a space-available basis.

OREGON

Tuition fees waived for courses on a space-available basis.

RHODE ISLAND

Tuition and general student fees are waived for credit courses on a space-available basis at the discretion of the institution.

SOUTH CAROLINA

Tuition fees are waived for courses, for credit or audit, on a space-available basis; students must meet admission standards of the institution, and must not be (or have a spouse who is) employed full-time.

SOUTH DAKOTA

Tuition fees are reduced for courses to an amount equal to one-fourth of resident tuition.

TENNESSEE

Tuition fees are waived for auditing courses on a space-available basis for students 60 and older; tuition fees are waived for enrolling in credit courses on a space-available basis for residents 65 and older.

TEXAS

Tuition fees are waived for auditing courses on a space-available basis.

UTAH

Tuition fees (but not quarterly registration fees) are waived for courses on a space-available basis.

VIRGINIA

Tuition fees are waived only for auditing courses on a space-available basis. If the student has a federal taxable income not exceeding $7,500, tuition fees are waived for courses taken for credit on a space-available basis. Regular admission procedures are required.

WASHINGTON

Depending on the institution, and for no more than two courses per term, tuition and general student fees are waived or reduced for courses taken for credit and waived entirely for courses taken for audit.

WISCONSIN

Tuition fees are waived for auditing courses; instructor's approval required.

ELDERHOSTEL

Need an excuse for traveling to a retirement place for a closer look? Consider enrolling in a week-long program at any of 850 colleges and universities that are part of the Elderhostel network. Many of the course topics—"Santa Fe: The City Different" offered at the College of Santa Fe, or "Arkansas Weather" scheduled at the University of Arkansas in Fayetteville, and "All About Asheville and Western North Carolina" given at the University of North Carolina at Asheville, for example—can orient you quickly to potential retirement destinations.

Admission Requirements: None but age. Hostelers must be at least 60 years old, or married to a participant who is. Companions over 50 years of age may accompany eligible participants.

Course Prerequisites: None but an enthusiastic, challenged intellect. No exams, no homework, no grades. Formal education or previous knowledge of the subject matter is not presumed.

Tuition and Accommodations: $215, all inclusive of registration, six nights double occupancy in a dormitory, all meals from Sunday supper through the following Saturday's breakfast, five days of classes, and extracurricular activities.

Where to Apply: Write Elderhostel (80 Boylston St., Suite 400, Boston, MA 02116) to get on their mailing list. Throughout the year, you'll receive three seasonal course catalogs and three issues of their newsletter.

DON'T PUT OFF YOUR WILL

It's human nature to avoid thinking about the need for a will. Seven out of every ten people die without one, and eight of ten who do have a will fail to keep it up-to-date. If you don't have a will when you die, the state where you live in your retirement years will write one for you according to its own statutes, and the assets you may have worked hard to accumulate will be distributed according to its laws.

Don't put off making a will because of imagined costs. A lawyer can tell you the basic fee in advance; it's usually $50 to $100 for a simple document. And it may save your heirs thousands.

Once you have a will, make a note to yourself in your calendar to review it every year. Births, marriages, deaths, hard feelings, the patching-up of hard feelings, plus changes in your finances, in your health, or in federal or state laws—any of these may affect your will. Regular, periodic review helps ensure that you won't forget to make needed adjustments.

If death and taxes are inevitable—as the old saying goes—so are taxes after death. But it isn't all bad. Since 1981, no estate smaller that $175,625 has been subject to any federal tax. State tax exemptions vary greatly and often change, another reason for keeping the document up-to-date.

Where should you keep your will? Put it in a safe place, but don't hide it behind a painting or under a rug. If you conceal it too well, a court may rule that you don't have one! Your lawyer should have a signed copy, and the original should be in a logical place, such as a safety-deposit box or your desk. Be sure your spouse, a close relative, or a friend knows where both the copies and the original are.

Finding the Right Lawyer

When you move from one state to another, you enter a new legal environment. Even if your will is legal in your new state (and it may not be), it might not do the best possible job. So when you resettle, see a lawyer in your new area to make certain your will is one your state will recognize. Some states, for example, require that the executor of a will be a resident of the state where the deceased lived. For a legal checkup, you might have to contact a family lawyer.

The law is a competitive field. In the past, lawyers and clients usually found each other in the Rotary Club, at a church supper, or on the golf course. Since 1977, when the Supreme Court struck down laws barring the legal profession from advertising, many lawyers have gotten quite adept at promoting themselves. Just look up "Lawyers" in a telephone book's Yellow Pages, and you'll be surprised by the techniques many firms borrow from consumer goods advertising. Specialists for 24-hour divorces, personal bankruptcy, workers' compensation, and personal injury claims abound. Somewhere hidden among the listings is a professional who can advise you. How do you find him or her?

- *Satisfied clients.* If a friend or neighbor has used a lawyer's services, ask what sort of matter the lawyer handled. Some lawyers, especially in large cities, specialize in a certain branch of law and aren't interested in taking on cases outside their specialty. They aren't family lawyers.

- *Lawyers referral service.* Most state bar associations have a referral service with a toll-free telephone number. Typically, the name you are given is an attorney who practices where you live, specializes in your legal problem, and is next up in the association's data base to be referred. You can have a first interview with him or her for a stated—and very modest—fee. In that interview, you can find out whether you'll need further legal services and, if so, you can decide whether you want to continue with the lawyer to whom you were referred. You will be under no obligation to do so if you do not want to.

- *Local bar association.* If the referral service lists no lawyer in your area, try the local bar association. If you don't find it in the telephone book, inquire for the president's name at the county courthouse. You can then ask him or her for the name of a good lawyer. Be sure to make it clear that you are asking, in their capacity as president of the local association, for the name of a reliable attorney who can perform the kind of service you are seeking.

Don't talk about your legal problems to strangers. (Lawyer referral services and presidents of bar associations are professional exceptions to this rule.) People who don't know you personally aren't likely to have your best interest at heart. Be particularly wary of any recommendation that is made without your asking for it.

FINDING THE RIGHT DOCTOR

Chances are good that you'll have to choose a new physician at some point; even if you don't move after retirement, your doctor might. Finding a replacement for the person in whom you've put so much trust isn't always easy.

Give some thought to the kind of doctor you are most comfortable with. Do you want to place complete faith in your physician? Or do you have questions about your treatment? Do you like a cooperative arrangement, in which you and your doctor work as a team? It's very important to most people that they have a doctor who will listen to their complaints, worries, and concerns, rather than one who may make patients feel that they're questioning the doctor's authority.

If you're planning to move, you might ask your present doctor if he or she knows anything about the doctors in the area where you are going. Or you can get names from the nearest hospital at the new location, from friends you make, from medical societies, and from new neighbors.

When you have decided whom you want to contact, call that doctor's office, saying that you are a prospective patient, and ask to speak to the doctor briefly. You may have to agree to call back, but making connection with a professional voice is an important step. If you can't arrange this, if the doctor is "too busy," you probably ought to go to the next name on your list. You need a physician who is readily accessible.

When you do make contact, tell the doctor enough about yourself so that he or she has a good idea of who you are and what your problems may be. If the doctor sounds "right" to you, you could ask about fees, house calls (yes, they are again being made when necessary),

---

RELOCATION RESOURCES

Surveying retirement places for whether they have the kind of medical care you'll need doesn't necessarily mean a long period of letter writing to chambers of commerce or county medical boards. A library's reference section has several sources to help you with this task.

Finding specialized hospital services. The best source is the American Hospital Association's annual *Guide to the Health Care Field.* Organized by state and by city, the guide provides a variety of information about every hospital in the United States, including address and telephone number, control (public, private, investor owned, federal, city, state), length of stay (short term, long term), and which ones are certified for Medicare participation and accredited by the Joint Commission on Accreditation of Hospitals.

More importantly, the guide indicates which of 54 specialized facilities are available in each hospital. Cardiac intensive care, volunteer services, physical therapy, hemodialysis, podiatric service, psychiatric outpatient service, blood bank, home care, and health promotion, for example, are several important facilities not obtainable everywhere.

Verifying medical credentials. It is up to the states to license and regulate professions. Kentucky licenses watchmakers and auctioneers but not psychologists; Maine certifies tree surgeons and movie projectionists but not occupational therapists; Arkansas licenses insect exterminators but not opticians. Fortunately, physicians and dentists must be certified before they can practice in any state.

Quacks practice everywhere, however, because impressive-looking credentials aren't difficult to obtain. One California firm, recently shut down by the postal service, furnished a medical degree—complete with transcript, diploma, and letters of recommendation—to anyone for $28,000. For $5, another firm mailed out "Outstanding Service" citations. Experts testifying in a recent House of Representatives hearing estimated that 1 of 50 "doctors" are doing a thriving business with fraudulent credentials, and that 3 out of 5 of their patients are over 65.

Check the dentist's background in the *American Dental Directory.* Check the doctor's background in the *Directory of Medical Specialists.* Both sources are updated each year, are organized by state and by city. What to look for: medical or dental school attended, year graduated (you're not looking for a health care professional who is about to retire), specializations, and board certifications.

and emergencies. Or you may wish to save some of these questions for a personal visit. It is important to establish through the initial phone call or visit that you and the doctor will be at ease with each other.

Evaluate the doctor's attitude. If he or she doesn't want to bother with you now, you will probably get that don't-bother-me treatment sooner or later when dealing with specific problems. Make sure that

- You can openly discuss your feelings and personal concerns about sexual and emotional problems.
- The doctor isn't vague, impatient, or unwilling to answer all your questions about the causes and treatment of your physical problems.
- The doctor takes a thorough history on you and asks about past physical and emotional problems, family medical history, medication you are taking, and other matters affecting your health.

- The doctor doesn't always attribute your problems to getting older, and that he or she doesn't automatically prescribe drugs rather than deal with real causes of your medical problems.
- The doctor has an associate to whom you can turn should your doctor retire or die.

Talk with the doctor about the transfer of your medical records. Some doctors like to have them, especially if there is any specific medical problem or chronic condition. Other doctors prefer not to see them, and to develop new records.

Even if you feel fine, arrange to have a physical or at least a quick checkup. This is more for the doctor's benefit than for yours, but it will help you, too. Should an emergency occur, the doctor will have basic information about you and some knowledge of your needs, and you will avoid the stress of trying to work with a doctor who has to learn about you in an emergency.

FOR RETIRED MILITARY

Forty of the retirement places profiled in this book have at least one base or post where your military ID card gives you the privileges of exchange and commissary shopping.

Albuquerque, NM
Kirtland Air Force Base

Athens, GA
Athens Naval Supply Corps School

Austin, TX
Bergstrom Air Force Base
Camp Mabry

Biloxi–Gulfport, MS
Gulfport Naval Construction Battalion Center
Keesler Air Force Base

Boise, ID
Gowen Field

Burlington, VT
Ethan Allen Firing Range
Camp Johnson

Cape Cod, MA
Coast Guard Air Station Cape Cod*

Cape May, NJ
Coast Guard Training Center Cape May*

Charleston, SC
Charleston Air Force Base
Charleston Naval Base
Coast Guard Base Charleston*

Charlottesville, VA
Judge Advocate General School

Colorado Springs, CA
Fort Carson
Peterson Air Force Base
U.S. Air Force Academy

Flagstaff, AZ
Navajo Army Depot

Fort Walton Beach, FL
Eglin Air Force Base
Hurlburt Field

Hilton Head–Beaufort, SC
Parris Island Marine Corps Recruiting Depot

Kauai, HI
Naval Missile Range Facility

Las Cruces, NM
White Sands Missile Range

Las Vegas, NV
Indian Springs Air Force Auxiliary Field
Nellis Air Force Base

Lexington, KY
Bluegrass Army Depot

Madison, WI
Truax Field

Melbourne–Titusville–Palm Bay, FL
Cape Canaveral Air Force Station
Patrick Air Force Base

Miami–Hialeah, FL
Coast Guard Air Station Miami*
Coast Guard Base Miami*
Homestead Air Force Base

Myrtle Beach, SC
Myrtle Beach Air Force Base

Oak Harbor–Whidbey Island, WA
Whidbey Island Naval Air Station

Ocean County, NJ
Lakehurst Naval Air Engineering Center

Orlando, FL
Orlando Naval Training Center

Oscoda–Huron Shore, MI
Wurtsmith Air Force Base

Panama City, FL
Panama City Naval Coastal System Center*
Tyndall Air Force Base

Phoenix, AZ
Gila Bend Air Force Auxiliary Field
Luke Air Force Base
Williams Air Force Base

Port Angeles–Strait of Juan de Fuca, WA
Coast Guard Air Station Port Angeles*

Portsmouth–Dover–Durham, NH
Pease Air Force Base
Portsmouth Naval Shipyard

St. Petersburg–Clearwater, FL
Coast Guard Air Station Clearwater*
Coast Guard Station St. Petersburg*

Salinas–Seaside–Monterey, CA
Fort Hunter Liggett*
Fort Ord
Monterey Naval Postgraduate School*
Presidio of Monterey*

San Antonio, TX
Brooks Air Force Base
Fort Sam Houston
Kelly Air Force Base
Lackland Air Force Base
Randolph Air Force Base

San Diego, CA
Camp Pendleton
Coast Guard Air Station San Diego*
Coronado Naval Amphibious Base*
Miramar Naval Air Station
North Island Naval Air Station
San Diego Marine Corps Recruiting Depot*
San Diego Naval Regional Medical Center*
San Diego Naval Station
San Diego Naval Training Center

San Luis Obispo, CA
Camp San Luis Obispo

Santa Rosa–Petaluma, CA
Coast Guard Training Center Petaluma*
Skaggs Island Naval Security Group

Traverse City–Grand Traverse Bay, MI
Coast Guard Air Station Traverse City*

Tucson, AZ
Davis-Monthan Air Force Base

Virginia Beach–Norfolk, VA
Camp Elmore*
Coast Guard Support Center, Portsmouth*
Little Creek Naval Amphibious Base
Norfolk Naval Base
Oceana Naval Air Station
Portsmouth Naval Shipyard

Yuma, AZ
Yuma Marine Corps Air Station
Yuma Proving Ground

Sources: Army and Air Force Exchange Service, Coast Guard Non-Appropriated Fund Activities, Marine Corps Exchange Service, and Navy Resale System, 1987.

*Exchange only

Housing :

Market Values,
Property
Taxes,
and Utility Bills

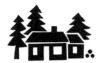 # INTRODUCTION: Housing

"It's like a sex drive," Martin Mayer quoted a well-known housing economist in his book *The Builders*, ". . . to own my own home on my own piece of land." It may well be. And it may well be true that people can't get too much housing, as real estate salespeople and homebuilders tell themselves when they want to endow their professions with recession-proof respectability.

But when you retire, even though the need to own your own address and the land it's on is as strong as ever, you may find you've finally got too much housing indeed. The phenomenon is called "overhousing," and it crops up when your children grow up, leave home, and scatter like tumbleweeds in the wind.

There's no mistaking the signs. Bedrooms are full of furniture but closed off, the creaking and settling you once heard at night when everything was still are now heard all the time, and those bills for property taxes, insurance, and upkeep on the family's sentimental shrine are as high as they ever were, and they still have to be paid.

Overhousing isn't just an empty-nester symptom. If you plan to see the country after you retire, your empty home and its yard running to weeds will worry you when you're supposed to be enjoying yourself. What's more, your home is your biggest asset; seven of every ten retired persons in this country own their homes, and 85 percent of these people have paid off their mortgages. Might your home's market value, which has appreciated over the years, be turned into cash and put to better use?

Certainly developers, investors, and marketers think so. "Move over, baby boomers," *Builder*, a construction trade magazine, announces. "Make way for your elders, who will constitute housing's hottest market for the rest of the century." If you're 55 to 65, you're now part of the "go-go" market for adults-only housing developments. If you're 65 to 75, you're a "go slow" customer for newfangled congregate housing. And if you're over 75, stop worrying; "no go" continuing-care facilities are springing up everywhere.

While these types of housing are attracting many residents, the seven alternatives for more independent living are the same and as plentiful as they ever were for retired people: *buying* a smaller house, condominium, or mobile home; or *renting* an apartment, smaller home, condominium, or mobile home.

TYPICAL HOUSING CHOICES . . .

If the burdens of overhousing lead you to put the old ark up for sale, heed the advice of other retired persons and scale down your housing needs when you scout for another address. *Buying down* to smaller, less expensive shelter can not only give you more income —it can boost your leisure time, too.

If you're thinking of buying down in a distant retirement place, it helps to know in advance what kinds of typical housing choices are there, what the average rent would be for an apartment, and since most relocating retired end up buying a single-family house, how much that would cost.

Single Houses

Older adults are no different from everyone else in the kind of roof they prefer overhead. Surveys by the National Association of Home Builders as well as the U.S. League of Savings Institutions show a common detached house is the overwhelming favorite.

If you open the front door of this typical American home, you'll find yourself in a structure that was built in 1965 and has a single-level, 1,600-square-foot floor plan enclosing six rooms (three bedrooms, one bath, a living room, and a complete kitchen); an insulated attic and storm windows to conserve the heat from the gas-fired, warm-air furnace; and no basement. This house is kept cool during hot spells by a central air-conditioning unit. It is also connected to city water and sewerage lines.

Single Houses in the Retirement Places

Most to Fewest	Percentage of All Year-round Units
Houghton Lake, MI	85%
Canton–Lake Tawakoni, TX	84
Franklin County, TN	84
Fredericksburg, TX	83
Cape Cod, MA	81
Crossville, TN	80
Door County, WI	80
Burnet–Marble Falls–Llano, TX	79
Mountain Home–Bull Shoals, AR	79
Roswell, NM	79
131 Retirement Places Average	**66**
United States Average	**61**
Lake Havasu City–Kingman, AZ	51
Maui, HI	51
Ocean City–Assateague Island, MD	50
Yuma, AZ	50
Las Vegas, NV	49
Reno, NV	49
Bradenton, FL	48
West Palm Beach–Boca Raton–Delray Beach, FL	44
Miami–Hialeah, FL	43
Fort Lauderdale–Hollywood–Pompano Beach, FL	42
Naples, FL	42

Source: U.S. Bureau of the Census, *1980 Census of Population and Housing.*

So much for the national composite. Among the 59 million single houses in the United States, a buyer can choose from many building styles—Cape Cods, Cape Annes and Queen Annes, mountain A-frames, American and Dutch colonials, desert adobes, cabins of peeled pine log, Greek revivals, Puget Sounds, catslides, saltboxes, exotic glass solaria, futuristic earth berms, Victorians, plantation cottages, ubiquitous split-levels, and California bungalows.

But in retirement places, the number of single homes you'll actually find among the other options—apartments, condominiums, and mobile homes—varies considerably.

Condominiums

Condominium was nothing more than an obscure Latin word before a new legal form of housing tenure was imported from Puerto Rico to the U.S. mainland in 1960. Under the arrangement, you could own outright an apartment, townhouse, or single house in a multiple-unit development. As an owner, you were subject to property taxes and could sell, lease, bequeath, and furnish that legally described cube of air space independently of other unit owners.

What's more, you owned the elevators, heating plant, streets, parking spaces, garden landscaping, tennis courts, swimming pool, lights, and walkways in common with the rest of the development's residents.

Throughout the 1970s, condominiums were marketed to young people making their way out of the rental market and older adults who wanted to unload large houses for smaller ones. While the construction boom has subsided in many sections of the country, the fact that the number of condos grew from nothing in 1960 to more than 3 million today certainly vouches for their appeal.

Condo housing ranges all the way from units in high-rise buildings and low-rise garden apartments to

The Most Condominiums

Retirement Place	Percentage of All Year-round Units
Maui, HI	32%
West Palm Beach–Boca Raton–Delray Beach, FL	30
Naples, FL	29
Ocean City–Assateague Island, MD	29
Fort Lauderdale–Hollywood–Pompano Beach, FL	28
Sarasota, FL	18
Hilton Head–Beaufort, SC	17
Fort Myers–Cape Coral, FL	14
Kauai, HI	13
Miami–Hialeah, FL	13
St. Petersburg–Clearwater, FL	13

Source: U.S. Bureau of the Census, *1980 Census of Population and Housing.*

Nationally, condominiums make up slightly less than 3 percent of year-round housing units; in 29 retirement places, they account for less than 1 percent.

row townhouse developments and even mobile-home parks. In several Florida metropolitan areas, in San Diego, and in resorts like Hilton Head–Beaufort and Maui, condos outnumber single homes in the "for sale" market. In more rural retirement places, condos are a negligible part of the housing mix.

Mobile Homes

The big plus of mobile homes is that they are the cheapest kind of housing you can buy. That they are affordable doesn't mean mobile homes resemble the drafty, 300-square-foot trailers that housed many defense workers during World War II or the somewhat larger tin cans built during the 1950s that were parked in enclaves beyond the railroad tracks.

Mobile homes now average 14 feet by 70 feet, offering nearly 1,000 square feet of living space. A 70-foot-long Double Wide can enclose three bedrooms, two ceramic-tiled baths, a living room, a dining room, and a full kitchen. These mobile homes are typically marketed complete: appliances, furniture, draperies, and carpeting are included in the price, as are the built-in plumbing, heating, air-conditioning, and electrical systems.

Outside, owners landscape with grass, trees, and shrubberies. When carports, porches, sheds, patios, and pitched shake roofs are added to the basic structures, sharp-eyed tax assessors sometimes mistake them for conventional houses.

The only time the mobile home is mobile is when it leaves the factory and is trucked in one or more sections to a concrete foundation on the owner's property or at one of 24,000 trailer parks in the country. When it gets there, the wheels, axle, and towing tongue are taken off. After that, the only element that hints of its origins as a trailer is the welded I-beam chassis, which becomes hidden structural reinforcement once the unit is winched onto the concrete pad and plumbed. When it's in place, the mobile home becomes more or less permanent; no more than 3 percent of them will ever be jacked up and rolled off to a new site.

Mobile homes are a big part of the Sun Belt housing mix. Last year, half of all newly built mobile homes were trucked to just eight states: California, Florida, Georgia, Louisiana, North Carolina, Oklahoma, South Carolina, and Texas. You'll search long and hard for a mobile-home park in Hawaii, the less rural parts of New England, and larger cities where the high cost of land offsets any savings from buying a mobile home.

Renting an Apartment

It can happen. One day you're out with a real estate broker scouting for a condo or small home and you spot an immaculate, stately old building near downtown with flowers in front and no sign but one: Apartment for Rent. The next day you're a tenant. Unlike younger newcomers who usually rent after

The Most Mobile Homes

Retirement Place	Percentage of All Year-round Units
Lake Havasu City–Kingman, AZ	39%
Clear Lake, CA	32
Yuma, AZ	30
Athens–Cedar Creek Lake, TX	23
Bradenton, FL	22
Deming, NM	22
Ocala, FL	22
Prescott, AZ	21
Bend, OR	20
Red Bluff–Sacramento Valley, CA	20
Southport, NC	20

Source: U.S. Bureau of the Census, *1980 Census of Population and Housing*.

Nationally, mobile homes make up 5 percent of year-round housing units; in Cape Cod, Massachusetts, and in Kauai and Maui, Hawaii, they account for less than 1 percent.

relocating, most retired persons buy. But renting may be smart for the short term; it allows you to remain flexible, since you need not stay in an apartment beyond the term of the lease if you decide to buy or to relocate to a different retirement place.

Renting is also cheaper. Rents haven't gone up as fast as the costs of owning. Other pluses: you don't need to come up with a large down payment; taxes, insurance, repairs, and sometimes utilities are the landlord's headaches. What's more, vacancy rates are predicted to climb as more and more renters buy. In some overbuilt Sun Belt retirement places—San Antonio and San Diego, for example—landlords are offering month-to-month arrangements or leases with six months free rent.

Retirement Places Rated defines an apartment as simply a rental unit in a structure with two or more rental units; this definition includes rental duplexes, triplexes, and fourplexes. Don't be put off by the image of impersonal blocks of large, high-rise tower complexes near a place's central business district. Only 1 out of 50 apartments is in a building of 13 stories or more,

The Most Apartments

Retirement Place	Percentage of All Year-round Units
Miami–Hialeah, FL	28%
Ann Arbor, MI	27
Iowa City, IA	27
Madison, WI	25
Athens, GA	24
Austin, TX	22
Lexington, KY	22
Blacksburg, VA	21
Bloomington–Brown County, IN	21
San Diego, CA	21
State College, PA	21

Source: U.S. Bureau of the Census, *1980 Census of Population and Housing*.

Nationally, apartments in buildings with two or more rental units make up 18 percent of all year-round housing. In Canton–Lake Tawakoni, Texas; Clayton–Clarkesville, Georgia; Houghton Lake, Michigan; New Paltz–Ulster County, New York; and Southport, North Carolina, they account for 1 percent or less.

and only 1 out of 10 is in a building higher than 3 stories. Make note: apartments make up a large chunk of housing, not only in bigger retirement places, but in smaller places dominated by state universities.

. . . AND TYPICAL HOUSING PRICES

If you sell your home, you'll likely realize enough cash to buy another home, perhaps a smaller one. Or you might buy a mobile home or condo. You might even rent, investing the money from the sale of your old home to provide retirement income.

Of course, if you decide to buy, what you buy and where you buy it greatly influences the price you pay. At the national level, prices are lowest for mobile homes, rise for resale condominiums, move higher for resale detached homes, higher still for new condominiums, and then peak for new homes.

Housing Winners and Losers

That three of the seven costliest retirement places for housing are in New England shouldn't surprise you if you've followed newspaper accounts of the housing inflation that's been going on there since the recession bottomed out in late 1982.

Although sky-high shelter costs don't always mean desirable housing, they do offer a clue to the pitch of supply and demand in desirable locations. The irony is that not only are house prices in choice Yankee Belt and Pacific Beach locations beyond the reach of most households elsewhere in the U.S., they're out of reach for most *local* households, too.

Six of the top places for inexpensive housing, on the other hand, are found in Rio Grande Country, the Texas Interior, or they are tucked into lesser-known rural pockets of the Mid-South. Could it be that these spots, in their own way, may see the same kind of late 1970s California-style inflation that New England is experiencing today? It's hardly likely. The circumstances of too much land for too few people are at play here.

LEAST EXPENSIVE RETIREMENT PLACE	Score
Roswell, NM	4,399
McAllen–Edinburg–Mission, TX	4,609
Brownsville–Harlingen, TX	4,673
Deming, NM	4,744
Paris–Big Sandy, TN	5,122
Canton–Lake Tawakoni, TX	5,139
Crossville, TN	5,328

MOST EXPENSIVE RETIREMENT PLACE	Score
Maui, HI	14,303
Litchfield County, CT	13,245
Burlington, VT	12,668
Cape Cod, MA	12,014
Kauai, HI	11,911
Naples, FL	11,815
San Diego, CA	11,807

The price difference between a mobile home and a site-built house is almost entirely due to labor costs. It takes a small builder's crew 60 to 90 days to erect a typical three-bedroom tract house. A mobile home takes 80 to 100 hours at the factory. In 1985, when the average square-foot cost of building a conventional home was $45.18, exclusive of land, the cost of manufacturing a mobile home was $20.19 per square foot.

If you want to strike a compromise between small-scale living and the satisfaction of owning your own address, consider the condominium form of ownership. In a new condominium, you'll have less interior space to look after (1,250 square feet, on average, versus 1,700 square feet for a new single home). Moreover, the tax advantages of ownership are yours at a lower cost (on average, new condos cost 10 to 15 percent less than new single homes).

In 1986, according to the National Association of Realtors, an existing single house in the United States had a median sales price of $80,000, an increase of 29 percent since 1980. In six years, prices rose 91 percent in the rebounding East, 55 percent in the South, only 36 percent in the slower-growing Midwest, and 21 percent in the West, where values rose to historic heights in the late 1970s.

The following prices come from the *1980 Census of Population and Housing* and are boosted by regional inflation factors (reported by the National Association of Realtors) to reflect realistic 1986 market values. These prices are estimated *medians;* in other words, one half of the owners would take less and one half would ask for more if they had to sell immediately. Moreover, they are median prices for all owner-occupied housing

---

The Lot Factor

Any real estate broker touting a suburban ranch or condo can tick off the basic factors that figure into the sales price. Aside from seller's greed, the factors are quality of original construction, turnover rate in the neighborhood, current condition, and location. But these are of secondary importance to local supply and demand.

Cut off a slice of a tract development in suburban San Antonio and drop it in the middle of California's San Diego County and you can see supply and demand at work. The transplanted homes will more than double in value, not because they are roomier and built with better materials but because of the more intense competition for housing in much of Southern California. You can still find well-cared-for three-bedroom ranches in San Antonio for less than $100,000 and nearly identical homes in San Diego for $200,000. The location of the site, more than any other factor, is the best single determinant of a home's sales price.

Based on Federal Housing Administration data, the value of the lot on which a typical house is built represents 19 percent of the home's sales price. However, the percentage varies considerably depending on where this typical house is found. In Hawaii, the cost of the site is half the price of the home; in California, it's 32 percent. In Kansas, it's only 13 percent.

Land Costs as Percentage of House Prices

HIGHEST		LOWEST	
Hawaii	50%	Kansas	13%
California	32	Indiana	14
Connecticut	26	Georgia	15
Oregon	26	Michigan	15
Washington	26	Missouri	15
Nevada	25	South Carolina	15

Source: Federal Housing Administration, *Property Characteristics, 1-Family Homes, by State, 1986.*

Median Housing Prices in the Retirement Places

Lowest to Highest

Roswell, NM	$ 36,800
McAllen–Edinburg–Mission, TX	37,500
Brownsville–Harlingen, TX	38,300
Deming, NM	38,800
Houghton Lake, MI	40,000
Canton–Lake Tawakoni, TX	42,800
Oscoda–Huron Shore, MI	42,900
Paris–Big Sandy, TN	45,800
Clayton–Clarkesville, GA	47,000
Branson–Cassville–Table Rock Lake, MO	47,200
131 Retirement Places Average	***70,800***
United States Average	***80,000***
Salinas–Seaside–Monterey, CA	104,500
Burlington, VT	104,600
Cape Cod, MA	104,800
Friday Harbor–San Juan Islands, WA	105,400
Santa Rosa–Petaluma, CA	106,800
Kauai, HI	109,700
San Diego, CA	109,900
Naples, FL	110,300
Litchfield County, CT	114,500
Maui, HI	137,200

Source: Derived from U.S. Bureau of the Census, *1980 Census of Population and Housing,* and National Association of Realtors, *Existing Home Sales, 1986.*

The above figures have been rounded to the nearest $100.

---

units: single detached houses, condos, and mobile homes.

SHOPPING FOR PROPERTY TAXES

Being overhoused doesn't only mean finding yourself with a surplus of living space. You can be *financially* overhoused, too, especially when you pay property taxes on a home that has increased in value at a time when income has abruptly become fixed.

Just because you're getting older doesn't mean the tax assessor will take notice and graciously lower your home's tax bill. Property tax relief, in the states that offer it to older adults, usually comes after specific income tests. The only place in this country where persons over 65 can completely forget their property taxes is Alaska (a state, incidentally, with the lowest proportion of people over 65). Why not "shop" for favorable property taxes the way corporations do when they plan moves?

In recent years, homeowners who organized to fight confiscatory property taxes likened them to a ransom they were forced to pay to save their homes from the tax assessor's auction block. Using this analogy, New Yorkers buy their homes back every 36 years, since New York's average residential property tax rate is 2.8 percent of a home's market value. In Louisiana, the "ransom" period is 625 years because of an extremely low average rate of .16 percent. The difference in these figures illustrates the wide variation in property taxes around the country.

Property taxes can vary locally, too, and be madly confusing to property owners. In California, two homes on the same street with identical sales prices and physical characteristics can have substantially different, yet legally impeccable, tax bills if one of them was sold before the approval of Proposition 13 and the other after. In Texas, a home's value can be assessed at different levels at different times of the year by different assessors.

Although states don't set tax rates (that is done by more than 20,000 cities, townships, counties, school districts, hospital districts, sanitary districts, and other special districts), statewide average property tax rates are useful in estimating local tax bills. The following estimated tax bills are derived from the median price of housing in 131 retirement places, taxed at the particular state's average rate on the value of the house.

Property Tax Bills in the Retirement Places

Lowest to Highest

Fairhope–Gulf Shores, AL	$ 261
Roswell, NM	280
Deming, NM	295
Yuma, AZ	346
Las Cruces, NM	384
Biloxi–Gulfport, MS	417
Lake Havasu City–Kingman, AZ	421
Panama City, FL	421
Rehoboth Bay–Indian River Bay, DE	422
Lakeland–Winter Haven, FL	441
Ocala, FL	441
131 Retirement Places Average	**903**
United States Average	**1,050**
Bennington, VT	1,874
Litchfield County, CT	1,924
Monticello–Liberty, NY	1,985
New Paltz–Ulster County, NY	2,001
Columbia County, NY	2,054
Canandaigua, NY	2,086
Ann Arbor, MI	2,345
Cape May, NJ	2,357
Ocean County, NJ	2,412
Burlington, VT	2,438

Source: Retirement Places Rated estimates based on median market values multiplied by each state's effective property tax rate as detailed in the Advisory Commission on Intergovernmental Relations, Significant Features of Fiscal Federalism, 1986.

WHAT DIFFERENCE DOES AGE MAKE?

Scuff over the sawdust and around the empty nail kegs, the stacked sheetrock, and the crated fiberglass

---

In Some Places, Older Isn't Always Cheaper

Most of us live in homes built years ago that were bought, lived in, and sold by a succession of owners. We all confirm the "filtering theory" of housing, which states that houses filter down from their high-income original owners to middle-income buyers and finally to lower-income owners. To put it another way, high-income households tend to live in newer homes, and lower-income households occupy older homes.

Sounds obvious, doesn't it?

However, when the real estate sections of *Yankee* magazine, the *Boston Globe*, the *Hartford Courant*, *Down East Magazine*, the *New York Times Magazine*, and the *Washington Post* list antique Cape Cod–style homes and Georgian country mansions built in the last century for hundreds of thousands of dollars, you're looking at a big exception to this theory. Nowhere is this more apparent than in Connecticut's Litchfield County, the Amherst–Northampton area in western Massachusetts, Maryland's Eastern Shore, and Charlottesville, Virginia.

Nevertheless, the theory holds true for most of the country and for most of the retirement places, too. The older the housing, the lower the price.

---

shower stall in a newly framed ranch in a suburban housing development, and you might wonder why the builder is asking a bundle for something he's putting up so quickly.

They don't build them the way they used to. Wraparound porches are rarely found. A porch is now merely a recessed space at the home's entrance. The 10-foot interior ceiling common before World War II has been replaced by the 8-foot standard. The kind of formal stairway with well-turned balusters and waxed rails that Andy Hardy used to slide down are no longer necessary—most new homes are erected on a single level. Milled red oak fascias and moldings have become too expensive for common use; walls are envelopes of three-eighths gypsum board fastened to studs rather than the old "mud jobs" of plaster on lath; and solid six-panel interior doors have lost out to hollow-core flush doors of hemlock veneer.

On the other hand, the seasonal threat of damp and flooded cellars arises less often, simply because there aren't many cellars being excavated. Polyvinyl chloride and copper have replaced galvanized iron for water pipes; cast-iron radiators no longer interfere with furniture arrangement; knob-and-tube wiring has surrendered to safer electrical circuitry; and pressure-treated wood has eliminated termite and dry-rot risks along the sills. Indeed, 20 percent of a new home's breathtaking price is due to builders' using superior materials for some types of jobs, according to a recent Prudential Insurance Company study.

One useful indication of the quality of an area's

housing stock is the percentage of homes built before World War II (defined here as "old") and the percentage built since 1980 (defined here as "new"). Although an old house isn't necessarily on the verge of tumbling down, age can signal functional obsolescence and looming maintenance headaches. Clapboards do need scraping and repainting every few years, sewer drains must be snaked regularly, furnaces do wear out, and so do chimneys and roofs. These chores mean dollars and difficulties.

New and Old Housing in the Retirement Places

NEWEST	Percentage of Housing Built Since 1980
Naples, FL	47%
St. George–Zion, UT	42
Fort Myers–Cape Coral, FL	32
Ocean City–Assateague Island, MD	31
Austin, TX	29
West Palm Beach–Boca Raton– Delray Beach, FL	29
Melbourne–Titusville–Palm Bay, FL	28
Ocala, FL	28
Grass Valley–Truckee, CA	26
Phoenix, AZ	26
Southport, NC	26

OLDEST	Percentage of Housing Built Before World War II
Camden–Penobscot Bay, ME	58%
Bar Harbor–Frenchman Bay, ME	50
Canandaigua, NY	46
Columbia County, NY	46
Bennington, VT	43
Hanover, NH	43
Keene, NH	43
Amherst–Northampton, MA	37
Lancaster, PA	37
New Paltz–Ulster County, NY	37

Source: U.S. Bureau of the Census, 1980 Census of Population and Housing, 1980, and Housing Units Authorized by Building Permits and Public Contracts, 1980, and annual to date.

HOME ENERGY REQUIREMENTS

If you don't count the loan initiation fees and closing costs that new homeowners pay to float their mortgages, then fuel and electricity for the home were the fastest-rising of all items on the Consumer Price Index between 1967 and 1985. What was once a minor and predictable expense, amounting to less than 1 percent of a household's budget 20 years ago, may now amount to more than the cost of medical care or clothing, in spite of the recent drop in oil prices.

Three factors account for the $856 difference between the annual average residential utility bills in Hot Springs–Lake Ouachita, Arkansas, and Kauai, Hawaii: local climate, the form of energy used to keep interiors comfortable, and the energy's source.

Counting Hours

Texans say that their Gulf Coast is one long stretch where air conditioning, like food and water, is a basic necessity without which all humanity would go mad and die. Here, a meteorologist measuring humidity with a psychrometer whenever the temperature climbs over 80 degrees Fahrenheit will count nearly 2,500 hours every year when the instrument's bulb stays wet from moist air. New Delhi records similar numbers, and so does Kinshasa, capital of Zaire. These 2,500-odd hours are the equivalent of more than 200 days per year having uncomfortable, sweaty, 12-hour periods of high humidity.

In desert retirement locations such as Las Vegas, Phoenix, and Tucson, the days are much drier, but the number of hours there when the temperature is more than 80 degrees Fahrenheit is even greater than the number found on the Texas Gulf Coast. These hours were first counted by Defense Department building engineers in the late 1940s and updated in 1978 for a worldwide inventory of military installations. Not only are these hours useful for gauging how hot a given place is over time, but they also signal how often your home's air conditioner may be humming.

Counting Days

In 1915, Eugene P. Milener, an engineer with the Gas Company of Baltimore, made a discovery for which he received little recognition outside his industry. The amount of natural gas needed to keep houses warm can be accurately predicted for every degree that the outdoor temperature falls below 32 degrees. Natural gas utilities still use this measurement, called a "heating-degree day," to estimate consumption patterns among their customers.

Heating-degree days are the number of degrees the daily average temperature drops below 65. Heating your home isn't usually necessary when the temperature outdoors is more than 65, but furnaces are fired up when the outdoors gets colder. Thus, a heating-degree day indicates the number of degrees of heating required to keep a house at 65. If, for example, the temperature on a winter day is 35, that day has 30

Heating Needs: The Top 10 Cold-Weather Retirement Places

Retirement Place	Annual Heating-Degree Days
Eagle River, WI	9,339
Rhinelander, WI	8,783
Kalispell, MT	8,554
Houghton Lake, MI	8,347
Missoula, MT	7,931
Burlington, VT	7,876
Door County, WI	7,876
Madison, WI	7,730
Traverse City– Grand Traverse Bay, MI	7,698
Bennington, VT	7,681

Source: National Oceanic and Atmospheric Administration, Climatography of the United States, Series 81, no date.

Air-Conditioning Needs: The Top Hot-Weather Retirement Places	
Retirement Place	Annual Hours over 80° F
Yuma, AZ	3,185
Phoenix, AZ	2,815
McAllen–Edinburg–Mission, TX	2,527
Miami–Hialeah, FL	2,408
Lake Havasu City–Kingman, AZ	2,360
Las Vegas, NV	2,360
Fort Lauderdale–Hollywood–Pompano Beach, FL	2,342
Brownsville–Harlingen, TX	2,295
West Palm Beach–Boca Raton–Delray Beach, FL	2,276
Austin, TX	2,243
Tucson, AZ	2,243

Source: U.S. Department of Defense, *Engineering Weather Data*, 1978.

heating-degree days, meaning that 30 degrees of heating are called for.

In 1985, the average for annual heating-degree days (total heating-degree days over the year) in the United States was 4,643, ranging from none in the Hawaiian Islands at sea level to nearly 20,000 in the Brooks Range of Alaska. The number of annual heating-degree days in a given year tells you how cold it gets and also how often you'll need to run a home's heating system to keep the indoors comfortable.

Household Energy Geography

Can you recall the Korean War years when the rumbling of coal trucks along their delivery routes was a familiar urban street sound? Three-dollar-a-ton black anthracite was the dominant home heating fuel everywhere east of the Mississippi except for Florida and New England. The blue flame of piped-in natural gas, the dominant heating fuel today, was just starting to burn in new refrigerators, stoves, clothes dryers, and in new home furnaces. The electric utilities were just beginning to offer rate incentives to buyers of total-electric homes.

Coal today is largely gone from the home-energy scene. In spite of heavy marketing of airtight coal stoves as an auxiliary means of heating houses, the number of homes burning this fuel declined by more than 1 million over the past decade. The major options in urban retirement places, from most expensive to least in cost per million British thermal units (Btu), are electricity, piped-in natural gas, and fuel oil or kerosene. In the rural parts of some retirement places, there's bottled gas and wood.

Electricity. In 1950, the only place where most of the homes were total-electric was the small desert town of Las Vegas, seat of Nevada's Clark County. The power there was the cheapest in the country because it was generated by falling water at the new Boulder

Canyon hydroelectric project some 25 miles southeast. Power is still cheap in Las Vegas, relative to nuclear-generated or fossil fuel–generated power that residential customers pay for elsewhere in the country. So is the power that heats and lights homes in the Puget Sound area, the Oregon Cascades, and the Kentucky and Tennessee lakes region, places that also get their power from major hydroelectric projects.

Although most American homes are heated with natural gas, electricity is the dominant choice in new homes. Between 1970 and 1980, the number of total-electric homes tripled. The reason: it costs much less to wire a new house for electric resistance heat than to install a gas or oil furnace with piping and sheet-metal hot-air conduits. Total-electric homes predominate in 46 of the 131 retirement places. The Washington, DC–based Edison Electric Institute tracks average annual residential electricity consumption and prices, and the following are its figures for 1985:

- Typical consumption: 17,956 kilowatt-hours per year
- Typical bill: $1,324 per year
- Cost per million Btu: $20.99

Bottled Gas. Bottled, or liquified petroleum (LP), gas is derived from oil and sold in compressed or liquid form. Like residual fuel oil, it requires on-site storage tanks. Unlike piped-in natural gas and electricity, it offers the advantage of an on-hand supply in case of interrupted service. In rural retirement spots, particularly in the Ozarks, it is the fuel of choice for heat and even for running air conditioners and refrigerators.

Most mobile homes from New England to the Desert Southwest are also heated by bottled gas. While this fuel is more expensive than piped-in natural gas, in the future it may be cheaper—given the dramatic drop in the price of crude oil from which LP is derived. Below are figures from the Department of Energy, which monitors average household prices and consumption:

- Typical consumption: 1,145 gallons per year
- Typical bill: $993
- Cost per million Btu: $9.46

Natural Gas. In 54 retirement places, the major source for heating a house is a by-product of oil drilling that for many years flamed at the wellhead for lack of a market. Natural gas, a fossil fuel, has meant inexpensive heat for most householders, mainly because the federal government has regulated its interstate price. Even after deregulation, its price continues to drop.

Natural gas hasn't ever been cheap to residential customers at the ends of the continental transmission lines that start in Louisiana and Texas gas fields, however. Transportation costs explain why natural gas isn't preferred in Yankee Belt or Mid-Atlantic Metro Belt retirement places, where oil is the least expensive of fuels, or in the Pacific Northwest, where hydro-generated electricity costs the least. The American Gas Association provides the following figures:

- Typical consumption: 10,200 cubic feet per year
- Typical bill: $606
- Cost per million Btu: $5.94

Oil and Kerosene. Though their prices have tumbled recently because of worldwide overproduction, #2 heating oil and kerosene were the only items on the Consumer Price Index to sextuple in cost between 1967 and 1980. High cost is one reason that the number of homes heated with fuel oil or kerosene declined by more than 2 million during the 1970s. You won't find the price varying greatly by location, but you will find these distillates of imported crude to be the most common heating fuel in 27 retirement places, mainly in the Yankee Belt, the Mid-Atlantic Metro Belt, and in western North Carolina. The following figures are based on Department of Energy consumption figures and a late 1986 price of $0.76 a gallon for home heating oil:

- Typical consumption: 1,043 gallons per year
- Typical bill: $793 per year
- Cost per million Btu: $5.47

Wood. Anyone who feeds a wood stove has heard the homely proverb about this fuel: it warms you twice, first when you cut and stack it, and second when you watch it burn. From Rocky Mountain piñon to hickory and ash from Ozark forests, it is burned in 3 million homes. Among retirement places, more than one third of the homes in Hamilton–Bitterroot Valley, Montana, and Twain Harte–Yosemite, California, are heated with wood because it is cheap and available right outside a householder's door.

Nationally, the cost of a cord of good, seasoned hardwood varies a great deal. You can buy half a cord for $300 in Manhattan, or, with a little sweat and permission, you can gather fallen timber in local state forests gratis. The U.S. Forest Service determines energy content for various kinds of wood; consumption and price figures come from the U.S. Department of Energy:

- Typical consumption: 2.8 cords per year
- Typical bill: $350
- Cost per million Btu: $5.34 (mixed hardwood)

Keeping It Running

Utility bills for home heating and cooling, lighting, and running appliances cost $1,357 up in New Paltz–Ulster County, New York, but only $556 in Coeur d'Alene, Idaho. Why such a great difference?

The high number of annual heating-degree days in both places is a sign of long winters, certainly. But in New Paltz–Ulster County, the cost of natural gas plus the electricity bills mailed to Consolidated Edison's residential customers are among the country's highest. As for Coeur d'Alene, homes there are total-electric and get their bills from the Washington Water Power Company, the distributor of cheap hydro-generated power.

If your only retirement concern is dodging both winter heating and summer air-conditioning bills, head for Hawaii. Unfortunately, you'll still be writing big monthly checks to the local electric power company. There are few heated homes here, and air conditioning isn't necessary. But the cost of electricity to keep your water hot, food cool, lamps lit, and appliances running is about as high as it gets anywhere. Why? Because power is generated by imported fuel oil.

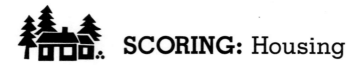 **SCORING:** Housing

Is housing less expensive in the North Woods than in New Appalachia or the Yankee Belt? When it comes to paying property taxes, would you be better off choosing the Ozark corner of Arkansas over Metropolitan South Florida? Might a move to Yuma, Arizona, in February haunt you in August when you realize how much air conditioning costs?

To help answer these questions, *Retirement Places Rated* tallies the three biggest dollar expenses of home-ownership: utility bills, property taxes, and mortgage payments. The total of these three equals the amount you can expect to pay each year for the basics of homeowning. It also represents each retirement place's score.

Property taxes and mortgage payments are based on the median value of owner-occupied units within each retirement place, as reported in the *1980 Census of Population and Housing*. These were owners' estimates of what their home, condominium, or mobile home would be worth if they decided to sell immediately. To show realistic prices for the first quarter of 1987, *Retirement Places Rated* updated these estimates with regional inflation factors reported by the National Association of Realtors.

Each place starts with a base score of zero. Points are added according to the following indicators:

1. *Utility bills.* Annual utility bills are estimated

for a home that uses natural gas for space heating, water heating, and cooking because this fuel is available everywhere and is the most frequently chosen in most of the retirement places. Also included in the utility bills are the costs of electricity for lighting, running appliances, and air conditioning based on local bills for 500 kilowatt-hours of monthly consumption as reported by the Department of Energy. In retirement places where total-electric homes predominate, utility bills reflect the annual cost of using 1,250 kilowatt-hours of electricity each month.

2. *Property taxes.* Property taxes are estimated by multiplying the median value of local housing by the state's average effective tax rate for residential property. In Cape Cod, for example, the tax bill of $1,646 is derived from a 1986 median home value of $104,800 times the effective residential property tax rate of 1.57 percent in Massachusetts.

3. *Mortgage Payments.* Annual mortgage payments are based on a 10 percent, 25-year mortgage on the median value of local housing units, after making a one-fifth down payment.

SCORING EXAMPLES

One way to compare housing costs is to look at three retirement places from different regions of the country: Roswell, New Mexico, in Rio Grande Country; San Antonio, Texas, a large metropolitan area in the Texas Interior; and Maui, Hawaii, in the Pacific Beaches region.

Roswell, New Mexico (#1)

With a median 1986 market value of $36,800, housing in Chaves County, New Mexico, is more affordable than in most retirement places. They say here that buffalo grass won't put up much resistance to developers. House lots are quite inexpensive in the open plains outside of Roswell, the county seat and historic cattle town.

This retirement place is more old than new. Just 1 home in 20 has been built since 1980, whereas 1 in 8 predates World War II. Most are single homes occupied by their owners. There are no condos to speak of, but the local percentage of rental apartments and mobile homes mean there are reasonable alternatives to buying a home. Utility bills in Roswell are $906, property taxes $280 (estimated from New Mexico's statewide

effective rate of .76 percent), and mortgage payments $3,213, totaling $4,399, the lowest homeowning costs of all the retirement places.

San Antonio, Texas (#21)

"The bank owns this one" isn't an uncommon phrase in San Antonio real estate advertising. Texas is surviving hard times brought on by the slump in the oil patch, and the consequences reach even this three-county metropolitan area dominated by defense employment.

Browse through a book of multiple listings, and you're struck by one thing: condomania hasn't hit San Antonio with the same force as it has elsewhere. Nearly all the photographs show brick or Texas-rock suburban ranches set back from the street on large lawns. Prices differ widely from the hundreds of thousands in Elm Creek to the low forties in some neighborhoods near Randolph Air Force Base and Fort Sam Houston. For an estimated $51,500 median price home in San Antonio, utility bills are $856, property taxes $680 (estimated from Texas's statewide effective rate of 1.32 percent), and mortgage payments $4,492, totaling $6,028, the lowest homeowning costs among retirement places with more than half a million people.

Maui, Hawaii (#131)

Thousands of miles to the west of San Antonio, the Pacific islands that make up Maui, Hawaii, have the highest basic homeowner costs of the 131 retirement places. The median market value of a Maui home is $137,200. It is likely to be a high-rise condominium, likely to have been built within the last ten years, and likely to be rented rather than owned by the people living in it. Maui has a greater percentage of year-round housing units that are condos than any other retirement place. Owing to the distance from stateside manufacturers and the astronomical cost of land, there aren't any mobile homes here. Also, unlike the freehold tenure common to most of the United States mainland, many homes here are built on ground leased for 99 years.

Even though most homes in Maui aren't air conditioned or heated, the bills from Maui Electric, Ltd., for using 500 kilowatt-hours of electricity just to cook, run appliances, and light your home in the evening come to $136 each month, or $1,636 a year. With Hawaii's exceptionally low effective rate of .51 percent, however, the property tax bill on this $137,200 dwelling comes to only $700 a year. But mortgage payments amount to nearly $11,967. Add them all together and you get homeowner costs of $14,303 a year.

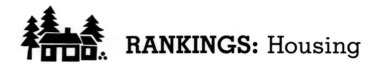

RANKINGS: Housing

Three criteria are used to rank retirement places for basic costs of owning a house over one year: (1) average utility bills, (2) property taxes, and (3) mortgage payments.

The sum of these three items represents the score for each retirement place. Places that receive a tie score are given the same rank and are listed in alphabetical order.

Retirement Places from Least to Most Expensive

Rank	Score	Rank	Score	Rank	Score
1. Roswell, NM	4,399	41. Front Royal, VA	7,082	83. Melbourne–Titusville–Palm Bay, FL	8,539
2. McAllen–Edinburg–Mission, TX	4,609	42. Lake Havasu City–Kingman, AZ	7,113	84. Las Vegas, NV	8,554
3. Brownsville–Harlingen, TX	4,673	43. Ocean City–Assateague Island, MD	7,152	85. Oak Harbor–Whidbey Island, WA	8,570
4. Deming, NM	4,744	44. Flagstaff, AZ	7,185		
5. Paris–Big Sandy, TN	5,122	45. Fredericksburg, TX	7,186	86. Bend, OR	8,576
				87. Medford–Ashland, OR	8,602
6. Canton–Lake Tawakoni, TX	5,139	46. Daytona Beach, FL	7,211	88. Hilton Head–Beaufort, SC	8,641
7. Crossville, TN	5,328	47. Kerrville, TX	7,304	89. Austin, TX	8,673
8. Franklin County, TN	5,520	48. Boise, ID	7,330	90. Eugene–Springfield, OR	8,699
9. Branson–Cassville–Table Rock Lake, MO	5,580	49. Rhinelander, WI	7,344		
9. Clayton–Clarkesville, GA	5,580	50. Hendersonville–Brevard, NC	7,356	91. Fort Collins–Loveland, CO	8,755
				92. Twain Harte–Yosemite, CA	8,874
11. Grand Lake–Lake Tenkiller, OK	5,653	51. Myrtle Beach, SC	7,378	93. Charlottesville, VA	9,002
12. Houghton Lake, MI	5,711	52. Tucson, AZ	7,418	94. Sarasota, FL	9,164
13. Las Cruces, NM	5,805	53. St. George–Zion, UT	7,442	95. Fort Myers–Cape Coral, FL	9,189
14. Springfield, MO	5,811	54. Bellingham, WA	7,447		
15. Yuma, AZ	5,849	55. Albuquerque, NM	7,473	96. Chapel Hill, NC	9,308
				97. Monticello–Liberty, NY	9,310
16. Hot Springs–Lake Ouachita, AR	5,852	56. Port Angeles–Strait of Juan de Fuca, WA	7,482	98. Amherst–Northampton, MA	9,312
17. Southport, NC	5,868	57. Colorado Springs, CO	7,506	99. Hanover, NH	9,475
18. Athens–Cedar Creek Lake, TX	5,903	58. Athens, GA	7,521	100. Columbia County, NY	9,546
19. Murray–Kentucky Lake, KY	5,907	59. Fort Walton Beach, FL	7,522		
20. Biloxi–Gulfport, MS	5,921	60. Petoskey–Straits of Mackinac, MI	7,534	101. New Paltz–Ulster County, NY	9,592
				102. Keene, NH	9,610
21. San Antonio, TX	6,028	61. St. Petersburg–Clearwater, FL	7,535	103. Iowa City, IA	9,704
22. Oscoda–Huron Shore, MI	6,073	62. Blacksburg, VA	7,548	104. Canandaigua, NY	9,752
23. Panama City, FL	6,127	63. Olympia, WA	7,673	105. Miami–Hialeah, FL	9,764
24. Kalispell, MT	6,466	64. Redding, CA	7,763		
25. Lakeland–Winter Haven, FL	6,483	65. Orlando, FL	7,780	106. West Palm Beach–Boca Raton–Delray Beach, FL	9,813
				107. Easton–Chesapeake Bay, MD	9,833
26. Hamilton–Bitterroot Valley, MT	6,485	66. Winchester, VA	7,835	108. Bennington, VT	9,992
27. Brunswick–Golden Isles, GA	6,492	67. Chico–Paradise, CA	7,839	109. San Luis Obispo, CA	10,016
28. Mountain Home–Bull Shoals, AR	6,494	67. Phoenix, AZ	7,839	110. State College, PA	10,086
29. Asheville, NC	6,501	69. Door County, WI	7,867		
30. Fayetteville, AR	6,546	70. Grand Junction, CO	7,884	111. Carson City–Minden, NV	10,125
				112. Laconia–Lake Winnipesaukee, NH	10,143
31. Red Bluff–Sacramento Valley, CA	6,556	71. Eagle River, WI	7,918	113. Madison, WI	10,159
32. Ocala, FL	6,594	72. Bar Harbor–Frenchman Bay, ME	7,919	114. Lancaster, PA	10,413
33. Burnet–Marble Falls–Llano, TX	6,612	73. Camden–Penobscot Bay, ME	7,938	115. North Conway–White Mountains, NH	10,470
34. Gainesville–Lake Lanier, GA	6,644	74. Missoula, MT	8,023		
35. Fairhope–Gulf Shores, AL	6,719	75. Bradenton, FL	8,038	116. Fort Lauderdale–Hollywood–Pompano Beach, FL	10,605
				117. Grass Valley–Truckee, CA	10,807
36. Rehoboth Bay–Indian River Bay, DE	6,745	76. Newport–Lincoln City, OR	8,074	118. Ann Arbor, MI	10,909
37. Bloomington–Brown County, IN	6,802	77. Lexington, KY	8,120	119. Friday Harbor–San Juan Islands, WA	11,003
38. Coeur d'Alene, ID	6,833	78. Clear Lake, CA	8,324	120. Salinas–Seaside–Monterey, CA	11,063
39. Prescott, AZ	6,899	79. Virginia Beach–Norfolk, VA	8,331		
40. Charleston, SC	7,023	80. Traverse City–Grand Traverse Bay, MD	8,343	121. Portsmouth–Dover–Durham, NH	11,146
		81. Reno, NV	8,406		
		82. Santa Fe, NM	8,518		

Rank	Score	Rank	Score	Rank	Score
122. Santa Rosa– Petaluma, CA	11,286	125. San Diego, CA	11,807	128. Cape Cod, MA	12,014
123. Cape May, NJ	11,494	126. Naples, FL	11,815	129. Burlington, VT	12,668
124. Ocean County, NJ	11,711	127. Kauai, HI	11,911	130. Litchfield County, CT	13,245
				131. Maui, HI	14,303

Retirement Places Listed Alphabetically

Retirement Place	Rank	Retirement Place	Rank	Retirement Place	Rank
Albuquerque, NM	55	Flagstaff, AZ	44	New Paltz–Ulster County, NY	101
Amherst–Northampton, MA	98	Fort Collins–Loveland, CO	91	Newport–Lincoln City, OR	76
Ann Arbor, MI	118	Fort Lauderdale–Hollywood–		North Conway–	
Asheville, NC	29	Pompano Beach, FL	116	White Mountains, NH	115
Athens, GA	58	Fort Myers–Cape Coral, FL	95	Oak Harbor–Whidbey Island, WA	85
		Fort Walton Beach, FL	59	Ocala, FL	32
Athens–Cedar Creek Lake, TX	18				
Austin, TX	89	Franklin County, TN	8	Ocean City–	
Bar Harbor–Frenchman Bay, ME	72	Fredericksburg, TX	45	Assateague Island, MD	43
Bellingham, WA	54	Friday Harbor–		Ocean County, NJ	124
Bend, OR	86	San Juan Islands, WA	119	Olympia, WA	63
		Front Royal, VA	41	Orlando, FL	65
Bennington, VT	108	Gainesville–Lake Lanier, GA	34	Oscoda–Huron Shore, MI	22
Biloxi–Gulfport, MS	20				
Blacksburg, VA	62	Grand Junction, CO	70	Panama City, FL	23
Bloomington–		Grand Lake–Lake Tenkiller, OK	11	Paris–Big Sandy, TN	5
Brown County, IN	37	Grass Valley–Truckee, CA	117	Petoskey–Straits of Mackinac, MI	60
Boise, ID	48	Hamilton–Bitterroot Valley, MT	26	Phoenix, AZ	67
		Hanover, NH	99	Port Angeles–	
Bradenton, FL	75			Strait of Juan de Fuca, WA	56
Branson–Cassville–		Hendersonville–Brevard, NC	50		
Table Rock Lake, MO	9	Hilton Head–Beaufort, SC	88	Portsmouth–Dover–Durham, NH	121
Brownsville–Harlingen, TX	3	Hot Springs–Lake Ouachita, AR	16	Prescott, AZ	39
Brunswick–Golden Isles, GA	27	Houghton Lake, MI	12	Red Bluff–Sacramento Valley, CA	31
Burlington, VT	129	Iowa City, IA	103	Redding, CA	64
				Rehoboth Bay–Indian River	
Burnet–Marble Falls–		Kalispell, MT	24	Bay, DE	36
Llano, TX	33	Kauai, HI	127		
Camden–Penobscot Bay, ME	73	Keene, NH	102	Reno, NV	81
Canandaigua, NY	104	Kerrville, TX	47	Rhinelander, WI	49
Canton–Lake Tawakoni, TX	6	Laconia–		Roswell, NM	1
Cape Cod, MA	128	Lake Winnipesaukee, NH	112	St. George–Zion, UT	53
				St. Petersburg–Clearwater, FL	61
Cape May, NJ	123	Lake Havasu City–Kingman, AZ	42		
Carson City–Minden, NV	111	Lakeland–Winter Haven, FL	25	Salinas–Seaside–Monterey, CA	120
Chapel Hill, NC	96	Lancaster, PA	114	San Antonio, TX	21
Charleston, SC	40	Las Cruces, NM	13	San Diego, CA	125
Charlottesville, VA	93	Las Vegas, NV	84	San Luis Obispo, CA	109
				Santa Fe, NM	82
Chico–Paradise, CA	67	Lexington, KY	77		
Clayton–Clarkesville, GA	9	Litchfield County, CT	130	Santa Rosa–Petaluma, CA	122
Clear Lake, CA	78	Madison, WI	113	Sarasota, FL	94
Coeur d'Alene, ID	38	Maui, HI	131	Southport, NC	17
Colorado Springs, CO	57	McAllen–Edinburg–Mission, TX	2	Springfield, MO	14
				State College, PA	110
Columbia County, NY	100	Medford–Ashland, OR	87		
Crossville, TN	7	Melbourne–Titusville–		Traverse City–	
Daytona Beach, FL	46	Palm Bay, FL	83	Grand Traverse Bay, MI	80
Deming, NM	4	Miami–Hialeah, FL	105	Tucson, AZ	52
Door County, WI	69	Missoula, MT	74	Twain Harte–Yosemite, CA	92
		Monticello–Liberty, NY	97	Virginia Beach–Norfolk, VA	79
Eagle River, WI	71			West Palm Beach–Boca Raton–	
Easton–Chesapeake Bay, MD	107	Mountain Home–Bull Shoals, AR	28	Delray Beach, FL	106
Eugene–Springfield, OR	90	Murray–Kentucky Lake, KY	19		
Fairhope–Gulf Shores, AL	35	Myrtle Beach, SC	51	Winchester, VA	66
Fayetteville, AR	30	Naples, FL	126	Yuma, AZ	15

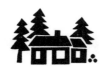

PLACE PROFILES: Housing

The following pages show housing features in each retirement place, dividing them into the categories of Local Choices, Typical Housing, Energy Requirements, and Annual Costs.

Data in the first category, Local Choices, show the mix of single detached houses, condominiums, mobile homes, and apartments (defined here as housing units in buildings with two or more rental units). These data are derived from the *1980 Census of Population and Housing*.

In the Typical Housing category, estimates on the median value for owner-occupied housing are derived from the *1980 Census of Population and Housing* and are adjusted for inflation using 1986 regional data from the National Association of Realtors quarterly publication *Existing Home Sales*. Property taxes are based on state-wide average residential rates taken from the 1986 issue of *Significant Features of Fiscal Federalism*, a publication of the Washington, DC–based Advisory Commission on Intergovernmental Relations. The percentages of housing units built before 1940 (defined as "old") and since 1980 (defined as "new") are estimated from the *1980 Census of Population and Housing* and from the Census Bureau's *Housing Permits and Construction*

Contracts for 1980, 1981, 1982, 1983, 1984, and 1985.

The heating season, listed under Energy Requirements, is given in terms of heating-degree days per year (see page 136 for explanation) and is taken from National Oceanic and Atmospheric Administration's *Climatography of the United States, Series 81*. The number of hours given for air conditioning represents the normal number of hours per year when the outside temperature climbs over 80 degrees Fahrenheit. These figures come from the Department of Defense manual *Engineering Weather Data*.

The dollar amounts given for Mortgage and Taxes are the annual sum of mortgage payments and property taxes. Utilities, too, are annual dollar amounts. Typical bills for residential natural gas by state are in *Gas Facts*, an annual report from the American Gas Association. The Energy Department's annual publication, *Typical Electric Bills*, details home electricity costs for each retirement place. To reflect realistic 1986 energy costs, data from these sources are adjusted for inflation using regional data from the Consumer Price Index for June 1986.

A star preceding a place's name highlights it as one of the best 15 places for homeowning costs.

Albuquerque, NM
Local Choices
62% houses, 2% condos, 6% mobile homes, 15% apartments (rent: $385)
Typical Housing
Median value: $67,500
Property taxes: $513
New: 16%   Old: 6%
Energy Requirements
Heating season: 4,292 degree days
Major source: Natural gas
Air conditioning: 1,130 hours
Annual Costs
Mortgage and taxes: $6,402
Utilities: $1,071

Score: 7,473
Rank: 55

Amherst–Northampton, MA
Local Choices
59% houses, 1% condos, 1% mobile homes, 12% apartments (rent: $300)
Typical Housing
Median value: $78,500
Property taxes: $1,233
New: 8%   Old: 37%
Energy Requirements
Heating season: 6,576 degree days
Major source: Oil
Air conditioning: 500 hours
Annual Costs
Mortgage and taxes: $8,082
Utilities: $1,230

Score: 9,312
Rank: 98

Ann Arbor, MI
Local Choices
53% houses, 3% condos, 2% mobile homes, 27% apartments (rent: $420)
Typical Housing
Median value: $84,300
Property taxes: $2,345
New: 8%   Old: 19%
Energy Requirements
Heating season: 6,306 degree days
Major source: Natural gas
Air conditioning: 511 hours
Annual Costs
Mortgage and taxes: $9,703
Utilities: $1,206

Score: 10,909
Rank: 118

Asheville, NC
Local Choices
71% houses, 1% condos, 11% mobile homes, 7% apartments (rent: $280)
Typical Housing
Median value: $56,100
Property taxes: $567
New: 10%   Old: 21%
Energy Requirements
Heating season: 4,237 degree days
Major source: Oil
Air conditioning: 610 hours
Annual Costs
Mortgage and taxes: $5,465
Utilities: $1,036

Score: 6,501
Rank: 29

Athens, GA
Local Choices
55% houses, 2% condos, 7% mobile homes, 24% apartments (rent: $310)
Typical Housing
Median value: $66,800
Property taxes: $722
New: 17%   Old: 10%
Energy Requirements
Heating season: 2,822 degree days
Major source: Natural gas
Air conditioning: 1,122 hours
Annual Costs
Mortgage and taxes: $6,553
Utilities: $968

Score: 7,521
Rank: 58

Athens–Cedar Creek Lake, TX
Local Choices
71% houses, 23% mobile homes, 3% apartments (rent: $275)
Typical Housing
Median value: $50,400
Property taxes: $665
New: 4%   Old: 10%
Energy Requirements
Heating season: 2,272 degree days
Major source: Natural gas
Air conditioning: 1,855 hours
Annual Costs
Mortgage and taxes: $5,063
Utilities: $840

Score: 5,903
Rank: 18

Austin, TX
Local Choices
60% houses, 2% condos, 4% mobile homes, 22% apartments (rent: $385)
Typical Housing
Median value: $78,500
Property taxes: $1,036
New: 29%   Old: 7%
Energy Requirements
Heating season: 1,737 degree days
Major source: Natural gas
Air conditioning: 2,243 hours
Annual Costs
Mortgage and taxes: $7,882
Utilities: $791

Score: 8,673
Rank: 89

Bar Harbor–Frenchman Bay, ME
Local Choices
76% houses, 1% condos, 9% mobile homes, 4% apartments (rent: $245)
Typical Housing
Median value: $69,700
Property taxes: $914
New: 4%   Old: 50%
Energy Requirements
Heating season: 7,240 degree days
Major source: Oil
Air conditioning: 137 hours
Annual Costs
Mortgage and taxes: $6,998
Utilities: $921

Score: 7,919
Rank: 72

Bellingham, WA
Local Choices
70% houses, 2% condos, 7% mobile homes, 11% apartments (rent: $385)
Typical Housing
Median value: $70,200
Property taxes: $709
New: 9%   Old: 25%
Energy Requirements
Heating season: 5,738 degree days
Major source: Total electric
Air conditioning: 40 hours
Annual Costs
Mortgage and taxes: $6,829
Utilities: $618

Score: 7,447
Rank: 54

Bend, OR
Local Choices
65% houses, 1% condos, 20% mobile homes, 6% apartments (rent: $430)
Typical Housing
Median value: $71,700
Property taxes: $1,592
New: 7%   Old: 11%
Energy Requirements
Heating season: 7,117 degree days
Major source: Total electric
Air conditioning: 375 hours
Annual Costs
Mortgage and taxes: $7,850
Utilities: $726

Score: 8,576
Rank: 86

Bennington, VT
Local Choices
67% houses, 1% condos, 8% mobile homes, 5% apartments (rent: $270)

Typical Housing
Median value: $80,400
Property taxes: $1,874
New: 7%   Old: 43%
Energy Requirements
Heating season: 7,681 degree days
Major source: Oil
Air conditioning: 335 hours
Annual Costs
Mortgage and taxes: $8,889
Utilities: $1,103

Score: 9,992
Rank: 108

Biloxi–Gulfport, MS
Local Choices
70% houses, 1% condos, 6% mobile homes, 11% apartments (rent: $315)
Typical Housing
Median value: $54,100
Property taxes: $417
New: 12%   Old: 10%
Energy Requirements
Heating season: 1,496 degree days
Major source: Natural gas
Air conditioning: 2,052 hours
Annual Costs
Mortgage and taxes: $5,139
Utilities: $782

Score: 5,921
Rank: 20

Blacksburg, VA
Local Choices
53% houses, 1% condos, 12% mobile homes, 21% apartments (rent: $370)
Typical Housing
Median value: $67,000
Property taxes: $670
New: 13%   Old: 11%
Energy Requirements
Heating season: 4,307 degree days
Major source: Natural gas
Air conditioning: 799 hours
Annual Costs
Mortgage and taxes: $6,515
Utilities: $1,033

Score: 7,548
Rank: 62

Bloomington–Brown County, IN
Local Choices
60% houses, 2% condos, 8% mobile homes, 21% apartments (rent: $300)
Typical Housing
Median value: $56,900
Property taxes: $694
New: 8%   Old: 16%
Energy Requirements
Heating season: 4,905 degree days
Major source: Natural gas
Air conditioning: 848 hours
Annual Costs
Mortgage and taxes: $5,654
Utilities: $1,148

Score: 6,802
Rank: 37

Boise, ID
Local Choices
70% houses, 2% condos, 7% mobile homes, 5% apartments (rent: $420)
Typical Housing
Median value: $69,000
Property taxes: $696
New: 13%   Old: 11%

Energy Requirements
Heating season: 5,833 degree days
Major source: Total electric
Air conditioning: 706 hours
Annual Costs
Mortgage and taxes: $6,712
Utilities: $618

Score: 7,330
Rank: 48

Bradenton, FL
Local Choices
48% houses, 12% condos, 22% mobile homes, 5% apartments (rent: $400)
Typical Housing
Median value: $70,600
Property taxes: $558
New: 20%   Old: 6%
Energy Requirements
Heating season: 597 degree days
Major source: Total electric
Air conditioning: 2,154 hours
Annual Costs
Mortgage and taxes: $6,714
Utilities: $1,324

Score: 8,038
Rank: 75

★ Branson–Cassville–Table Rock Lake, MO
Local Choices
77% houses, 1% condos, 15% mobile homes, 2% apartments (rent: $220)
Typical Housing
Median value: $47,200
Property taxes: $481
New: 2%   Old: 27%
Energy Requirements
Heating season: 4,406 degree days
Major source: Bottled gas
Air conditioning: 1,058 hours
Annual Costs
Mortgage and taxes: $4,599
Utilities: $981

Score: 5,580
Rank: 9

★ Brownsville–Harlingen, TX
Local Choices
65% houses, 2% condos, 7% mobile homes, 11% apartments (rent: $310)
Typical Housing
Median value: $38,300
Property taxes: $506
New: 18%   Old: 10%
Energy Requirements
Heating season: 650 degree days
Major source: Natural gas
Air conditioning: 2,295 hours
Annual Costs
Mortgage and taxes: $3,848
Utilities: $825

Score: 4,673
Rank: 3

Brunswick–Golden Isles, GA
Local Choices
70% houses, 2% condos, 8% mobile homes, 8% apartments (rent: $335)
Typical Housing
Median value: $56,900
Property taxes: $615
New: 11%   Old: 11%
Energy Requirements
Heating season: 1,331 degree days

Major source: Total electric
Air conditioning: 1,365 hours
Annual Costs
Mortgage and taxes: $5,580
Utilities: $912

Score: 6,492
Rank: 27

Burlington, VT
Local Choices
76% houses, 3% condos, 5% mobile
   homes, 12% apartments (rent: $325)
Typical Housing
Median value: $104,600
Property taxes: $2,438
New: 12%   Old: 29%
Energy Requirements
Heating season: 7,876 degree days
Major source: Oil
Air conditioning: 263 hours
Annual Costs
Mortgage and taxes: $11,565
Utilities: $1,103

Score: 12,668
Rank: 129

Burnet–Marble Falls–Llano, TX
Local Choices
79% houses, 1% condos, 13% mobile
   homes, 2% apartments (rent: $355)
Typical Housing
Median value: $55,500
Property taxes: $733
New: 5%   Old: 12%
Energy Requirements
Heating season: 2,163 degree days
Major source: Total electric
Air conditioning: 1,715 hours
Annual Costs
Mortgage and taxes: $5,577
Utilities: $1,035

Score: 6,612
Rank: 33

Camden–Penobscot Bay, ME
Local Choices
73% houses, 1% condos, 6% mobile
   homes, 5% apartments (rent: $255)
Typical Housing
Median value: $69,900
Property taxes: $916
New: 5%   Old: 58%
Energy Requirements
Heating season: 7,353 degree days
Major source: Oil
Air conditioning: 236 hours
Annual Costs
Mortgage and taxes: $7,017
Utilities: $921

Score: 7,938
Rank: 73

Canandaigua, NY
Local Choices
68% houses, 1% condos, 8% mobile
   homes, 5% apartments (rent: $275)
Typical Housing
Median value: $74,500
Property taxes: $2,086
New: 6%   Old: 46%
Energy Requirements
Heating season: 6,656 degree days
Major source: Natural gas
Air conditioning: 419 hours

Annual Costs
Mortgage and taxes: $8,587
Utilities: $1,165

Score: 9,752
Rank: 104

★ Canton–Lake Tawakoni, TX
Local Choices
84% houses, 10% mobile homes, 1%
   apartments (rent: $210)
Typical Housing
Median value: $42,800
Property taxes: $565
New: 3%   Old: 14%
Energy Requirements
Heating season: 2,272 degree days
Major source: Natural gas
Air conditioning: 1,855 hours
Annual Costs
Mortgage and taxes: $4,299
Utilities: $840

Score: 5,139
Rank: 6

Cape Cod, MA
Local Choices
81% houses, 3% condos, 5% apartments
   (rent: $315)
Typical Housing
Median value: $104,800
Property taxes: $1,646
New: 24%   Old: 14%
Energy Requirements
Heating season: 5,395 degree days
Major source: Oil
Air conditioning: 164 hours
Annual Costs
Mortgage and taxes: $10,789
Utilities: $1,225

Score: 12,014
Rank: 128

Cape May, NJ
Local Choices
65% houses, 3% condos, 2% mobile
   homes, 5% apartments (rent: $330)
Typical Housing
Median value: $89,900
Property taxes: $2,357
New: 22%   Old: 19%
Energy Requirements
Heating season: 4,946 degree days
Major source: Oil
Air conditioning: 508 hours
Annual Costs
Mortgage and taxes: $10,203
Utilities: $1,291

Score: 11,494
Rank: 123

Carson City–Minden, NV
Local Choices
54% houses, 7% condos, 16% mobile
   homes, 14% apartments (rent: $560)
Typical Housing
Median value: $97,600
Property taxes: $615
New: 9%   Old: 3%
Energy Requirements
Heating season: 5,753 degree days
Major source: Natural gas
Air conditioning: 574 hours
Annual Costs
Mortgage and taxes: $9,129

Utilities: $996
Score: 10,125
Rank: 111

Chapel Hill, NC
Local Choices
53% houses, 1% condos, 11% mobile
   homes, 20% apartments (rent: $390)
Typical Housing
Median value: $85,200
Property taxes: $860
New: 16%   Old: 10%
Energy Requirements
Heating season: 3,454 degree days
Major source: Total electric
Air conditioning: 977 hours
Annual Costs
Mortgage and taxes: $8,288
Utilities: $1,020

Score: 9,308
Rank: 96

Charleston, SC
Local Choices
58% houses, 2% condos, 8% mobile
   homes, 9% apartments (rent: $340)
Typical Housing
Median value: $64,100
Property taxes: $519
New: 15%   Old: 12%
Energy Requirements
Heating season: 1,904 degree days
Major source: Natural gas
Air conditioning: 1,252 hours
Annual Costs
Mortgage and taxes: $6,107
Utilities: $916

Score: 7,023
Rank: 40

Charlottesville, VA
Local Choices
61% houses, 1% condos, 5% mobile
   homes, 16% apartments (rent: $415)
Typical Housing
Median value: $81,400
Property taxes: $814
New: 14%   Old: 18%
Energy Requirements
Heating season: 4,162 degree days
Major source: Natural gas
Air conditioning: 826 hours
Annual Costs
Mortgage and taxes: $7,918
Utilities: $1,084

Score: 9,002
Rank: 93

Chico–Paradise, CA
Local Choices
63% houses, 1% condos, 14% mobile
   homes, 11% apartments (rent: $375)
Typical Housing
Median value: $71,400
Property taxes: $728
New: 12%   Old: 11%
Energy Requirements
Heating season: 2,865 degree days
Major source: Natural gas
Air conditioning: 1,410 hours
Annual Costs
Mortgage and taxes: $6,954
Utilities: $885

Score: 7,839
Rank: 67

★ Clayton–Clarkesville, GA

Local Choices
78% houses, 16% mobile homes, 1% apartments (rent: $225)
Typical Housing
Median value: $47,000
Property taxes: $508
New: 8% Old: 16%
Energy Requirements
Heating season: 3,672 degree days
Major source: Bottled gas
Air conditioning: 1,011 hours
Annual Costs
Mortgage and taxes: $4,612
Utilities: $968

Score: 5,580
Rank: 9

Clear Lake, CA

Local Choices
57% houses, 32% mobile homes, 3% apartments (rent: $365)
Typical Housing
Median value: $70,800
Property taxes: $722
New: 12% Old: 9%
Energy Requirements
Heating season: 2,460 degree days
Major source: Total electric
Air conditioning: 1,200 hours
Annual Costs
Mortgage and taxes: $6,895
Utilities: $1,429

Score: 8,324
Rank: 78

Coeur d'Alene, ID

Local Choices
69% houses, 13% mobile homes, 6% apartments (rent: $385)
Typical Housing
Median value: $64,500
Property taxes: $651
New: 11% Old: 14%
Energy Requirements
Heating season: 6,564 degree days
Major source: Total electric
Air conditioning: 363 hours
Annual Costs
Mortgage and taxes: $6,277
Utilities: $556

Score: 6,833
Rank: 38

Colorado Springs, CO

Local Choices
63% houses, 2% condos, 4% mobile homes, 17% apartments (rent: $365)
Typical Housing
Median value: $69,400
Property taxes: $680
New: 20% Old: 10%
Energy Requirements
Heating season: 6,473 degree days
Major source: Natural gas
Air conditioning: 644 hours
Annual Costs
Mortgage and taxes: $6,738
Utilities: $768

Score: 7,506
Rank: 57

Columbia County, NY

Local Choices
68% houses, 8% mobile homes, 4% apartments (rent: $240)
Typical Housing
Median value: $73,400
Property taxes: $2,054
New: 3% Old: 46%
Energy Requirements
Heating season: 6,888 degree days
Major source: Oil
Air conditioning: 420 hours
Annual Costs
Mortgage and taxes: $8,455
Utilities: $1,091

Score: 9,546
Rank: 100

★ Crossville, TN

Local Choices
80% houses, 2% condos, 9% mobile homes, 3% apartments (rent: $240)
Typical Housing
Median value: $47,500
Property taxes: $460
New: 10% Old: 11%
Energy Requirements
Heating season: 4,744 degree days
Major source: Total electric
Air conditioning: 1,150 hours
Annual Costs
Mortgage and taxes: $4,601
Utilities: $727

Score: 5,328
Rank: 7

Daytona Beach, FL

Local Choices
63% houses, 6% condos, 11% mobile homes, 9% apartments (rent: $360)
Typical Housing
Median value: $61,900
Property taxes: $489
New: 23% Old: 7%
Energy Requirements
Heating season: 897 degree days
Major source: Total electric
Air conditioning: 1,675 hours
Annual Costs
Mortgage and taxes: $5,887
Utilities: $1,324

Score: 7,211
Rank: 46

★ Deming, NM

Local Choices
62% houses, 22% mobile homes, 6% apartments (rent: $245)
Typical Housing
Median value: $38,800
Property taxes: $295
New: 1% Old: 15%
Energy Requirements
Heating season: 3,294 degree days
Major source: Natural gas
Air conditioning: 1,848 hours
Annual Costs
Mortgage and taxes: $3,676
Utilities: $1,068

Score: 4,744
Rank: 4

Door County, WI

Local Choices
80% houses, 1% condos, 6% mobile homes, 2% apartments (rent: $300)
Typical Housing
Median value: $63,500
Property taxes: $1,271
New: 14% Old: 33%
Energy Requirements
Heating season: 7,876 degree days
Major source: Oil
Air conditioning: 264 hours
Annual Costs
Mortgage and taxes: $6,813
Utilities: $1,054

Score: 7,867
Rank: 69

Eagle River, WI

Local Choices
78% houses, 5% mobile homes, 2% apartments (rent: $290)
Typical Housing
Median value: $63,500
Property taxes: $1,271
New: 12% Old: 20%
Energy Requirements
Heating season: 9,339 degree days
Major source: Bottled gas
Air conditioning: 436 hours
Annual Costs
Mortgage and taxes: $6,813
Utilities: $1,105

Score: 7,918
Rank: 71

Easton–Chesapeake Bay, MD

Local Choices
78% houses, 1% condos, 4% mobile homes, 4% apartments (rent: $340)
Typical Housing
Median value: $86,900
Property taxes: $1,094
New: 10% Old: 36%
Energy Requirements
Heating season: 4,299 degree days
Major source: Oil
Air conditioning: 635 hours
Annual Costs
Mortgage and taxes: $8,671
Utilities: $1,162

Score: 9,833
Rank: 107

Eugene–Springfield, OR

Local Choices
64% houses, 1% condos, 8% mobile homes, 13% apartments (rent: $390)
Typical Housing
Median value: $75,100
Property taxes: $1,668
New: 4% Old: 10%
Energy Requirements
Heating season: 4,739 degree days
Major source: Total electric
Air conditioning: 441 hours
Annual Costs
Mortgage and taxes: $8,220
Utilities: $479

Score: 8,699
Rank: 90

Fairhope–Gulf Shores, AL

Local Choices
78% houses, 1% condos, 13% mobile homes, 3% apartments (rent: $350)
Typical Housing
Median value: $63,700
Property taxes: $261
New: 18%   Old: 11%
Energy Requirements
Heating season: 1,573 degree days
Major source: Natural gas
Air conditioning: 1,514 hours
Annual Costs
Mortgage and taxes: $5,822
Utilities: $897

Score: 6,719
Rank: 35

Fayetteville, AR

Local Choices
71% houses, 8% mobile homes, 10% apartments (rent: $315)
Typical Housing
Median value: $56,900
Property taxes: $768
New: 8%   Old: 14%
Energy Requirements
Heating season: 3,938 degree days
Major source: Natural gas
Air conditioning: 966 hours
Annual Costs
Mortgage and taxes: $5,734
Utilities: $812

Score: 6,546
Rank: 30

Flagstaff, AZ

Local Choices
58% houses, 1% condos, 19% mobile homes, 10% apartments (rent: $495)
Typical Housing
Median value: $67,100
Property taxes: $477
New: 20%   Old: 5%
Energy Requirements
Heating season: 7,322 degree days
Major source: Natural gas
Air conditioning: 184 hours
Annual Costs
Mortgage and taxes: $6,334
Utilities: $851

Score: 7,185
Rank: 44

Fort Collins–Loveland, CO

Local Choices
63% houses, 4% condos, 8% mobile homes, 13% apartments (rent: $410)
Typical Housing
Median value: $81,200
Property taxes: $795
New: 16%   Old: 12%
Energy Requirements
Heating season: 6,599 degree days
Major source: Natural gas
Air conditioning: 647 hours
Annual Costs
Mortgage and taxes: $7,874
Utilities: $881

Score: 8,755
Rank: 91

Fort Lauderdale–Hollywood– Pompano Beach, FL

Local Choices
42% houses, 28% condos, 5% mobile homes, 14% apartments (rent: $470)
Typical Housing
Median value: $97,600
Property taxes: $771
New: 11%   Old: 2%
Energy Requirements
Heating season: 244 degree days
Major source: Total electric
Air conditioning: 2,342 hours
Annual Costs
Mortgage and taxes: $9,281
Utilities: $1,324

Score: 10,605
Rank: 116

Fort Myers–Cape Coral, FL

Local Choices
52% houses, 14% condos, 18% mobile homes, 6% apartments (rent: $415)
Typical Housing
Median value: $82,700
Property taxes: $653
New: 32%   Old: 3%
Energy Requirements
Heating season: 457 degree days
Major source: Total electric
Air conditioning: 1,863 hours
Annual Costs
Mortgage and taxes: $7,865
Utilities: $1,324

Score: 9,189
Rank: 95

Fort Walton Beach, FL

Local Choices
62% houses, 7% condos, 11% mobile homes, 8% apartments (rent: $340)
Typical Housing
Median value: $67,900
Property taxes: $537
New: 25%   Old: 3%
Energy Requirements
Heating season: 1,361 degree days
Major source: Total electric
Air conditioning: 1,788 hours
Annual Costs
Mortgage and taxes: $6,463
Utilities: $1,059

Score: 7,522
Rank: 59

★ Franklin County, TN

Local Choices
84% houses, 8% mobile homes, 2% apartments (rent: $210)
Typical Housing
Median value: $50,100
Property taxes: $486
New: 1%   Old: 19%
Energy Requirements
Heating season: 3,497 degree days
Major source: Total electric
Air conditioning: 1,056 hours
Annual Costs
Mortgage and taxes: $4,856
Utilities: $664

Score: 5,520
Rank: 8

Fredericksburg, TX

Local Choices
83% houses, 8% mobile homes, 2% apartments (rent: $340)
Typical Housing
Median value: $64,100
Property taxes: $846
New: 7%   Old: 30%
Energy Requirements
Heating season: 2,107 degree days
Major source: Natural gas
Air conditioning: 1,715 hours
Annual Costs
Mortgage and taxes: $6,434
Utilities: $752

Score: 7,186
Rank: 45

Friday Harbor–San Juan Islands, WA

Local Choices
78% houses, 3% condos, 8% mobile homes, 3% apartments (rent: $435)
Typical Housing
Median value: $105,400
Property taxes: $1,065
New: 16%   Old: 13%
Energy Requirements
Heating season: 5,609 degree days
Major source: Total electric
Air conditioning: 53 hours
Annual Costs
Mortgage and taxes: $10,261
Utilities: $742

Score: 11,003
Rank: 119

Front Royal, VA

Local Choices
74% houses, 1% condos, 6% mobile homes, 8% apartments (rent: $285)
Typical Housing
Median value: $63,000
Property taxes: $630
New: 8%   Old: 21%
Energy Requirements
Heating season: 4,375 degree days
Major source: Oil
Air conditioning: 679 hours
Annual Costs
Mortgage and taxes: $6,123
Utilities: $959

Score: 7,082
Rank: 41

Gainesville–Lake Lanier, GA

Local Choices
73% houses, 13% mobile homes, 6% apartments (rent: $290)
Typical Housing
Median value: $58,500
Property taxes: $632
New: 14%   Old: 12%
Energy Requirements
Heating season: 3,267 degree days
Major source: Total electric
Air conditioning: 1,077 hours
Annual Costs
Mortgage and taxes: $5,732
Utilities: $912

Score: 6,644
Rank: 34

Grand Junction, CO
Local Choices
67% houses, 2% condos, 12% mobile homes, 8% apartments (rent: $410)
Typical Housing
Median value: $71,200
Property taxes: $698
New: 23%   Old: 14%
Energy Requirements
Heating season: 5,605 degree days
Major source: Natural gas
Air conditioning: 988 hours
Annual Costs
Mortgage and taxes: $6,914
Utilities: $970

Score: 7,884
Rank: 70

★ Grand Lake–Lake Tenkiller, OK
Local Choices
76% houses, 14% mobile homes, 3% apartments (rent: $240)
Typical Housing
Median value: $49,800
Property taxes: $473
New: 3%   Old: 13%
Energy Requirements
Heating season: 3,587 degree days
Major source: Natural gas
Air conditioning: 1,399 hours
Annual Costs
Mortgage and taxes: $4,816
Utilities: $837

Score: 5,653
Rank: 11

Grass Valley–Truckee, CA
Local Choices
75% houses, 2% condos, 11% mobile homes, 5% apartments (rent: $435)
Typical Housing
Median value: $96,200
Property taxes: $982
New: 26%   Old: 12%
Energy Requirements
Heating season: 4,900 degree days
Major source: Total electric
Air conditioning: 647 hours
Annual Costs
Mortgage and taxes: $9,378
Utilities: $1,429

Score: 10,807
Rank: 117

Hamilton–Bitterroot Valley, MT
Local Choices
72% houses, 15% mobile homes, 5% apartments (rent: $280)
Typical Housing
Median value: $58,200
Property taxes: $664
New: 1%   Old: 29%
Energy Requirements
Heating season: 7,187 degree days
Major source: Natural gas
Air conditioning: 303 hours
Annual Costs
Mortgage and taxes: $5,741
Utilities: $744

Score: 6,485
Rank: 26

Hanover, NH
Local Choices
61% houses, 5% condos, 8% mobile homes, 10% apartments (rent: $275)
Typical Housing
Median value: $77,400
Property taxes: $1,563
New: 6%   Old: 43%
Energy Requirements
Heating season: 7,680 degree days
Major source: Oil
Air conditioning: 312 hours
Annual Costs
Mortgage and taxes: $8,312
Utilities: $1,163

Score: 9,475
Rank: 99

Hendersonville–Brevard, NC
Local Choices
74% houses, 1% condos, 12% mobile homes, 3% apartments (rent: $295)
Typical Housing
Median value: $65,600
Property taxes: $663
New: 12%   Old: 13%
Energy Requirements
Heating season: 4,266 degree days
Major source: Oil
Air conditioning: 610 hours
Annual Costs
Mortgage and taxes: $6,386
Utilities: $970

Score: 7,356
Rank: 50

Hilton Head–Beaufort, SC
Local Choices
58% houses, 17% condos, 15% mobile homes, 4% apartments (rent: $425)
Typical Housing
Median value: $78,500
Property taxes: $636
New: 8%   Old: 4%
Energy Requirements
Heating season: 1,941 degree days
Major source: Total electric
Air conditioning: 1,393 hours
Annual Costs
Mortgage and taxes: $7,482
Utilities: $1,159

Score: 8,641
Rank: 88

Hot Springs–Lake Ouachita, AR
Local Choices
69% houses, 3% condos, 8% mobile homes, 9% apartments (rent: $220)
Typical Housing
Median value: $48,900
Property taxes: $660
New: 4%   Old: 19%
Energy Requirements
Heating season: 2,729 degree days
Major source: Natural gas
Air conditioning: 1,643 hours
Annual Costs
Mortgage and taxes: $4,922
Utilities: $930

Score: 5,852
Rank: 16

★ Houghton Lake, MI
Local Choices
85% houses, 9% mobile homes, 1% apartments (rent: $240)
Typical Housing
Median value: $40,000
Property taxes: $1,112
New: 3%   Old: 10%
Energy Requirements
Heating season: 8,347 degree days
Major source: Natural gas
Air conditioning: 218 hours
Annual Costs
Mortgage and taxes: $4,600
Utilities: $1,111

Score: 5,711
Rank: 12

Iowa City, IA
Local Choices
52% houses, 1% condos, 7% mobile homes, 27% apartments (rent: $335)
Typical Housing
Median value: $83,500
Property taxes: $1,361
New: 9%   Old: 21%
Energy Requirements
Heating season: 6,404 degree days
Major source: Natural gas
Air conditioning: 615 hours
Annual Costs
Mortgage and taxes: $8,648
Utilities: $1,056

Score: 9,704
Rank: 103

Kalispell, MT
Local Choices
67% houses, 18% mobile homes, 5% apartments (rent: $325)
Typical Housing
Median value: $57,800
Property taxes: $659
New: 6%   Old: 21%
Energy Requirements
Heating season: 8,554 degree days
Major source: Natural gas
Air conditioning: 26 hours
Annual Costs
Mortgage and taxes: $5,705
Utilities: $761

Score: 6,466
Rank: 24

Kauai, HI
Local Choices
71% houses, 13% condos, 5% apartments (rent: $415)
Typical Housing
Median value: $109,700
Property taxes: $559
New: 17%   Old: 15%
Energy Requirements
Heating season: 0 degree days
Major source: Total electric
Air conditioning: 1,091 hours
Annual Costs
Mortgage and taxes: $10,125
Utilities: $1,786

Score: 11,911
Rank: 127

Keene, NH
Local Choices
66% houses, 7% mobile homes, 9% apartments (rent: $295)
Typical Housing
Median value: $78,100
Property taxes: $1,578
New: 7%   Old: 43%
Energy Requirements
Heating season: 6,969 degree days
Major source: Oil
Air conditioning: 335 hours
Annual Costs
Mortgage and taxes: $8,394
Utilities: $1,216
Score: 9,610
Rank: 102

Kerrville, TX
Local Choices
67% houses, 14% mobile homes, 7% apartments (rent: $345)
Typical Housing
Median value: $65,300
Property taxes: $862
New: 8%   Old: 15%
Energy Requirements
Heating season: 2,399 degree days
Major source: Natural gas
Air conditioning: 1,715 hours
Annual Costs
Mortgage and taxes: $6,558
Utilities: $746
Score: 7,304
Rank: 47

Laconia–Lake Winnipesaukee, NH
Local Choices
63% houses, 3% condos, 8% mobile homes, 9% apartments (rent: $270)
Typical Housing
Median value: $83,100
Property taxes: $1,678
New: 15%   Old: 36%
Energy Requirements
Heating season: 7,315 degree days
Major source: Oil
Air conditioning: 398 hours
Annual Costs
Mortgage and taxes: $8,927
Utilities: $1,216
Score: 10,143
Rank: 112

Lake Havasu City–Kingman, AZ
Local Choices
51% houses, 2% condos, 39% mobile homes, 3% apartments (rent: $480)
Typical Housing
Median value: $59,300
Property taxes: $421
New: 21%   Old: 3%
Energy Requirements
Heating season: 2,425 degree days
Major source: Total electric
Air conditioning: 2,360 hours
Annual Costs
Mortgage and taxes: $5,593
Utilities: $1,520
Score: 7,113
Rank: 42

Lakeland–Winter Haven, FL
Local Choices
66% houses, 2% condos, 16% mobile homes, 7% apartments (rent: $330)
Typical Housing
Median value: $55,800
Property taxes: $441
New: 13%   Old: 10%
Energy Requirements
Heating season: 678 degree days
Major source: Total electric
Air conditioning: 1,759 hours
Annual Costs
Mortgage and taxes: $5,312
Utilities: $1,171
Score: 6,483
Rank: 25

Lancaster, PA
Local Choices
55% houses, 1% condos, 5% mobile homes, 10% apartments (rent: $270)
Typical Housing
Median value: $89,900
Property taxes: $1,376
New: 8%   Old: 37%
Energy Requirements
Heating season: 5,283 degree days
Major source: Oil
Air conditioning: 654 hours
Annual Costs
Mortgage and taxes: $9,223
Utilities: $1,190
Score: 10,413
Rank: 114

★ Las Cruces, NM
Local Choices
60% houses, 1% condos, 17% mobile homes, 8% apartments (rent: $355)
Typical Housing
Median value: $50,500
Property taxes: $384
New: 16%   Old: 9%
Energy Requirements
Heating season: 3,194 degree days
Major source: Natural gas
Air conditioning: 1,848 hours
Annual Costs
Mortgage and taxes: $4,787
Utilities: $1,018
Score: 5,805
Rank: 13

Las Vegas, NV
Local Choices
49% houses, 5% condos, 11% mobile homes, 20% apartments (rent: $510)
Typical Housing
Median value: $81,900
Property taxes: $516
New: 22%   Old: 1%
Energy Requirements
Heating season: 2,601 degree days
Major source: Total electric
Air conditioning: 2,360 hours
Annual Costs
Mortgage and taxes: $7,658
Utilities: $896
Score: 8,554
Rank: 84

Lexington, KY
Local Choices
62% houses, 1% condos, 4% mobile homes, 22% apartments (rent: $340)
Typical Housing
Median value: $74,600
Property taxes: $709
New: 8%   Old: 19%
Energy Requirements
Heating season: 4,729 degree days
Major source: Natural gas
Air conditioning: 954 hours
Annual Costs
Mortgage and taxes: $7,217
Utilities: $903
Score: 8,120
Rank: 77

Litchfield County, CT
Local Choices
70% houses, 2% condos, 1% mobile homes, 7% apartments (rent: $295)
Typical Housing
Median value: $114,500
Property taxes: $1,924
New: 10%   Old: 36%
Energy Requirements
Heating season: 6,150 degree days
Major source: Oil
Air conditioning: 344 hours
Annual Costs
Mortgage and taxes: $11,915
Utilities: $1,330
Score: 13,245
Rank: 130

Madison, WI
Local Choices
55% houses, 1% condos, 1% mobile homes, 25% apartments (rent: $345)
Typical Housing
Median value: $84,600
Property taxes: $1,692
New: 8%   Old: 21%
Energy Requirements
Heating season: 7,730 degree days
Major source: Natural gas
Air conditioning: 485 hours
Annual Costs
Mortgage and taxes: $9,075
Utilities: $1,084
Score: 10,159
Rank: 113

Maui, HI
Local Choices
51% houses, 32% condos, 11% apartments (rent: $660)
Typical Housing
Median value: $137,200
Property taxes: $700
New: 22%   Old: 10%
Energy Requirements
Heating season: 0 degree days
Major source: Total electric
Air conditioning: 1,414 hours
Annual Costs
Mortgage and taxes: $12,667
Utilities: $1,636
Score: 14,303
Rank: 131

★ McAllen–Edinburg–Mission, TX
Local Choices
67% houses, 1% condos, 10% mobile homes, 9% apartments (rent: $270)
Typical Housing
Median value: $37,500
Property taxes: $495
New: 16%   Old: 8%
Energy Requirements
Heating season: 696 degree days
Major source: Natural gas
Air conditioning: 2,527 hours
Annual Costs
Mortgage and taxes: $3,770
Utilities: $839

Score: 4,609
Rank: 2

Medford–Ashland, OR
Local Choices
67% houses, 1% condos, 13% mobile homes, 9% apartments (rent: $400)
Typical Housing
Median value: $72,000
Property taxes: $1,598
New: 5%   Old: 13%
Energy Requirements
Heating season: 4,930 degree days
Major source: Total electric
Air conditioning: 630 hours
Annual Costs
Mortgage and taxes: $7,876
Utilities: $726

Score: 8,602
Rank: 87

Melbourne–Titusville–Palm Bay, FL
Local Choices
63% houses, 7% condos, 11% mobile homes, 10% apartments (rent: $365)
Typical Housing
Median value: $75,800
Property taxes: $599
New: 28%   Old: 2%
Energy Requirements
Heating season: 611 degree days
Major source: Total electric
Air conditioning: 2,088 hours
Annual Costs
Mortgage and taxes: $7,215
Utilities: $1,324

Score: 8,539
Rank: 83

Miami–Hialeah, FL
Local Choices
43% houses, 13% condos, 2% mobile homes, 28% apartments (rent: $405)
Typical Housing
Median value: $88,700
Property taxes: $701
New: 13%   Old: 6%
Energy Requirements
Heating season: 206 degree days
Major source: Total electric
Air conditioning: 2,408 hours
Annual Costs
Mortgage and taxes: $8,440
Utilities: $1,324

Score: 9,764
Rank: 105

Missoula, MT
Local Choices
56% houses, 1% condos, 14% mobile homes, 10% apartments (rent: $375)
Typical Housing
Median value: $73,500
Property taxes: $838
New: 3%   Old: 19%
Energy Requirements
Heating season: 7,931 degree days
Major source: Natural gas
Air conditioning: 303 hours
Annual Costs
Mortgage and taxes: $7,254
Utilities: $769

Score: 8,023
Rank: 74

Monticello–Liberty, NY
Local Choices
67% houses, 8% mobile homes, 8% apartments (rent: $260)
Typical Housing
Median value: $70,900
Property taxes: $1,985
New: 4%   Old: 32%
Energy Requirements
Heating season: 6,556 degree days
Major source: Oil
Air conditioning: 623 hours
Annual Costs
Mortgage and taxes: $8,169
Utilities: $1,141

Score: 9,310
Rank: 97

Mountain Home–Bull Shoals, AR
Local Choices
79% houses, 1% condos, 13% mobile homes, 2% apartments (rent: $270)
Typical Housing
Median value: $54,200
Property taxes: $732
New: 2%   Old: 9%
Energy Requirements
Heating season: 3,852 degree days
Major source: Total electric
Air conditioning: 966 hours
Annual Costs
Mortgage and taxes: $5,461
Utilities: $1,033

Score: 6,494
Rank: 28

Murray–Kentucky Lake, KY
Local Choices
77% houses, 11% mobile homes, 3% apartments (rent: $240)
Typical Housing
Median value: $54,000
Property taxes: $513
New: 0.3%   Old: 14%
Energy Requirements
Heating season: 3,893 degree days
Major source: Total electric
Air conditioning: 1,160 hours
Annual Costs
Mortgage and taxes: $5,227
Utilities: $680

Score: 5,907
Rank: 19

Myrtle Beach, SC
Local Choices
64% houses, 4% condos, 16% mobile homes, 4% apartments (rent: $340)
Typical Housing
Median value: $66,700
Property taxes: $540
New: 22%   Old: 8%
Energy Requirements
Heating season: 2,023 degree days
Major source: Total electric
Air conditioning: 1,204 hours
Annual Costs
Mortgage and taxes: $6,358
Utilities: $1,020

Score: 7,378
Rank: 51

Naples, FL
Local Choices
42% houses, 29% condos, 13% mobile homes, 7% apartments (rent: $390)
Typical Housing
Median value: $110,300
Property taxes: $871
New: 47%   Old: 1%
Energy Requirements
Heating season: 345 degree days
Major source: Total electric
Air conditioning: 1,890 hours
Annual Costs
Mortgage and taxes: $10,491
Utilities: $1,324

Score: 11,815
Rank: 126

New Paltz–Ulster County, NY
Local Choices
66% houses, 1% condos, 6% mobile homes, 1% apartments (rent: $295)
Typical Housing
Median value: $71,500
Property taxes: $2,001
New: 5%   Old: 37%
Energy Requirements
Heating season: 7,447 degree days
Major source: Oil
Air conditioning: 460 hours
Annual Costs
Mortgage and taxes: $8,235
Utilities: $1,357

Score: 9,592
Rank: 101

Newport–Lincoln City, OR
Local Choices
66% houses, 3% condos, 15% mobile homes, 6% apartments (rent: $365)
Typical Housing
Median value: $67,100
Property taxes: $1,491
New: 9%   Old: 15%
Energy Requirements
Heating season: 5,235 degree days
Major source: Total electric
Air conditioning: 296 hours
Annual Costs
Mortgage and taxes: $7,348
Utilities: $726

Score: 8,074
Rank: 76

North Conway–White Mountains, NH
Local Choices
78% houses, 2% condos, 6% mobile homes, 4% apartments (rent: $275)
Typical Housing
Median value: $86,100
Property taxes: $1,740
New: 9%   Old: 35%
Energy Requirements
Heating season: 7,612 degree days
Major source: Oil
Air conditioning: 398 hours
Annual Costs
Mortgage and taxes: $9,254
Utilities: $1,216

Score: 10,470
Rank: 115

Oak Harbor–Whidbey Island, WA
Local Choices
74% houses, 1% condos, 11% mobile homes, 7% apartments (rent: $380)
Typical Housing
Median value: $80,400
Property taxes: $812
New: 13%   Old: 8%
Energy Requirements
Heating season: 5,380 degree days
Major source: Total electric
Air conditioning: 53 hours
Annual Costs
Mortgage and taxes: $7,828
Utilities: $742

Score: 8,570
Rank: 85

Ocala, FL
Local Choices
66% houses, 2% condos, 22% mobile homes, 4% apartments (rent: $325)
Typical Housing
Median value: $55,800
Property taxes: $441
New: 28%   Old: 5%
Energy Requirements
Heating season: 700 degree days
Major source: Total electric
Air conditioning: 1,824 hours
Annual Costs
Mortgage and taxes: $5,312
Utilities: $1,282

Score: 6,594
Rank: 32

Ocean City–Assateague Island, MD
Local Choices
50% houses, 29% condos, 7% mobile homes, 4% apartments (rent: $350)
Typical Housing
Median value: $58,900
Property taxes: $743
New: 31%   Old: 15%
Energy Requirements
Heating season: 4,303 degree days
Major source: Oil
Air conditioning: 461 hours
Annual Costs
Mortgage and taxes: $5,884
Utilities: $1,268

Score: 7,152
Rank: 43

Ocean County, NJ
Local Choices
73% houses, 8% condos, 3% mobile homes, 6% apartments (rent: $345)
Typical Housing
Median value: $92,000
Property taxes: $2,412
New: 15%   Old: 8%
Energy Requirements
Heating season: 5,128 degree days
Major source: Oil
Air conditioning: 586 hours
Annual Costs
Mortgage and taxes: $10,441
Utilities: $1,270

Score: 11,711
Rank: 124

Olympia, WA
Local Choices
64% houses, 1% condos, 11% mobile homes, 10% apartments (rent: $425)
Typical Housing
Median value: $70,900
Property taxes: $716
New: 12%   Old: 12%
Energy Requirements
Heating season: 5,530 degree days
Major source: Total electric
Air conditioning: 117 hours
Annual Costs
Mortgage and taxes: $6,900
Utilities: $773

Score: 7,673
Rank: 63

Orlando, FL
Local Choices
64% houses, 4% condos, 8% mobile homes, 14% apartments (rent: $385)
Typical Housing
Median value: $70,700
Property taxes: $559
New: 25%   Old: 5%
Energy Requirements
Heating season: 704 degree days
Major source: Total electric
Air conditioning: 1,675 hours
Annual Costs
Mortgage and taxes: $6,729
Utilities: $1,051

Score: 7,780
Rank: 65

Oscoda–Huron Shore, MI
Local Choices
77% houses, 9% mobile homes, 5% apartments (rent: $270)
Typical Housing
Median value: $42,900
Property taxes: $1,191
New: 4%   Old: 14%
Energy Requirements
Heating season: 7,506 degree days
Major source: Natural gas
Air conditioning: 219 hours
Annual Costs
Mortgage and taxes: $4,930
Utilities: $1,143

Score: 6,073
Rank: 22

Panama City, FL
Local Choices
64% houses, 4% condos, 13% mobile homes, 7% apartments (rent: $315)
Typical Housing
Median value: $53,400
Property taxes: $421
New: 25%   Old: 4%
Energy Requirements
Heating season: 1,388 degree days
Major source: Total electric
Air conditioning: 1,908 hours
Annual Costs
Mortgage and taxes: $5,076
Utilities: $1,051

Score: 6,127
Rank: 23

★ Paris–Big Sandy, TN
Local Choices
78% houses, 12% mobile homes, 2% apartments (rent: $225)
Typical Housing
Median value: $45,800
Property taxes: $444
New: 3%   Old: 20%
Energy Requirements
Heating season: 3,882 degree days
Major source: Total electric
Air conditioning: 1,160 hours
Annual Costs
Mortgage and taxes: $4,435
Utilities: $687

Score: 5,122
Rank: 5

Petoskey–Straits of Mackinac, MI
Local Choices
75% houses, 2% condos, 8% mobile homes, 5% apartments (rent: $280)
Typical Housing
Median value: $55,700
Property taxes: $1,549
New: 9%   Old: 33%
Energy Requirements
Heating season: 7,669 degree days
Major source: Natural gas
Air conditioning: 301 hours
Annual Costs
Mortgage and taxes: $6,411
Utilities: $1,123

Score: 7,534
Rank: 60

Phoenix, AZ
Local Choices
61% houses, 6% condos, 8% mobile homes, 14% apartments (rent: $485)
Typical Housing
Median value: $73,300
Property taxes: $520
New: 26%   Old: 3%
Energy Requirements
Heating season: 1,552 degree days
Major source: Natural gas
Air conditioning: 2,815 hours
Annual Costs
Mortgage and taxes: $6,915
Utilities: $924

Score: 7,839
Rank: 67

Port Angeles–Strait of Juan de Fuca, WA

Local Choices
70% houses, 1% condos, 15% mobile homes, 7% apartments (rent: $365)
Typical Housing
Median value: $70,500
Property taxes: $712
New: 8%   Old: 16%
Energy Requirements
Heating season: 5,842 degree days
Major source: Total electric
Air conditioning: 0 hours
Annual Costs
Mortgage and taxes: $6,864
Utilities: $618

Score: 7,482
Rank: 56

Portsmouth–Dover–Durham, NH

Local Choices
61% houses, 1% condos, 8% mobile homes, 8% apartments (rent: $320)
Typical Housing
Median value: $92,400
Property taxes: $1,867
New: 10%   Old: 34%
Energy Requirements
Heating season: 7,089 degree days
Major source: Oil
Air conditioning: 220 hours
Annual Costs
Mortgage and taxes: $9,930
Utilities: $1,216

Score: 11,146
Rank: 121

Prescott, AZ

Local Choices
67% houses, 2% condos, 21% mobile homes, 3% apartments (rent: $385)
Typical Housing
Median value: $63,300
Property taxes: $449
New: 24%   Old: 10%
Energy Requirements
Heating season: 4,956 degree days
Major source: Natural gas
Air conditioning: 925 hours
Annual Costs
Mortgage and taxes: $5,969
Utilities: $930

Score: 6,899
Rank: 39

Red Bluff–Sacramento Valley, CA

Local Choices
64% houses, 20% mobile homes, 6% apartments (rent: $350)
Typical Housing
Median value: $58,200
Property taxes: $594
New: 12%   Old: 14%
Energy Requirements
Heating season: 2,688 degree days
Major source: Natural gas
Air conditioning: 1,515 hours
Annual Costs
Mortgage and taxes: $5,671
Utilities: $885

Score: 6,556
Rank: 31

Redding, CA

Local Choices
62% houses, 19% mobile homes, 9% apartments (rent: $400)
Typical Housing
Median value: $73,700
Property taxes: $751
New: 12%   Old: 7%
Energy Requirements
Heating season: 2,610 degree days
Major source: Natural gas
Air conditioning: 1,515 hours
Annual Costs
Mortgage and taxes: $7,177
Utilities: $586

Score: 7,763
Rank: 64

Rehoboth Bay–Indian River Bay, DE

Local Choices
68% houses, 4% condos, 19% mobile homes, 2% apartments (rent: $310)
Typical Housing
Median value: $59,400
Property taxes: $422
New: 14%   Old: 20%
Energy Requirements
Heating season: 4,303 degree days
Major source: Oil
Air conditioning: 456 hours
Annual Costs
Mortgage and taxes: $5,604
Utilities: $1,141

Score: 6,745
Rank: 36

Reno, NV

Local Choices
49% houses, 9% condos, 10% mobile homes, 20% apartments (rent: $570)
Typical Housing
Median value: $79,200
Property taxes: $499
New: 13%   Old: 7%
Energy Requirements
Heating season: 6,022 degree days
Major source: Natural gas
Air conditioning: 647 hours
Annual Costs
Mortgage and taxes: $7,410
Utilities: $996

Score: 8,406
Rank: 81

Rhinelander, WI

Local Choices
74% houses, 11% mobile homes, 3% apartments (rent: $285)
Typical Housing
Median value: $58,600
Property taxes: $1,172
New: 10%   Old: 25%
Energy Requirements
Heating season: 8,783 degree days
Major source: Natural gas
Air conditioning: 436 hours
Annual Costs
Mortgage and taxes: $6,285
Utilities: $1,059

Score: 7,344
Rank: 49

★ Roswell, NM

Local Choices
79% houses, 7% mobile homes, 6% apartments (rent: $320)
Typical Housing
Median value: $36,800
Property taxes: $280
New: 5%   Old: 13%
Energy Requirements
Heating season: 3,697 degree days
Major source: Natural gas
Air conditioning: 1,617 hours
Annual Costs
Mortgage and taxes: $3,493
Utilities: $906

Score: 4,399
Rank: 1

St. George–Zion, UT

Local Choices
67% houses, 6% condos, 15% mobile homes, 5% apartments (rent: $395)
Typical Housing
Median value: $72,600
Property taxes: $631
New: 42%   Old: 9%
Energy Requirements
Heating season: 3,425 degree days
Major source: Total electric
Air conditioning: 789 hours
Annual Costs
Mortgage and taxes: $6,963
Utilities: $479

Score: 7,442
Rank: 53

St. Petersburg–Clearwater, FL

Local Choices
65% houses, 13% condos, 9% mobile homes, 13% apartments (rent: $375)
Typical Housing
Median value: $66,700
Property taxes: $527
New: 16%   Old: 6%
Energy Requirements
Heating season: 551 degree days
Major source: Total electric
Air conditioning: 1,881 hours
Annual Costs
Mortgage and taxes: $6,345
Utilities: $1,190

Score: 7,535
Rank: 61

Salinas–Seaside–Monterey, CA

Local Choices
59% houses, 4% condos, 4% mobile homes, 16% apartments (rent: $485)
Typical Housing
Median value: $104,500
Property taxes: $1,065
New: 8%   Old: 13%
Energy Requirements
Heating season: 2,959 degree days
Major source: Natural gas
Air conditioning: 14 hours
Annual Costs
Mortgage and taxes: $10,178
Utilities: $885

Score: 11,063
Rank: 120

San Antonio, TX
Local Choices
69% houses, 1% condos, 3% mobile homes, 14% apartments (rent: $335)
Typical Housing
Median value: $51,500
Property taxes: $680
New: 14%   Old: 11%
Energy Requirements
Heating season: 1,570 degree days
Major source: Natural gas
Air conditioning: 2,004 hours
Annual Costs
Mortgage and taxes: $5,172
Utilities: $856

Score: 6,028
Rank: 21

San Diego, CA
Local Choices
54% houses, 8% condos, 5% mobile homes, 21% apartments (rent: $465)
Typical Housing
Median value: $109,900
Property taxes: $1,121
New: 14%   Old: 8%
Energy Requirements
Heating season: 1,507 degree days
Major source: Natural gas
Air conditioning: 130 hours
Annual Costs
Mortgage and taxes: $10,707
Utilities: $1,100

Score: 11,807
Rank: 125

San Luis Obispo, CA
Local Choices
62% houses, 2% condos, 12% mobile homes, 10% apartments (rent: $465)
Typical Housing
Median value: $93,700
Property taxes: $956
New: 16%   Old: 10%
Energy Requirements
Heating season: 2,472 degree days
Major source: Natural gas
Air conditioning: 329 hours
Annual Costs
Mortgage and taxes: $9,131
Utilities: $885

Score: 10,016
Rank: 109

Santa Fe, NM
Local Choices
61% houses, 3% condos, 10% mobile homes, 11% apartments (rent: $410)
Typical Housing
Median value: $78,400
Property taxes: $596
New: 18%   Old: 13%
Energy Requirements
Heating season: 6,007 degree days
Major source: Natural gas
Air conditioning: 686 hours
Annual Costs
Mortgage and taxes: $7,433
Utilities: $1,085

Score: 8,518
Rank: 82

Santa Rosa–Petaluma, CA
Local Choices
69% houses, 3% condos, 7% mobile homes, 9% apartments (rent: $455)
Typical Housing
Median value: $106,800
Property taxes: $1,089
New: 12%   Old: 13%
Energy Requirements
Heating season: 3,065 degree days
Major source: Natural gas
Air conditioning: 770 hours
Annual Costs
Mortgage and taxes: $10,401
Utilities: $885

Score: 11,286
Rank: 122

Sarasota, FL
Local Choices
56% houses, 18% condos, 13% mobile homes, 7% apartments (rent: $425)
Typical Housing
Median value: $82,400
Property taxes: $651
New: 21%   Old: 3%
Energy Requirements
Heating season: 527 degree days
Major source: Total electric
Air conditioning: 2,154 hours
Annual Costs
Mortgage and taxes: $7,835
Utilities: $1,329

Score: 9,164
Rank: 94

Southport, NC
Local Choices
73% houses, 1% condos, 20% mobile homes, 1% apartments (rent: $325)
Typical Housing
Median value: $49,200
Property taxes: $497
New: 26%   Old: 6%
Energy Requirements
Heating season: 2,433 degree days
Major source: Total electric
Air conditioning: 683 hours
Annual Costs
Mortgage and taxes: $4,786
Utilities: $1,082

Score: 5,868
Rank: 17

★ Springfield, MO
Local Choices
75% houses, 4% mobile homes, 11% apartments (rent: $275)
Typical Housing
Median value: $49,600
Property taxes: $506
New: 8%   Old: 20%
Energy Requirements
Heating season: 4,570 degree days
Major source: Natural gas
Air conditioning: 964 hours
Annual Costs
Mortgage and taxes: $4,830
Utilities: $981

Score: 5,811
Rank: 14

State College, PA
Local Choices
57% houses, 1% condos, 7% mobile homes, 21% apartments (rent: $305)
Typical Housing
Median value: $87,900
Property taxes: $1,344
New: 8%   Old: 27%
Energy Requirements
Heating season: 6,132 degree days
Major source: Oil
Air conditioning: 351 hours
Annual Costs
Mortgage and taxes: $9,008
Utilities: $1,078

Score: 10,086
Rank: 110

Traverse City–Grand Traverse Bay, MI
Local Choices
74% houses, 1% condos, 11% mobile homes, 6% apartments (rent: $360)
Typical Housing
Median value: $62,000
Property taxes: $1,724
New: 14%   Old: 22%
Energy Requirements
Heating season: 7,698 degree days
Major source: Natural gas
Air conditioning: 308 hours
Annual Costs
Mortgage and taxes: $7,136
Utilities: $1,207

Score: 8,343
Rank: 80

Tucson, AZ
Local Choices
56% houses, 4% condos, 11% mobile homes, 14% apartments (rent: $420)
Typical Housing
Median value: $70,300
Property taxes: $499
New: 17%   Old: 5%
Energy Requirements
Heating season: 1,707 degree days
Major source: Natural gas
Air conditioning: 2,243 hours
Annual Costs
Mortgage and taxes: $6,630
Utilities: $788

Score: 7,418
Rank: 52

Twain Harte–Yosemite, CA
Local Choices
75% houses, 16% mobile homes, 2% apartments (rent: $390)
Typical Housing
Median value: $82,000
Property taxes: $836
New: 15%   Old: 11%
Energy Requirements
Heating season: 4,800 degree days
Major source: Bottled gas
Air conditioning: 647 hours
Annual Costs
Mortgage and taxes: $7,989
Utilities: $885

Score: 8,874
Rank: 92

Virginia Beach–Norfolk, VA
Local Choices
59% houses, 1% condos, 5% mobile
  homes, 17% apartments (rent: $415)
Typical Housing
Median value: $74,500
Property taxes: $745
New: 15%   Old: 11%
Energy Requirements
Heating season: 3,488 degree days
Major source: Natural gas
Air conditioning: 990 hours
Annual Costs
Mortgage and taxes: $7,247
Utilities: $1,084

Score: 8,331
Rank: 79

West Palm Beach–Boca Raton–
  Delray Beach, FL
Local Choices
44% houses, 30% condos, 5% mobile
  homes, 9% apartments (rent: $420)

Typical Housing
Median value: $89,200
Property taxes: $705
New: 29%   Old: 4%
Energy Requirements
Heating season: 299 degree days
Major source: Total electric
Air conditioning: 2,276 hours
Annual Costs
Mortgage and taxes: $8,484
Utilities: $1,329

Score: 9,813
Rank: 106

Winchester, VA
Local Choices
72% houses, 7% mobile homes, 8%
  apartments (rent: $330)
Typical Housing
Median value: $69,400
Property taxes: $694
New: 11%   Old: 23%
Energy Requirements
Heating season: 4,679 degree days
Major source: Oil

Air conditioning: 679 hours
Annual Costs
Mortgage and taxes: $6,751
Utilities: $1,084

Score: 7,835
Rank: 66

★ Yuma, AZ
Local Choices
50% houses, 2% condos, 30% mobile
  homes, 7% apartments (rent: $400)
Typical Housing
Median value: $48,800
Property taxes: $346
New: 12%   Old: 5%
Energy Requirements
Heating season: 1,005 degree days
Major source: Total electric
Air conditioning: 3,185 hours
Annual Costs
Mortgage and taxes: $4,602
Utilities: $1,247

Score: 5,849
Rank: 15

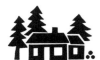 ET CETERA: Housing

YOUR $125,000 DECISION

Prior to 1987, capital gains were taxed up to a maximum of 20 percent. The new Tax Reform Law now treats capital gains as ordinary income taxable up to a maximum of 38.5 percent during 1987 and 28 percent in subsequent years. Your house is a capital asset, and if you sell it at a profit, your capital gains are taxable in the year you sell. A loss on the sale, however, isn't deductible.

There are two important exceptions to this rule that can help you put off the payment of taxes or eliminate them altogether: the "rollover" available to sellers of any age and the one-time exclusion, which can be taken advantage of only by sellers 55 and over.

The Rollover. If you sell your house at a profit, the tax on the profit may be postponed if, within two years from the date you sell, you buy another house and pay as much or more than the sale price of your old house. This time limit works forward and backward: you can buy the new house as long as 24 months before or 24 months after you sell your old house. If you anticipate retiring, this rule allows you to buy a vacation home up to two years before you sell your principal residence and claim the rollover when you move into the vacation home for full-time living.

If the price of your new home is less than the sale price of your old one, part of the profit will be taxable during the year. The profit will also be taxable during the year in which you sold in the event that you don't

buy a new principal residence but instead rent an apartment or house.

The rollover can be used over and over again until the day you sell your home and don't buy another. When that happens, the taxes are due on all the accumulated profits realized in all your principal residences sold over prior years. That is an ideal time to claim the one-time exclusion.

The Exclusion. If either you or your spouse are 55 by the day you sell your home at a profit, and you've owned and used the home as your principal residence for at least three of the five years ending on the day the property is sold, you can elect to exclude up to $125,000 of profit from tax altogether ($62,500 for married persons filing separately).

The exclusion can be claimed only once, so don't use it to shelter a paltry gain if you anticipate an even larger gain later on. Also, if you sell your house and buy another, you can postpone all or part of your gain anyway. If you take the exemption and later wish you hadn't, you can revoke your decision within three years after filing your return for the year the sale occurred or within two years of the time the tax for that year was paid, whichever is later.

Remember, too, that once the exclusion is claimed by a married couple, it cannot be claimed again by either spouse. Divorced or widowed persons who jointly used the exemption with their previous spouses are branded for life in the eyes of the IRS.

HOME-EQUITY CONVERSION: LIVING "ON THE HOUSE"

If you're over 65 and own a home, you're likely to possess an asset that has appreciated dramatically since 1970. Economists put the total value of homes owned by people over 65 in the United States at more than $600 billion.

Home-equity conversion, or reverse-equity plans, are designed to help older house-rich and cash-poor homeowners unlock the value of their home and convert it into additional retirement income without being forced to move. Unlike common home-equity loans available to most homeowners, you don't have to show sufficient monthly income for a commercial bank's approval. Some plans involve actual transfer of title to the property; others do not. Some provide income for only a specified period; others provide income for life.

Deciding which plan is best takes careful thought; interested homeowners should seek the advice of an attorney for help in weighing the benefits and liabilities of specific plans. The following are three major variations:

A **Reverse Appreciation Mortgage** (RAM) is a loan paid out in monthly installments to the homeowner by a lender, thereby creating a debt (hence the word *mortgage*) that increases each month. The house must be free of any mortgage or lien, since the amount of the loan is determined by the price the home would fetch if the property were put up for sale. The loan comes due at the end of the term or when the owner dies or decides to sell the property. The RAM is repaid out of money from the sale of the house or from other resources.

A **sale-leaseback** lets you stay in your home for the rest of your life as long as you're physically able. You sell your house to an investor who leases the property back to you at a fixed rent for as long as you can or want to live in the house. You receive a down payment and a monthly mortgage payment from the investor, who is responsible for taxes, maintenance, and insurance on the property. The investor takes full possession of the property when you choose to move out of the house or in the event of your death.

Deferred payment loans are home-improvement loans offered most often by city governments or neighborhood housing service agencies. They are generally open to all ages and charge low or no interest. The loan comes due when the owner dies or sells the property. In either case, the deferred loan is then paid out of cash from the sale of the house or at the estate settlement.

For a list of publications relating to home-equity con-

version, send a stamped, self-addressed envelope to:

National Center for Home Equity Conversion
110 East Main Street, Room 605
Madison, WI 53703

PROPERTY TAXES

Although the dollar amount of your home's recent property tax bills may seem to ratchet upward with each reassessment, there is some slight comfort in knowing that the rate at which your home is being taxed is actually going down.

Over the past ten years, while the prices of existing homes were rising, the average effective property tax rates dropped from 2 percent of these values to less than 1.25 percent nationwide. Economists expect the downward trend to continue.

Nowhere in the United States can you own a home and entirely escape property taxes (except in Alaska, but you have to be 65). But homeowners in certain states (like Louisiana, where the statewide average property tax rate is .15 percent) shoulder less of a burden than do homeowners in other states (such as New York, which has an average tax rate of 2.8, or almost 20 times that of Louisiana).

Exemptions

When you shop for low property taxes around the country, adopt a circumspect attitude when you hear of places that give retired people additional property tax relief. Are any of these benefits, by themselves, worth a move? Read on.

Homestead exemptions are specific dollar amounts deducted by local assessors when they compute your bill. In Hawaii, for example, homeowners over 60 get an exemption of $40,000; when they turn 70, the exemption increases to $50,000. All homeowners in Florida receive a $25,000 exemption if they are permanent residents. According to the Washington, D.C.–based Advisory Commission on Intergovernmental Relations, 17 states grant exemptions to *all* homeowners:

Alabama	Louisiana
California	Massachusetts
Florida	(local option)
Georgia	Minnesota
Hawaii	Mississippi
Idaho	Nebraska
Illinois	New Jersey
Indiana	Oregon
Iowa	Texas

Nine states allow special exemptions or credits to *older homeowners* without any income qualifications: Alaska, Hawaii, Idaho, Illinois, Kentucky, New Jersey, South Carolina, Texas, and West Virginia.

Do the exemptions in these states translate into much hard cash? Except in Alaska—where you can forget property taxes once you turn 65—not really. Based on statewide average property tax rates, you'll save $204 in Hawaii, ($255 if you're over 70), $90 in Illinois, $152 in Kentucky, $162 in South Carolina, and $136 in West Virginia.

The bottom line? Property tax exemptions can be an extra benefit in retirement, but if you're planning a move, you'd do well to put other considerations, such as energy costs and house prices, first.

Deferrals

Nine states allow older persons to legally postpone payment of all or part of their property taxes. In property tax deferral programs, the state pays the tax for the retired homeowner and puts a lien on the property, secured by its sale value. Interest is charged each year on the amount postponed. The tax-deferral loan comes due when the home is sold, given away, or when the owner dies, in which case the heirs or estate must pay what's due.

State Property Tax Deferral Programs

State	Minimum Age	Maximum Income	Interest Rate
California	62	$24,000	Yield on state investments
Colorado	65	None	8%
Georgia	62	15,000	Local bank rates
Illinois	65	10,000	6%
Michigan	65	10,000	No interest
Oregon	62	17,500	6%
Texas	65	None	6%
Utah	65	8,000	6%
Washington	61	15,000	8%

Source: National Conference of State Legislatures, *State Tax Policy & Senior Citizens: A Legislator's Guide,* 1985.

Six states—Florida, Iowa, Massachusetts, New Hampshire, Tennessee, and Virginia—that do not have statewide property tax deferral programs permit it at local option. Wisconsin passed property tax deferral legislation in 1981, but the state hasn't implemented the program.

A SINGLE-HOUSE MISCELLANY

Each year, the Federal Housing Authority reports on the characteristics of existing single-family homes whose mortgages it insures. Here's a geography of nine of these features.

Lot Size. Imagine a house lot with 85 feet of frontage and 100 feet of depth. The 8,500 square feet it encloses is the average lot size for a resale house in the United States. Resale houses sitting on lots over half an acre (21,780 square feet) are more frequently found in Connecticut, Georgia, Maine, New Hampshire, and North Carolina than in the other states.

Construction and Exterior. In frame construction, the wood frame supports the floors and roof; in masonry construction, the exterior masonry wall serves as the support. Except in the Texas Interior, masonry construction using local stone has virtually disappeared in new houses. Concrete-block masonry construction, however, is a common technique in Arizona and Florida, where either spray-paint or stucco is used on the exterior. Everywhere else, the majority of new houses are of frame construction.

Aluminum siding is the preferred exterior in Maryland and Ohio; wood is the choice in Georgia, Maine, Massachusetts, New Hampshire, and Washington. Exteriors of brick or stucco are preferred in California, Louisiana, Nevada, Oklahoma, South Carolina, and Texas.

Stories. The word *story* originally referred to tiers of stained-glass or painted windows that described a special event. The common definition today is "the space between the floor and the ceiling, roof, or the floor above, in the case of a multistory home." It has nothing to do with the height of a house; a house that appears from the outside to be two stories may actually be a single story with a cathedral ceiling. Two thirds of existing houses in this country have only one story. However, in Arizona, California, Florida, Louisiana, Mississippi, New Mexico, Oklahoma, and Texas single-story houses constitute more than 90 percent of resale homes. Multistory resale homes, on the other hand, predominate in the District of Columbia, Maine, Maryland, Massachusetts, New Jersey, New York, and Pennsylvania.

Basements. The basement is an area of full-story height below the first floor that is not meant for year-round living. Only 15 percent of new houses have basements; they've become too expensive to excavate. In seven states, however, two out of three resale houses have a full basement, reflecting a pattern of locating the furnace below grade and a preference for extra living space. These states are Connecticut, Iowa, Maine, Massachusetts, Minnesota, New Hampshire, and Wisconsin.

Most resale houses have no basements at all. More than two thirds of the houses in Arizona, Florida, Louisiana, Mississippi, New Mexico, and Texas simply rest on a concrete slab poured on the ground. In Alabama, Arkansas, North Carolina, Oregon, South Carolina, and Tennessee, a majority of existing houses have a crawl space (an unfinished accessible space below the first floor that is usually less than full-story height).

Bathrooms. Bathrooms are either full (a tub or shower stall, a sink, and a toilet) or half (just a sink and a toilet). Just one of five resale homes have both a full bathroom and a half bathroom. In Hawaii, Mississippi, New Hampshire, New Mexico, North Carolina, and South Carolina, however, more than one third of resale homes have both full and half bathrooms.

Garages and Carports. Garages, as everyone knows, are completely enclosed shelters for automobiles; carports are roofed shelters that aren't completely enclosed. Six out of ten houses, new and old, have garages; one in ten have only carports. Only in Arizona, Hawaii, Louisiana, and Mississippi is this pattern reversed.

Fireplaces. Flueless, imitation fireplaces, like dinettes and rumpus rooms, are memories of the 1950s. Nearly half of new American homes now have a working fireplace and chimney. Resale homes with a fireplace can be found most frequently in the northern timber states of Idaho, Minnesota, Montana, Oregon, and Washington, and also in North Carolina and Pennsylvania.

Swimming Pools. You won't find new houses built on speculation with in-ground swimming pools anywhere. Builders have learned that few buyers shop for shelter *and* a swimming pool at the same time. Among resale homes, less than 2 percent have them. You're most likely to find them in Arizona, California, Nevada, and surprisingly, Maine and New York.

Enclosed Porches. A porch is a covered addition or recessed space at the entrance of a home. Main Street lookouts, they have disappeared from new home markets. You'll find enclosed porches on 8 percent of resale homes in this country. In Connecticut, Iowa, Maine, Massachusetts, New Jersey, and New York, more than 20 percent of these homes have them.

Resale Houses and New Houses

If a single, detached house is your preference, consider the pluses and minuses of resale houses versus new houses.

In most markets, resale homes are less expensive than equivalent new homes and are available in broader price ranges, with more architectural styles and locations in town. Resale homes usually have had their minor defects, often unforseen when the home was new, corrected by the seller. But the age of the structure may signal problems. Repairs to the roof, floor coverings, appliances, and mechanical systems, which have depreciated over the years, may be necessary during the first two years you own the house. More importantly, as a neighborhood matures, some homes are maintained better than others and price disparities develop, which can affect your own home's value.

New houses in new, homogeneous neighborhoods portend more rapid appreciation in value over equivalent resale houses. You can have a new house covered by an extended homeowner warranty to protect you from major structural defects. If timing permits, you also can "customize" the house with options and extras and have the opportunity to select colors, appliance brands, and technological features such as heating and air-conditioning systems. But the drawback to new homes in many communities is their 10 to 20 percent price premium over equivalent resale homes.

Buying a new home is more complicated, too, since many more decisions have to be made about finish details and landscaping, all of which may mean frequent site visits to confer with the builder.

Duplexes

If you're a first-time investor considering a home for rental income, a duplex (a house divided into apartments for two households) often is a better buy than single house because of a better relation between price and income. A duplex might be bought for 8 to 10 times its annual rental income, where a single house might cost 13 to 15 times what it could bring in rent.

You might consider buying a duplex, renting one of the apartments, and occupying the other yourself. This is particularly attractive in college towns. From Ann Arbor, Michigan, to State College, Pennsylvania, college towns have more rental properties and renters than other retirement places. Aside from the income and depreciation you would have from the rental unit, if you live alone, congenial tenants—perhaps a graduate student and family—can watch the house should you want to do some traveling. You can also trade lower rent for maintenance help.

A MOBILE-HOME MISCELLANY

According to Foremost Insurance Company surveys, the average age of a mobile-home owner is climbing past middle age, and persons over 60 now comprise 33 percent of the market. Mobile homes made up one third of all new housing purchased in the United States last year. Living in one makes sense if you are on a limited budget. It also presents two major problems: (1) this type of housing doesn't appreciate in value everywhere and (2) owners are subject to sometimes arbitrary eviction from mobile-home parks.

Are Mobile Homes Investments?

Whether real estate salespeople tout houses, condos, townhouses, or mobile homes, they've all learned the five factors that influence price tags: quality of original construction, the neighborhood's turnover rate, supply and demand for housing, current upkeep, and location.

With these factors at work in the housing market, mobile homes, like automobiles, tend to go down in value as they get older. During the 1970s, according to the American Institute of Real Estate Appraisers, the typical mobile home in a typical park depreciated 10 percent the first year and between 5 and 6 percent each year thereafter.

But this wasn't the case in all parts of the country. In seven states, all but two of them in the West, mobile homes appreciated at a modest annual rate during the 1970s, according to a survey from the Foremost Insurance Company. These states are Alaska, Arizona, California, Florida, New Jersey, Oregon, and Washington. In the central states, values kept pace with new home costs. In the eastern third of the country, however, mobile homes declined in value from the moment they were first winched onto a permanent pad.

Do mobile homes make good investments?

Yes, if you want to live in Florida, New Jersey, Arizona, or the Pacific Coast states but can't afford to buy a house or a condominium in the competitive real estate markets there. While the appreciation in mobile homes lags behind that of conventional houses, you still have a good chance to make money when you sell.

Perhaps, if you have your sights set on a destination in the Rocky Mountain states, the Ozarks, northern Michigan, or Texas but can't afford conventional housing. Search carefully for a well-managed park near popular resorts or natural outdoor endowments.

No, if you're headed for the southeastern states, Pennsylvania, New York, or New England and have enough money to buy conventional housing. Mobile homes here have a history of depreciating when prices for existing site-built homes have gone up.

Tenant Rights for Mobile-Home Owners

Except in New Mexico, the Uniform Residential Landlord and Tenant Act doesn't protect mobile-home owners who rent space in a mobile-home park. In most states, a park owner can evict you for any reason. The park owner rarely gives leases and can demand sharp rent increases and a variety of costly fees once you've spent money moving your mobile home to the park. You may be forced to sell at a loss if the park owner tells you to get out and no other park has space for your home.

Twelve states have passed "just cause" laws to protect mobile-home owners from being arbitrarily evicted from mobile-home parks, according to a survey by the American Mobilehome Association. Just causes for eviction include nonpayment of rent, being tried and convicted of a crime, violation of reasonable park rules, or conversion of park land to other uses. The states are

Arizona	Oregon
California	New Jersey
Colorado	New Mexico
Florida	New York
Illinois	Utah
Nevada	Washington

A CONDO MISCELLANY

Condominiums are pushed to people making their way out of the rental market and older persons drawn to maintenance-free living at a lower cost, often in adults-only developments. While the construction boom has faded in certain parts of the country, the fact that condominiums accounted for 15 percent of all new housing units during the 1970s certainly vouches for their appeal.

Ten Negatives

The complaints reported by the Urban Land Institute 15 years ago in an extensive survey of condominium residents are still being raised today. Among them are

- noisy children and undesirable neighbors
- pets
- parking problems
- poor association management
- ticky-tacky construction
- dishonest salespeople
- renters in other units
- thin party walls
- long rows of identically designed houses
- unneeded and overpromoted recreation facilities

If you are thinking of condominium living in your retirement, these complaints are a guide to judging condominium developments. Ask questions of the association and the broker. What are the restrictions on pets? Children? How are they enforced? Does each unit have an assigned parking space? Are there rules in the association's bylaws limiting the number of rental units? What is the average tenure of the unit owners? Of the renters? Are any units set aside for time shares? Is their number restricted?

As a retired person, you are one of the two major targets of condominium marketing. The other is the young person or family buying their first home. Both groups want lower costs, freedom from house and yard maintenance in a ready-made environment, social life, and recreation facilities, all with the tax advantages of ownership. There isn't any reason the two groups can't live together harmoniously in the same development. In well-managed condominiums they do. But in other developments, the mix can prove unhappy.

Legal Protection for Condo Buyers

Many state legislatures recognize that consumers have little protection at the point of purchasing a condominium. Ten states have enacted comprehensive statutes to deal with condominium ownership based on the Uniform Condominium Act (1980) drawn up by the National Conference of Commissioners on Uniform State Laws. The states are

Maine	New Mexico
Minnesota	North Carolina
Missouri	Pennsylvania
Nebraska	Rhode Island
New Hampshire	Virginia

The act covers owners' associations, developers' activities, eminent domain, separate titles and taxation, and safeguards for condominium buyers. Among its provisions are

- The developer must provide you with a Public Offering Statement, accurately and fully disclosing a schedule for completion of all construction, the total number of condominium units, the bylaws of the owners' association, copies of any contracts or leases that you must sign, a current balance sheet and projected one-year budget for the owners' association, and a statement of the monthly common assessments you'll have to pay.
- After signing a purchase agreement, you still have 15 days to cool off, after which you can either cancel the agreement without penalty or accept conveyance of the property.
- If you buy a condominium without first being given the Public Offering Statement, you are entitled to receive from the developer an amount equal to 10 percent of the sales price of the unit you bought.
- The developer and real estate agent must guarantee that the unit you are buying is free from defective materials, is built according to sound engineering and construction standards, and conforms to local codes.

CAVEAT EMPTOR: SUBDIVISION LOTS

Every year real estate developers ring up billions of dollars in interstate land sales. During the 1970s, one

of the results of this lucrative business was to leave a million Americans with real estate they didn't want and couldn't sell. Many of these buyers who found themselves holding title to swampland or desert were retired persons looking for a spot to put up a vacation home or permanent residence.

Buying out-of-state land is always risky, especially if the buyer doesn't visit the property. Even if you do see the homesite before buying, it may be very difficult to be sure the developer will actually follow through on promised amenities. The slick promotional brochure will describe golf courses, landscaped parks, swimming pools, clubhouses, and marinas, but any promise not clearly outlined in the sales contract isn't enforceable. What you consider to be a sound retirement investment may turn out to be no more of a sure thing than the prospects at the $2 window at the track.

"You can always resell your lot if you change your mind," the salesperson will tell you. "In fact, the developer will buy it back from you." What is not revealed is that the price you are paying for the lot has already been inflated to nearly twice its real value to cover the advertising and other initial sales costs. Where do you suppose the money comes from for the fancy literature, the gourmet dinners fed to prospective buyers, the free trips often proffered to hot prospects who want to see what they're buying? Right out of that earnest money you're about to write a check for, that's where! So even if you do successfully resell your lot, you may take a heavy loss on the transaction.

A Land Buyer's Rights

Federal legislation amended in 1984 to protect the land buyer applies to brokers and developers who subdivide land into 100 or more lots and sell or advertise them in more than one state. Some of the provisions are:

- The buyer has seven calendar days to back out of any sales agreement. A legal or legitimate reason isn't necessary for the cancellation.
- A buyer who fails to receive a property report before signing a purchase agreement may cancel the agreement up to two years from the time of signing.
- A buyer who doesn't receive a warranty deed within 180 days of signing a purchase agreement may, in most cases, cancel the agreement.
- Buyers who legally revoke their contracts are entitled to a refund.
- For a period up to three years after signing the purchase contract, the buyer may sue the seller if he:

  Sells property without giving the property report to the buyer before he signs the contract

Sells any property when the property report contains any false facts or omits a material fact

Provides or distributes promotional material that is inconsistent with material in the property report

The federal Office of Interstate Lands Sales Registration (OILSR) maintains records on 17,000 multilot developments that are promoted in interstate commerce. If you want to do a little homework on real estate investment before making any commitment, OILSR publishes a booklet "Before Buying Land, Get the Facts," available free by writing:

Office of Interstate Lands Sales Registration
Room 6278
451 Seventh Street, S.W.
Washington, DC 20410

AN APARTMENT MISCELLANY

The kind of apartment building you choose to live in definitely makes a difference in your monthly costs. In larger cities where apartments are a significant part of the housing mix, rents for a typical four-room, 850-square-foot unit are higher in high-rise elevator buildings (U.S. median $489) than in walk-ups or elevator

Apartment Rent in the Retirement Places

LOWEST	Monthly Median
Canton–Lake Tawakoni, TX	$210
Franklin County, TN	210
Branson–Cassville–Table Rock Lake, MO	220
Hot Springs–Lake Ouachita, AR	220
Clayton–Clarkesville, GA	225
Paris–Big Sandy, TN	225
Columbia County, NY	240
Crossville, TN	240
Grand Lake–Lake Tenkiller, OK	240
Houghton Lake, MI	240
Murray–Kentucky Lake, KY	240

HIGHEST	Monthly Median
Maui, HI	$660
Reno, NV	570
Carson City–Minden, NV	560
Las Vegas, NV	510
Flagstaff, AZ	495
Phoenix, AZ	485
Salinas–Seaside–Monterey, CA	485
Lake Havasu City–Kingman, AZ	480
Fort Lauderdale–Hollywood–Pompano Beach, FL	470
San Diego, CA	465
San Luis Obispo, CA	465

Source: U.S. Bureau of the Census, 1980 Census of Population and Housing.

These figures represent rents for an apartment in a building with two or more rental units boosted by regional Consumer Price Index inflation factors to show realistic 1986 figures. All figures are rounded to the nearest $5.

buildings of three stories or fewer (U.S. median $432), according to a 1986 Institute of Real Estate Management survey. The least expensive kind of building is the garden apartment, defined as a group of low-rise apartment buildings on a large landscaped lot under one manager. The national monthly rental for this kind of building is $429.

You'll find the annual turnover rate, defined as newly occupied apartments as a percentage of all the apartments in the building in a year's time, also varies by the kind of building. Around the country, high-rise elevator buildings have the lowest turnover rate (U.S. median 33 percent), whereas the turnover rate in walk-ups and elevator buildings of three or fewer stories is half again that rate (U.S. median 47 percent). The kind of apartment building with the most transient population is the garden apartment, in which 57 percent of the tenants moved in within the previous 12 months.

The Rule of 156

One useful way of determining the rent for a house is to divide its market value by 156. Using this rule plus the prices of houses given in the Place Profiles, it isn't difficult to figure roughly what it would cost you to rent a house in a given retirement area, assuming that the landlord has realistic expectations for the rate of return on property.

In Maui, Hawaii, the rent would be about $880; in Cape Cod, $670; in Roswell, New Mexico, $236. The rule of 156 may seem unfair to landlords, since there is only an 8 percent return from which maintenance and taxes must be paid. Bear in mind, however, that landlords rarely buy houses for the rental income they may bring; rather, they buy them for their market appreciation and rent them during the interim merely to cover expenses.

Renters' Legal Rights

Seventeen states have enacted landlord-tenant laws based on the Uniform Residential Landlord and Tenant Act (1972), a piece of model legislation drawn up by the National Conference of Commissioners on Uniform State Laws. These states are

Alaska	Montana
Arizona	Nebraska
Connecticut	New Mexico
Florida	Oklahoma
Hawaii	Oregon
Iowa	Tennessee
Kansas	Virginia
Kentucky	Washington
Michigan	

The landlord-tenant act defines rights and obligations of both parties to a lease on an apartment or house, and it also specifies the way disputes can be resolved. Among its provisions are the following:

- If your dispute with a landlord leads you to

complain to the local housing board, join a tenants' group, or bring suit against the landlord, your landlord may not retaliate by cutting services, raising your rent, or evicting you.

- If the landlord doesn't make needed repairs, and the cost of the repairs isn't more than $100 or half the rent, whichever is greater, you may make repairs and deduct the expense from your monthly rent.
- After you vacate the apartment or house, any money you've deposited as security must be returned. If there are any deductions from the deposit for damages or other reasons, these deductions must be itemized.
- If the landlord doesn't live up to the terms of the lease, you may recover damages in small-claims court.

NUCLEAR HOT SPOTS

Would you mind living near a nuclear power plant? Given the record of the industry after 1,000 reactor years of commercial operation in this country, even proponents of nuclear power would admit that fears about a catastrophic meltdown or low-level environmental contamination are legitimate.

Because of a lower demand for electricity, construction and regulatory delays, skyrocketing costs, and concerns about reactor safety after the Three Mile Island and Chernobyl incidents, the growth of nuclear power has slowed considerably. Utility planners are simply unwilling to take the risk of investing billions in a 12- to 14-year process of building a nuclear plant and then face the possibility of not being allowed to operate it. As a result, plans for 76 power plants have been canceled over the past decade, and not one nuclear plant has been ordered since 1978.

During 1986, the 400 billion kilowatt-hours produced by nuclear reactors accounted for 16 percent of total U.S. electrical output. In South Carolina, 66 percent of electricity consumed comes from nuclear power; in Maine, 56 percent; in Connecticut and Nebraska, 50 percent or more.

Atomic Retirement Places

Retirement Place	Nuclear Power Plants	Generating Capacity (Megawatts)
Miami–Hialeah, FL	2	2,586
Ocean County, NJ	1	650
Phoenix, AZ	3	3,810
Portsmouth–Dover–Durham, NH	1	1,150
San Luis Obispo, CA	2	2,190
San Diego, CA	3	2,586
Southport, NC	2	1,642

Source: Atomic Industrial Forum, 1987.

The following list ranks, in order of their total generating capacity, the 34 states in which nuclear power plants are found. The generating capacity, or power output, for a typical reactor is 1,000 megawatts (1 million kilowatts) of electricity, or enough to supply the needs of a city of 600,000 people at any given moment. Each plant is either operating or under construction as of February 1987. The date of operation —actual or planned—is also given for each unit, along with its county location.

1. Illinois: 12,815 megawatts total capacity
DE WITT COUNTY: Clinton #1 (1987). GRUNDY COUNTY: Dresden #2 (1970), Dresden #3 (1971). LA SALLE COUNTY: La Salle #1 (1984), La Salle #2 (1984). LAKE COUNTY: Zion #1 (1973), Zion #2 (1974). OGLE COUNTY: Byron #1 (1985), Byron #2 (1987). ROCK ISLAND COUNTY: Quad Cities #1 (1972), Quad Cities #2 (1972). WILL COUNTY: Braidwood #1 (1987), Braidwood #1 (1988).

2. Pennsylvania: 8,009 megawatts total capacity
BEAVER COUNTY: Beaver Valley #1 (1976), Beaver Valley #2 (1987). LUZERNE COUNTY: Susquehanna #1 (1983), Susquehanna #2 (1985). MONTGOMERY COUNTY: Limerick #1 (1986), Limerick #2 (1990). YORK COUNTY: Peach Bottom #2 (1974), Peach Bottom #3 (1974).

3. Alabama: 7,279 megawatts total capacity
HOUSTON COUNTY: Farley #1 (1977), Farley #2 (1981). JACKSON COUNTY: Bellefonte #1 (1994), Bellefonte #2 (1996). MORGAN COUNTY: Browns Ferry #1 (1974), Browns Ferry #2 (1975), Browns Ferry #3 (1977).

4. South Carolina: 6,435 megawatts total capacity
DARLINGTON COUNTY: Robinson #2 (1971). FAIRFIELD COUNTY: Summer #1 (1984). OCONEE COUNTY: Oconee #1 (1973), Oconee #2 (1974). Oconee #3 (1974). YORK COUNTY: Catawba #1 (1985), Catawba #2 (1986).

5. California: 5,694 megawatts total capacity
SACRAMENTO COUNTY: Rancho Seco #1 (1976). SAN DIEGO COUNTY: San Onofre #1 (1968), San Onofre #2 (1983), San Onofre #3 (1984). SAN LUIS OBISPO COUNTY: Diablo Canyon #1 (1985), Diablo Canyon #1 (1986).

6. New York: 5,623 megawatts total capacity
OSWEGO COUNTY: Nine Mile Point #1 (1969), Nine Mile Point #2 (1987). SUFFOLK COUNTY: Fitzpatrick (1975), Shoreham (indefinite). WAYNE COUNTY: Ginna (1970). WESTCHESTER COUNTY: Indian Point #2 (1973), Indian Point #3 (1976).

7. North Carolina: 4,842 megawatts total capacity
BRUNSWICK COUNTY: Brunswick #1 (1977), Brunswick #2 (1975). MECKLENBURG COUNTY: McGuire #1 (1981), McGuire #2 (1984). WAKE COUNTY: Harris #1 (1987).

8. Texas: 4,800 megawatts total capacity
MATAGORDA COUNTY: South Texas #1 (1987), South Texas #2 (1989). SOMERVELLE COUNTY: Comanche Peak #1 (1989), Comanche Peak #2 (1989).

9. Tennessee: 4,650 megawatts total capacity
HAMILTON COUNTY: Sequoyah #1 (1981), Sequoyah #2 (1982). RHEA COUNTY: Watts Bar #1 (indefinite), Watts Bar #2 (indefinite).

10. Michigan: 4,076 megawatts total capacity
BERRIEN COUNTY: Cook #1 (1975), Cook #2 (1978). CHARLEVOIX COUNTY: Big Rock Point (1965). MONROE COUNTY: Fermi #2 (1987). VAN BUREN COUNTY: Palisades (1971).

11. New Jersey: 3,922 megawatts total capacity
OCEAN COUNTY: Oyster Creek (1969). SALEM COUNTY: Hope Creek (1987), Salem #1 (1977), Salem #2 (1981).

12. Florida: 3,856 megawatts total capacity
CITRUS COUNTY: Crystal River #3 (1977). DADE COUNTY: Turkey Point #3 (1972), Turkey Point #4 (1973). ST. LUCIE COUNTY: St. Lucie #1 (1976), St. Lucie #1 (1983).

Nuclear Power Plants in the United States

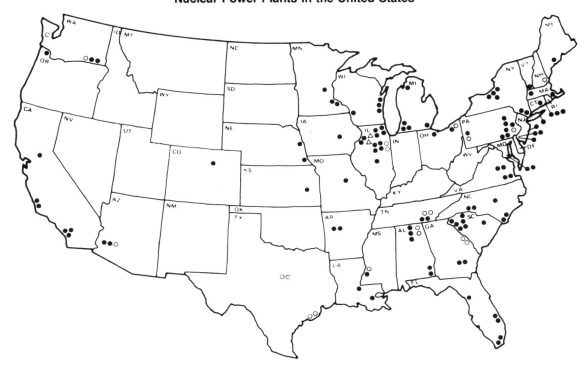

Key
- ● Reactors With Operating License
- ○ Reactors With Construction Permit
- △ Reactors On Order

105	Reactors operable	91,538 MWe
20	Reactors with construction permits	23,320 MWe
2	Reactors on order	2,240 MWe
127	Total	117,098 MWe

Source: Atomic Industrial Forum, Inc., January 1, 1987.

---

13. Arizona: 3,810 megawatts total capacity
MARICOPA COUNTY: Palos Verde #1 (1986), Palos Verde #2 (1986), Palos Verde #3 (1987).

14. Georgia: 3,800 megawatts total capacity
APPLING COUNTY: Hatch #1 (1976), Hatch #2 (1979). BURKE COUNTY: Vogtle #1 (1987), Vogtle #2 (1988).

15. Virginia: 3,414 megawatts total capacity
LOUISA COUNTY: North Anna #1 (1978), North Anna #2 (1980). SURRY COUNTY: Surry #1 (1972), Surry #2 (1973).

16. Ohio: 3,270 megawatts total capacity
LAKE COUNTY: Perry #1 (1987), Perry #2 (indefinite). OTTAWA COUNTY: Davis-Besse #1 (1977).

17. Connecticut: 3,262 megawatts total capacity
MIDDLESEX COUNTY: Haddam Neck (1968). NEW LONDON COUNTY: Millstone #1 (1970), Millstone #2 (1975), Millstone #3 (1986).

18. Mississippi: 2,500 megawatts total capacity
CLAIBORNE COUNTY: Grand Gulf #1 (1985), Grand Gulf #2 (indefinite).

19. Louisiana: 2,044 megawatts total capacity
ST. CHARLES PARISH: WATERFORD #3 (1985). WEST FILICIANA PARISH: RIVER BEND #1 (1986).

20. Washington: 1,960 megawatts total capacity
BENTON COUNTY: Hanford Nuclear (1966), WPPSS #2 (1984).

21. Arkansas: 1,762 megawatts total capacity
POPE COUNTY: Arkansas Nuclear #1 (1974), Arkansas Nuclear #2 (1980).

22. Maryland: 1,650 megawatts total capacity
CALVERT COUNTY: Calvert Cliffs #1 (1975), Calvert Cliffs #2 (1977).

23. Minnesota: 1,605 megawatts total capacity
GOODHUE COUNTY: Prairie Island #1 (1973), Prairie Island #2 (1974). WRIGHT COUNTY: Monticello (1971).

24. Wisconsin: 1,555 megawatts total capacity
KEWAUNEE COUNTY: Kewaunee (1974). MANITOWOC COUNTY: Point Beach #1 (1970), Point Beach #2 (1972). VERNON COUNTY: LaCrosse (1969).

25. Nebraska: 1,246 megawatts total capacity
NAMAHA COUNTY: Cooper (1974). WASHINGTON COUNTY: Fort Calhoun #1 (1973).

26. Kansas: 1,150 megawatts total capacity
COFFEE COUNTY: Wolfe Creek (1985).

27. New Hampshire: 1,150 megawatts total capacity
ROCKINGHAM COUNTY: Seabrook #1 (1987).

28. Oregon: 1,130 megawatts total capacity
COLUMBIA COUNTY: Trojan (1976).

29. Missouri: 1,120 megawatts total capacity
CALLAWAY COUNTY: Callaway (1984).

30. Massachusetts: 845 megawatts total capacity
FRANKLIN COUNTY: Yankee (1961). PLYMOUTH COUNTY: Pilgrim #1 (1972).

31. Maine: 825 megawatts total capacity
LINCOLN COUNTY: Maine Yankee (1972).

32. Iowa: 545 megawatts total capacity
LINN COUNTY: Arnold (1975).

33. Vermont: 514 megawatts total capacity
WINDHAM COUNTY: Vermont Yankee (1972).

34. Colorado: 330 megawatts total capacity
WELD COUNTY: Fort St. Vrain (1979).

Leisure Living :
Common Denominators, Performing Arts, and the Outdoors

INTRODUCTION: Leisure Living

You may have heard stories similar to these: a couple, rebounding from South Florida's pleasant winter but hellish summer, moved up the Atlantic Coast to Myrtle Beach, South Carolina. "It seemed as if half our waking hours were spent waiting in line," they recalled. "Wait an hour to tee off at the par-three golf course, wait in line for tickets to a concert, wait in our car for the traffic jam on the Palmetto Expressway to unravel. The place is too crowded."

Another couple, after a dull two years in a Desert Southwest retirement community, reestablished themselves in their New England hometown. "Forget it," they said. "We'll regret leaving the climate and the low cost of living, but we'll never miss sitting and playing bridge, sitting and talking, sitting and watching cable TV, and bestirring ourselves for an occasional rodeo, barbecue, and square dance."

These stories aren't uncommon among retired persons who make a geographic move. Many discover their dreamed-about life in a distant paradise is a thudding letdown and pack up and either move to a new haven or return home. Is their choice of location to blame? Not entirely.

The routine that starts with first grade and lasts through formal schooling and 10,000 working days abruptly ends with retirement. Unless you've developed specific hobbies and established your leisure goals long before your last day at a full-time job, you may be hard put to take advantage of the final quarter of your life no matter where you decide to live it.

If you're a joiner, rest assured you'll have things to do and people to do them with for a long, long time. In Roswell, New Mexico, for example, the Four "I's" (retired persons hailing from Illinois, Iowa, Indiana, and Idaho) meet regularly, as do Florida Club members (newcomers who resettle after a disappointing Florida stint) in North Carolina; everywhere you'll find Knife & Fork clubs and local chapters for Rotary, Kiwanis, American Association of Retired Persons, and National Association of Retired Federal Employees; in Metropolitan South Florida, there are clubs for ex-teachers, ex–police officers, ex-Seabees, Catholics, and even clubs for people suffering from the same disease.

But natural and man-made leisure activities aren't distributed in the geography with fairness; some places have more indoor and outdoor things going for them than others. Many of these attractions are doubly important if you want to make the most of your leisure time—especially if you want to balance "fun and games" with culture, and culture with the great outdoors.

COMMON DENOMINATORS

When it comes to clam digging, hang gliding, alpine skiing, river rafting, or just growing good tomatoes, a few parts of the country are better than all the others simply because of the fortunate circumstances of geography.

But you'll find more-conventional activities everywhere: golfing at a public course on a weekday when the greens fees are cheaper; browsing among the quiet stacks at a public library; team bowling in the din at a local tenpin center; moviegoing at a downtown picture palace or at a suburban shopping mall off the interstate; or dining out in a quality restaurant.

You might call these familiar activities "common denominators." They are found everywhere. On a per capita basis, though, their supply varies considerably from place to place.

Counting Stars: Good Restaurants

In the United States, the most ubiquitous retail establishment is the one where you can sit down and order something to eat. Of the dollars' persons over 55 budget for food, one third are spent dining out, so if you enjoy an occasional dinner splurge you might as well go to a worthwhile eatery instead of a local diner or a portion-controlled Casa de la Maison House where distantly prepared frozen packs of beef Wellington and veal cordon bleu are microwaved, dished out, and "menued" at ten times what the chef paid for them.

To learn whether any of the retirement places have restaurants more than just a cut or two above average, *Retirement Places Rated* consulted the seven-volume *Mobil Travel Guide*, which since 1958 has rated restaurants across the country. The ratings are derived from two sources: customer comments and inspection reports of field representatives who dine anonymously at establishments throughout the year.

Restaurants are judged by the quality of their food, service, and ambience. Ratings range from one star for a "good, better than average" restaurant to five stars for "one of the best in the country." Only a handful of restaurants receive the coveted five stars in any given year; of the 12 top-rated restaurants in the United States for 1986, one is located in each of three retirement places.

To gauge access to good restaurants, *Retirement Places Rated* divides the local population by the total number of quality stars awarded establishments in each retirement place. Three 2-star restaurants and four 3-star restaurants, for example, would yield 18 quality stars. Even though small places like Santa Fe,

163

New Mexico, and Door County, Wisconsin, have fewer rated restaurants than glitzy Miami–Hialeah or Las Vegas, they can still boast at least one Mobil quality star for every 2,000 people.

Access to Good Food

BEST RETIREMENT PLACES	Restaurants/ Quality Stars	Residents per Star
Eagle River, WI	9/16	1,063
Petoskey–Straits of Mackinac, MI	12/20	1,215
North Conway–White Mountains, NH	9/22	1,464
Door County, WI	12/18	1,550
Santa Fe, NM	21/54	1,787
Bar Harbor–Frenchman Bay, ME	14/25	1,800
Cape Cod, MA	42/82	2,085
Newport–Lincoln City, OR	7/17	2,329
Camden–Penobscot Bay, ME	7/15	2,340
Kalispell, MT	12/20	2,800
Hilton Head–Beaufort, SC	11/26	3,127
Ocean City–Assateague Island, MD	5/11	3,145
Grand Lake–Lake Tenkiller, OK	6/17	3,724
Grass Valley–Truckee, CA	7/19	3,779
Rhinelander, WI	5/8	4,075

Source: Rand McNally & Company, *Mobil Travel Guide*, 1986, and Woods & Poole Economics, Inc., population forecasts.

Thirteen retirement places have restaurants not rated by *Mobil Travel Guide:* Athens–Cedar Creek Lake, Texas; Burnet–Marble Falls–Llano, Texas; Canton–Lake Tawakoni, Texas; Deming, New Mexico; Franklin County, Tennessee; Fredericksburg, Texas; Friday Harbor–San Juan Islands, Washington; Gainesville–Lake Lanier, Georgia; Kauai, Hawaii; Maui, Hawaii; Monticello–Liberty, New York; Oscoda–Huron Shore, Michigan; Southport, North Carolina.

Counting Holes: Public Golf Courses

According to the Interior Department's latest *Outdoor Recreation Survey*, the percentage of persons between 55 and 64 who play golf regularly is greater than that in any other age group.

You've got three options if you're in search of a golf outing on an idle, sunny weekend: the *private* course, typically part of a country club open only to members and guests; a private *daily-fee* operation open to all players for a fee; and a *municipal* course operated by any tax-supported agency such as a city, county, school, or park district.

If you can afford to join a private country club with an 18-hole course, the dues you pay buy one big benefit besides the use of the swimming pool and tennis courts. You belong to the fortunate 14 percent of golfers who don't have to kill time waiting to tee off at crowded public courses. On the other hand, if you're one of 12 million golfers in the country who regularly plays a round at a daily-fee or municipal course, only six of every ten of the nation's courses are open to you.

Because public regulation golf is an excellent indicator of other leisure options in a retirement place, *Retirement Places Rated* counts not the number of municipal and daily-fee courses but their total number of holes per capita. Eagle River, Wisconsin, and Brunswick–Golden Isles, Georgia, have one municipal course each, for example. But there are 36 holes at the

course in Georgia, and only 9 at the one in the North Woods.

Access to Public Golf

BEST RETIREMENT PLACES	Courses/Holes	Residents per Golf Hole
Myrtle Beach, SC	29/612	206
Door County, WI	7/117	238
North Conway–White Mountains, NH	9/117	275
Monticello–Liberty, NY	13/207	312
Eagle River, WI	5/54	315
Houghton Lake, MI	5/63	325
Petoskey–Straits of Mackinac, MI	3/72	338
Burnet–Marble Falls–Llano, TX	5/99	367
Southport, NC	7/126	375
Hilton Head–Beaufort, SC	10/207	393

WORST RETIREMENT PLACES	Courses/Holes	Residents per Golf Hole
Columbia County, NY	1/9	6,689
Athens–Cedar Creek Lake, TX	1/9	5,878
Santa Fe, NM	1/18	5,361
Virginia Beach–Norfolk, VA	10/171	5,172
Colorado Springs, CO	4/72	5,121
Red Bluff–Sacramento Valley, CA	1/9	5,089
Albuquerque, NM	5/108	4,502
Miami–Hialeah, FL	20/423	4,383
San Antonio, TX	13/297	4,378
Ocean County, NJ	6/90	4,214

Source: National Golf Foundation, unpublished data, and Woods & Poole Economics, Inc., population forecasts.

The national average is 2,227 persons per public golf hole; in the 129 retirement places that have public golf, the average is one hole for every 1,647 persons.

Public golf is played at *daily-fee* operations open to all players for a fee and *municipal* courses operated by any tax-supported agency, such as a city, county, school, or park district. Canton–Lake Tawakoni, Texas, and Winchester, Virginia, have no public golf facilities.

Counting Lanes: Tenpin Bowling

The sound of a hardwood ball striking hardwood pins was sometimes mistaken for a thunderclap in early 19th-century America. The sport has been around a long, long time indeed, and along with all its variations—skittles, fivepins, ninepins, tenpins, candlepins, duckpins, and bocce—is probably played by more people in the world than any other game (with the exception of soccer).

In the United States, the dominant variation is tenpins, and nearly 70 million people take a turn at it once or twice a year. But if the 8,300 bowling centers had to depend solely on this kind of casual participation, many might quickly convert to tanning salons or Jazzercise studios for a steadier income. The credit for keeping the alleys in business goes to the American Bowling Congress (ABC), to which 4.3 million men belong, and the Women's International Bowling Congress (WIBC), with 3.7 million women members, which promote tournaments throughout the country.

The sport is highly recommended for older adults. Dr. Morris Fishbein, once editor of the *Journal of the American Medical Association*, told *Family Health* magazine that, aside from relieving the postural backache that comes from sitting too long, the physical exercise and the challenge of making the ball knock down all those pins at once "produce better coordination of vision and mind with practically all the muscles of the body."

Another plus for older newcomers is the ready-made social contacts that are part of formal bowling competition. Whether you're in Daytona Beach, Deming, or Door County, you'll find team bowling. With 1.5 million teams in 133,000 leagues around the country, what better odds can there be for meeting a group that's right for you?

Nearly every tenpin bowling center in this country is certified by the ABC for tournament competition. To rate each retirement place for bowling, *Retirement Places Rated* counts the number of certified lanes rather than the number of bowling centers to derive a per capita access score. Bennington, Vermont, for example, and Bradenton, Florida, each have two ABC centers. There are 88 certified lanes in the Metropolitan South Florida retirement place and only 28 in its Yankee Belt counterpart. Yet Bennington gets a higher rating than Bradenton because there are more lanes for the local population.

Access to Certified Bowling

BEST RETIREMENT PLACES	Bowling Centers/ Lanes	Residents per Lane
Canandaigua, NY	5/106	594
Rhinelander, WI	4/42	776
Door County, WI	4/34	821
Oak Harbor–Whidbey Island, WA	3/56	836
Columbia County, NY	4/66	985
Madison, WI	23/386	916
Hamilton–Bitterroot Valley, MT	3/28	925
Eagle River, WI	2/18	944
Kalispell, MT	6/58	966
Mountain Home– Bull Shoals, AR	3/46	985
Petoskey–Straits of Mackinac, MI	1/24	1,013
Houghton Lake, MI	2/20	1,025
Coeur d'Alene, ID	4/68	1,041
Naples, FL	5/114	1,047
Port Angeles– Strait of Juan de Fuca, WA	5/50	1,066

Source: American Bowling Congress, unpublished 1986 data, and Woods & Poole Economics, Inc., population forecasts.

The national average is one lane for every 1,583 persons; in the 119 retirement places that have ABC–certified lanes, it is one lane for every 2,209 persons.

Twelve retirement places have no ABC-certified lanes: Athens–Cedar Creek Lake, Texas; Burnet–Marble Falls–Llano, Texas; Camden–Penobscot Bay, Maine; Canton–Lake Tawakoni, Texas; Clayton–Clarkesville, Georgia; Franklin County, Tennessee; Friday Harbor–San Juan Islands, Washington; Hanover, New Hampshire; Kauai, Hawaii; Keene, New Hampshire; North Conway–White Mountains, New Hampshire; Southport, North Carolina.

Counting Theaters: The Movies

The number of people over 55 who regularly catch a commercial film tripled during the 1970s. This may seem odd, since moviemakers tend to forget that older adults are part of audience demographics when new picture ideas are scrutinized for marketability. Aside

from there being more people over 55 each year, another reason for increased attendance is the afternoon deep-discount ticket policy at movie houses in suburban shopping malls.

You may recall the 1940s when moviegoing was a routine family activity. Remember when John Huston won two Academy Awards—best director and best screenplay—for *The Treasure of Sierra Madre*? And his father, Walter, was named best supporting actor for his portrayal of the old prospector in the same film? Jane Wyman won an Oscar for her role in *Johnny Belinda; Hamlet* was best picture, and its star, Laurence Olivier, best actor.

The year was 1948, a time when moviegoing was the American thing to do of an evening, any evening. Popcorn was regularly swept up from the aisles between shows, the next John Wayne or Spencer Tracy film was announced on a large easel in the lobby, usherettes took you to your seat with a red-lensed flashlight, and you always got a MovieTone or Warner-Pathé newsreel with the show. There were 18,631 movie houses back then. Never again would there be so many. Most were neighborhood establishments, with a few downtown palaces for "premieres" and first-run screenings.

Retirement Places Rated divides the local population by the number of commercial four-wall (as opposed to drive-in) theaters to determine local access to movies. Many of these movie houses are of the multiscreen,

Access to Movie Theaters

BEST RETIREMENT PLACES	Theaters	Residents per Theater
Cape May, NJ	11	8,027
Friday Harbor–San Juan Islands, WA	1	9,800
Bend, OR	7	10,086
Monticello–Liberty, NY	6	10,750
Oak Harbor–Whidbey Island, WA	4	11,700
Cape Cod, MA	14	12,214
Canton–Lake Tawakoni, TX	3	12,300
St. George–Zion, UT	3	12,367
Missoula, MT	6	12,883
Bellingham, WA	9	12,967

WORST RETIREMENT PLACES	Theaters	Residents per Theater
Hendersonville–Brevard, NC	1	94,000
Gainesville–Lake Lanier, GA	1	81,000
Lancaster, PA	5	77,520
Lake Havasu City–Kingman, AZ	1	75,400
Fort Walton Beach, FL	2	67,300
Keene, NH	1	66,000
Ocala, FL	3	61,000
Columbia County, NY	1	60,200
Bradenton, FL	3	59,367
Virginia Beach–Norfolk, VA	15	58,960

Source: U.S. Bureau of the Census, *1982 Census of Selected Services*, 1985, and Woods & Poole Economics, Inc., population forecasts.

The national average is 33,813 persons per movie theater; in the 125 retirement places that have at least one theater, it is 32,318.

Six retirement places have no movie theaters: Athens–Cedar Creek Lake, Texas; Clayton–Clarkesville, Georgia; Crossville, Tennessee; Deming, New Mexico; Houghton Lake, Michigan; and Southport, North Carolina.

Access to Public Library Resources

BEST RETIREMENT PLACES	Libraries/Volumes	Residents per 1,000 Volumes
Oak Harbor– Whidbey Island, WA	1/438,433	107
Amherst– Northampton, MA	18/721,317	194
Keene, NH	21/316,301	209
Door County, WI	1/132,060	211
North Conway–White Mountains, NH	12/145,269	222
Camden– Penobscot Bay, ME	10/153,260	229
Cape May, NJ	3/380,634	232
Laconia–Lake Winnipesaukee, NH	10/191,790	239
Olympia, WA	1/607,000	254
Friday Harbor–San Juan Islands, WA	3/38,384	255

WORST RETIREMENT PLACES	Libraries/Volumes	Residents per 1,000 Volumes
Kalispell, MT	1/14,426	3,882
Crossville, TN	1/13,805	2,311
Orlando, FL	13/445,793	2,061
Grand Lake– Lake Tenkiller, OK	3/32,500	1,948
San Diego, CA	37/1,192,804	1,837
Fort Walton Beach, FL	3/79,485	1,693
West Palm Beach– Boca Raton– Delray Beach, FL	11/488,774	1,625
Oscoda–Huron Shore, MI	3/18,000	1,556
Colorado Springs, CO	11/237,354	1,553
Franklin County, TN	1/21,653	1,524
Paris–Big Sandy, TN	2/31,000	1,477

Source: Various state library data, American Library Association, *American Library Directory,* 1985, and Woods & Poole Economics, Inc., population forecasts.

Cinema Six variety found in shopping malls, but most are still the single-screen Bijou or Strand kind of neighborhood theater.

Counting Books: Local Public Libraries

One common denominator that's almost always run by local government is the public library, perhaps the vital center of any place's intellectual life. Besides books, most libraries have collections of recordings, slides, filmstrips, magazines, and other items that may be borrowed for free. Many have programs for older adults that go far beyond the traditional mission of acquiring books and periodicals and loaning them for a few weeks to patrons.

There are more than 8,500 public libraries in the United States, 5,000 of which are branch libraries of a city, county, or regional library system. From all this, you might expect libraries to be the most plentiful of leisure-living institutions. They aren't. Nearly a quarter of the *Retirement Places Rated* locations have only one library.

Libraries and library books are concentrated in larger places. San Diego's 1.2 million volumes are shelved in one main building and 36 neighborhood branches; Miami's 26 libraries house 2.5 million books. But the size of the collection tells only half the story.

Measured by the number of people for every 1,000 public library books, the supply per person is greater in smaller places, especially college towns and towns in New England where the public library is well into its second century of operation.

THE PERFORMING ARTS

How do you measure the cultural goings-on in another place? If you loved your hometown's symphony, will you, after surfacing in a retirement place, be forced to settle for shaded seats at the annual outdoor Country Harmonica Blowoff?

This is no imaginary concern. Recent Harris polls show that, for every ten older adults who have access to the performing arts, four want to take advantage of the opportunity regularly.

Back to our point: if you exchange a big place for a smaller one, dirty air for clean, cold seasons for warm sun, the costly for the economical, do you also risk trading the lively arts for a cultural desert?

Campus and Civic Auditorium Bookings

Well before a touring pianist, European boys' choir, or visiting New York contemporary dance troupe comes to town for a date at the local performing arts center, it is typically booked by a nonprofit college or community concert association.

Does this mean you'll find the performing arts only in a big city blessed with an expensive concert hall and a nonprofit community concert association bankrolled by philanthropists, managed by paid professionals, and attended by season member-subscribers? Not necessarily.

The enormous attendance growth at fine arts concerts since 1970 is due not to turning up the volume and variety of performances in big cities but to increased popular interest in the fine arts in smaller cities and towns. And a good part of the interest comes from older fans. Among the *Retirement Places Rated* destina-

---

Are There Any Lively Arts Out There?

Quick, identify the retirement place whose performing arts series booked the following musical events during the 1985–86 season:

October 14—Kalidoskopio of Greece
November 15—De Falla Guitar Trio
February 20—Linda Maxey, marimba
March 31—Peter Nero, piano

Answer: Grand Junction, in the midst of Colorado's forested western slope. Concerts are given in the Grand Junction High School Auditorium (capacity 1,500). The town's symphony orchestra plays an additional 11 dates during the year. So much for the notion that performing arts find little appreciation in small places.

Performing Arts Calendar: 20 Outstanding Retirement Places

Retirement Place	Dates
Phoenix, AZ	415
San Diego, CA	387
Miami–Hialeah, FL	266
St. Petersburg–Clearwater, FL	251
Ann Arbor, MI	232
Fort Lauderdale–Hollywood–Pompano Beach, FL	224
San Antonio, TX	210
Virginia Beach–Norfolk, VA	190
Orlando, FL	169
Sarasota, FL	148
Austin, TX	143
Albuquerque, NM	136
Lexington, KY	120
Madison, WI	120
Salinas–Seaside–Monterey, CA	117
Fort Myers–Cape Coral, FL	116
West Palm Beach–Boca Raton–Delray Beach, FL	107
Colorado Springs, CO	97
Bloomington–Brown County, IN	85
Burlington, VT	84

Source: ABC Leisure Magazines, *Musical America: 1986 International Directory of the Performing Arts*, 1986.

Forty-seven retirement places have neither resident ensembles nor auditorium bookings reported in *Musical America*.

tions, 80 benefit from college and community arts series that regularly book touring artists, according to the latest edition of *Musical America*.

Resident Ensembles

Besides taking in the touring attractions, residents in some retirement places have the additional option of attending performances of resident ensembles, defined here as local opera companies that belong to Opera America and local orchestras that are members of the American Symphony Orchestra League.

Opera. Twenty-seven retirement places have live opera. Boise, Biloxi–Gulfport, Madison, and Miami–Hialeah may not have much else in common but they all belong to this select group. The image of horned helmets, silvery shields, and unintelligible singing is a low-brow cliche. Fans boast that operatic stagecraft is the most demanding of the performing arts because of the unique commingling of instruments and voice with theater and dance; if you're introduced to a good production, they say, you'll be hooked for life.

A few numbers confirm opera's growing appeal: from the 650 performing groups in the 1969–70 season, the number of opera groups swelled to 1,000 a dozen years later, and audiences doubled to 11 million during the same period.

Most of these opera groups are community clubs, choruses, and college workshops. But 130 have annual budgets exceeding $100,000. Full-scale opera productions that use professional orchestra and bring the world's leading singers to the stage are a costly business. In 1986, only 10 companies nationwide were of the "grand opera" scale, meaning their annual budgets were more than $3 million. Two of these operas are in San Diego and Santa Fe.

Symphony Orchestras. Orchestras are more common than opera companies. Sixty-six retirement places have at least one. Their music can be heard everywhere, from woodsy state parks to high-school auditoriums, and from philharmonic halls to impressive new civic arts centers to small-town bandboxes and pavilions. San Antonio and San Diego have "major" symphonies; that is, orchestras with budgets over $3.25 million.

OUTDOOR ASSETS

For older adults, one "destination pull" that may outweigh all the urban "origin push" factors associated with crime, congestion, and cost of living is the lure of the great outdoors. To be sure, the "great outdoors" takes in a wide range of possibilities. It might mean lying on a Gulf Coast beach, tramping the Appalachian Trail, flycasting for Rocky Mountain rainbow, daysailing on Chesapeake Bay, or just getting away from it all to a cabin on the edge of a Pacific Northwest wilderness area.

Well before the time comes for shedding job obligations, many people have already identified from past family vacations the places where, when they retire, their own ideal of the great outdoors will be right outside their door.

The Water Draw

Maryland watermen tell mainland tourists who come to offshore Chesapeake Bay fishing villages for the oysters and soft-shell crabs that the true length of estuarine shore reached by the Bay's tide would total more than 8,000 miles if all the kinks and bends were flattened out.

They say in Michigan's Roscommon County that the locals tend to live away from Houghton Lake, the state's biggest inland body of water, while the transplanted retired folks who've migrated up from Detroit or Cleveland or Chicago unerringly light on the shore like loons there for the duration.

And Oklahomans vaunt the state's prized collection of lakes. If you could tip the state a bit to the south, they say, the water would flow out and flood Texas for a good while.

No behaviorist has ever explained exactly what it is about a large body of water that attracts people who can live anywhere they want. Just being able to view a mirror surface at sunset or stroll barefoot along a strand of talcum-fine sand or enjoy cool breezes off the lapping waves when the weather is hot doesn't tell the whole story.

In 1981, sociologists at the University of Wisconsin tried to isolate which features of the environment determined migration among older adults. One was a mild average temperature for January and for June. Another was the extent of resort development, indicated by the number of people working in the recreation-services sector of the local economy. The third feature was water.

Was there any correlation between the migration of retired people on the one hand and mild temperatures, resort development, and water on the other? Yes and no. Water, whether found in streams, rivers, lakes, or along ocean and Great Lakes coasts, didn't play nearly as great a part in attracting older adults as did a mild climate and resort development. In fact, certain Arizona, Nevada, and New Mexico counties that were desert-dry attracted retired people at a faster rate than "wet" counties in other parts of the country. Just water in itself wasn't a sufficient magnet for migration, the research showed. Without mild climate and commercial development, retired people as a general rule aren't searching for sandy beaches and alpine lakes.

Nonetheless, you'll spot bodies of inland water in 9 out of 10 of the 131 *Retirement Places Rated* retirement locations. Aside from being a basic necessity for supporting life, water is regarded by most people as a scenic amenity; many regard it as a recreational amenity—as long as there is enough of it to fish in, boat on, or swim in without enduring snowmelt-cold temperatures. What's Petoskey without the Straits of Mackinac?

Or Cape Cod minus the Atlantic Ocean? Four out of five Americans today live within 100 miles of a coastline; by the end of this century, the Department of the Interior predicts three out of four will live within 50 miles. Not surprisingly, 47 *Retirement Places Rated* havens have an ocean or Great Lakes coastline.

Large Areas of Inland Water

Retirement Place	Inland Water Area	Percentage of Total Surface Area
Friday Harbor–San Juan Islands, WA	89.3 sq mi	33%
Brownsville–Harlingen, TX	262.9	23
Fort Myers–Cape Coral, FL	238.0	23
Melbourne–Titusville–Palm Bay, FL	299.0	23
Camden–Penobscot Bay, ME	103.0	22
Easton–Chesapeake Bay, MD	67.7	21
Bar Harbor–Frenchman Bay, ME	392.8	20
St. Petersburg–Clearwater, FL	70.8	20
Ocean City–Assateague Island, MD	110.0	19
Hilton Head–Beaufort, SC	112.5	16
Eagle River, WI	150.5	15
Ocean County, NJ	113.8	15
Laconia–Lake Winnipesaukee, NH	66.9	14
Panama City, FL	123.8	14
Burlington, VT	81.1	13

Source: U.S. Bureau of the Census, unpublished area–measurement data, 1985.

Inland water area includes ponds and lakes of surface area greater than than 40 acres; streams, canals, and rivers if width is one-eighth mile or more; water along irregular Great Lakes and ocean coastlines if bays, inlets, and estuaries are between 1 and 10 miles wide. Seven retirement places have no inland water: Albuquerque, New Mexico; Athens, Georgia; Deming, New Mexico; Fredericksburg, Texas; Front Royal, Virginia; Kerrville, Texas; and Las Cruces, New Mexico.

Counting Acres: The Public Lands

Of all the outdoor activities that older adults take to most frequently, the leading ones—pleasure driving, walking, picnicking, sightseeing, bird-watching, nature walking, and fishing—might arguably be more fun in the country's splendid system of federal- and state-run public recreation areas.

National Forests. Some 22 million of the National Forest System's 186 million acres are in *Retirement Places Rated* retirement areas. Although various parts of the national forests are classified as "wilderness," "primitive," "scenic," "historic," or "recreation" areas, the main purpose of the system is silviculture: growing wood, harvesting it carefully, and preserving naturally beautiful areas from the depredations of amateur chain saws, burger palaces, miniature golf, and condomania.

In rainy Deschutes National Forest near Bend, Oregon, for example, the harvest is Douglas fir; in the widespread components of Mark Twain National Forest in the Ozarks of southern Missouri, the crop is mainly local hardwoods of blackjack oak and hickory; in Pisgah National Forest, in western North Carolina, the trees are virgin oak, beech, and black walnut.

Within the forest system are more than a quarter of a million miles of paved roads, built not just for 18-wheel logging trucks but for everyone. They lead to a wide variety of recreation developments: some 400 privately operated resorts, marinas, and ski lodges, plus fishing lakes and streams, campgrounds, and hiking trails.

Large Areas of National Forest Lands

Retirement Place	Percentage of Land Area in . . .	National Forests
Hamilton–Bitterroot Valley, MT	73%	Bitterroot, Lolo
Medford–Ashland, OR	70	Klamath, Rogue River, Umpqua
Kalispell, MT	53	Flathead, Kootenai, Lolo
Bend, OR	50	Deschutes
Eugene–Springfield, OR	49	Siuslaw, Umpqua, Willamette
Clayton–Clarkesville, GA	45	Chattahoochee
Missoula, MT	42	Bitterroot, Flathead, Lolo
Twain Harte–Yosemite, CA	42	Calaveras Bigtree, Stanislaus
Prescott, AZ	38	Coconino, Kaibab, Prescott, Tonto

Source: U.S. Department of Agriculture, *Land Areas of the National Forest System,* 1986.

National Parks. Where multiple use is the philosophy behind national forests, the National Park System preserves irreplaceable geographic and historic treasures for public recreation. This has been its mission ever since Congress created Yellowstone National Park in adjacent western corners of the old Montana and Wyoming territories "as a public park or pleasuring ground for the benefit and enjoyment of the people" back in 1872.

Today, the collection of national parks, preserves, monuments, memorials, battlefields, seashores, riverways, and trails makes up the oldest and largest national park system in the world. Seven million of the National Park System's 79 million acres are found in *Retirement Places Rated* areas.

National Wildlife Refuges. Simply put, wildlife refuges protect native flora and fauna from people. This purpose is unchanged since 1903, when Theodore Roosevelt created the first refuge, Florida's Pelican Island, to save mangrove-nesting egrets from human poachers in search of plumage for women's hats.

Most of the 436 refuges are open for wildlife activities, particularly photography and nature observation. In certain of the refuges and at irregular times, fishing and hunting are permitted, depending on the size of the refuge's wild populations.

You don't necessarily have to move to the sticks to be close to nature. One third of the land area of Clark County, Nevada, (where Las Vegas is the seat of government) is dedicated to wildlife refuges; and Fort Myers–Cape Coral, Florida, has four refuges on 5,635 acres—Caloosahatchee, J. N. ''Ding'' Darling, Matlacha Pass, and Pine Island.

State Recreation Areas. Beaches, forests, historical sites, parks, natural or man-made lakes—all are parts of the 10 million acres of state-run recreation areas. The facilities are often equal in quality to the federal public lands, and in most states older visitors get a break on entrance fees.

State recreation areas range from small day-use

	Large Areas of National Park Lands	
Retirement Place	**Percentage of Land Area in . . .**	**National Parks**
Miami–Hialeah, FL	48%	Big Cypress National Preserve, Biscayne National Park, Everglades National Park
Naples, FL	34	Big Cypress National Preserve, Everglades National Park
Twain Harte–Yosemite, CA	30	Yosemite National Park
Port Angeles–Strait of Juan de Fuca, WA	29	Olympic National Park
Bellingham, WA	28	North Cascades National Park, Ross Lake National Recreation Area
Kalispell, MT	19	Glacier National Park
Lake Havasu City–Kingman, AZ	15	Grand Canyon National Park, Lake Mead National Recreation Area
Front Royal, VA	15	Appalachian Trail, Shenandoah National Park
Cape Cod, MA	14	Cape Cod National Seashore
Las Vegas, NV	11	Lake Mead National Recreation Area

Source: National Park Service, unpublished master deed listing, 1986.

parks in wooded areas or on beaches, offering little more than picnic tables and rest rooms, to large rugged parks and forests with developed hiking trails and campsites, and big-time destination resorts complete with golf courses, swimming pools, tennis courts and full-time recreation staffs.

SCORING: Leisure Living

If you are a hiker, golfer, birder, reader, bowler, moviegoer, and symphony lover, will you enjoy yourself more in Bend, Blacksburg, or Burlington?

Burlington, most likely. But there's the rub.

One can argue that ranking retirement places by their collections of leisure-living assets can't be done with total fairness. A Florida boater, hauling his smoky outboard motor out for a tune-up, may care nothing for the announced dates of a local civic concert series. Likewise, an older Cape Cod couple lolling on the beach may never know the joys of Wisconsin ice fishing, nor would they ever regret the loss.

When it comes to recreation, there are far too many differences in taste to develop a rating system that suits all preferences. Having said that, we can also say that it is possible to measure the supply of selected amenities in retirement places from coast to coast. It's certainly done all the time in chamber-of-commerce brochures and state-tourism promotion kits. Travelers, too, make their own comparisons in casual conversa-

tion. Hearsay may hold that winter living in the flatwoods of northern Michigan is as dull and lonesome today as it was for the many natives who quit the area for the city generations ago or that there's little in the way of peaceful outdoor recreation in sunbaked Orlando.

Retirement Places Rated tries a more objective approach. We neither judge the quality of music by local symphonies and opera companies nor critique museum and library collections. Neither do we push the recreation benefits of the desert over seashore or forest environs. Rather, we simply indicate the presence or absence of local assets that most of us would agree enhance retirement living.

Each place starts with a base score of zero, to which points are added according to the following criteria.

Common Denominators

Points are awarded on the basis of how accessible five common amenities are to residents in each place.

Access to these items is rated AA, A, B, or C (AA indicates the best access and C the worst), and the place is awarded points accordingly: 400 points for an AA rating, 300 points for A, 200 points for B, and 100 points for C.

1. *Good restaurants.*

A retirement place gets a rating of:	If there is one quality star for every:
AA	5,000 or fewer people
A	5,001 to 10,000 people
B	10,001 to 20,000 people
C	20,001 or more people

2. *Public golf courses.*

A retirement place gets a rating of:	If there is one public golf hole for every:
AA	750 or fewer people
A	751 to 1,500 people
B	1,501 to 2,250 people
C	2,251 or more people

3. *Bowling lanes.*

A retirement place gets a rating of:	If there is one lane for every:
AA	1,250 or fewer people
A	1,251 to 1,750 people
B	1,751 to 2,500 people
C	2,501 or more people

4. *Movie theaters.*

A retirement place gets a rating of:	If there is one theater for every:
AA	20,000 or fewer people
A	20,001 to 27,500 people
B	27,501 to 40,000 people
C	40,001 or more people

5. *Public libraries.*

A retirement place gets a rating of:	If there are 1,000 volumes for every:
AA	430 or fewer people
A	431 to 630 people
B	631 to 900 people
C	901 or more people

Performing Arts Calendar

1. *Campus and civic auditorium bookings.* In the calendar year, each date booked for touring fine arts groups to perform at local auditoriums is worth 10 points. Phoenix's 256 such dates, for example, are good for 2,560 points.

2. *Resident Ensembles.* In the calendar year, each performance date for local opera companies and symphony orchestras is worth an additional 10 points. The 146 total performance dates for Ann Arbor's one opera and five symphony orchestras, for example, contribute 1,460 points to its score.

Outdoor Assets

1. *Coastlines.* Each mile of general coastline, whether on the ocean or on the Great Lakes, gets 10 points. For example, the 55 miles of Pacific coastline on the western edge of San Diego earn this place 550 points.

2. *Inland water area.* The percentage of a place's total surface area that is classified as inland water is multiplied by 50. In Franklin County, Tennessee, 23.7 of the 567 square miles of surface area are inland water. That works out to 4.18 percent inland water, or 209 points.

3. *National forests, parks, and wildlife refuges.* The percentage of a place's land area that is set aside for national forests, parks, and wildlife refuges is multiplied by 50. St. George–Zion, Utah, has 1,550,720 total acres, 33.85 percent of which comprises the Dixie National Forest (394,393 acres) and Zion National Park (130,602 acres), giving that Desert Southwest retirement place 1,693 points.

4. *State recreation areas.* The percentage of a place's land area that is set aside for state recreation areas is multiplied by 50. Columbia County, New York, has 414,656 total acres. It also has four components of the New York State Park System, totaling 6,808 acres. This works out to 1.64 percent state park acreage, or 82 points.

SCORING EXAMPLES

A Sun Belt capital, a rustic resort in western Montana, and a small New England college area illustrate the different routes by which retirement places arrive at their leisure-living ratings.

San Diego, California (#2)

Just because one place possesses a greater number of leisure-time amenities than another place doesn't always mean it's better. For example, tiny Rhinelander, Wisconsin, has a greater supply of bowling lanes, movie theaters, public golf, good restaurants, and library volumes per capita than does giant San Diego. Rhinelander's score for these common denominators is 1,900; San Diego's is 600. True, there are more choices in densely populated places. But there are also more people to use them. No wonder it is dryly said in Southern California that much of one's time is spent waiting in line.

San Diego's big outdoor asset is its 55 miles of Pacific shoreline from Border Field Beach at the Mexican border all the way up to San Clemente. That plus San Diego County's more than 52 square miles of lakes and reservoirs, 16 state parks and beaches, a national forest, a national wildlife refuge, and a national monument contribute another 1,227 points.

It is in the performing arts that San Diego really shines. The San Diego Symphony Orchestra performs almost every other day at Symphony Hall. Operas are regularly staged at the Civic Theater and at the Old Globe Theater in Balboa Park. Suburban La Jolla is a center for chamber music. Together the 387 performance dates at various local campus and civic auditoriums add another 3,870 points to San Diego's leisure-living score.

Kalispell, Montana (#3)

"To Hell with Heaven's Gate" read many a Kalispell bumper sticker in 1979. More than a few locals were protesting the disruption caused by a large Hollywood production unit on location here for the filming of a story of 19th-century immigrant settlers battling powerful cattlemen. A year later, after being released and then quickly withdrawn, the film—Heaven's Gate—became the biggest flop in moviemaking, costing United Artists nearly $40 million.

The movie's only good character, some critics said, was its ruggedly beautiful scenery. Kalispell, the county seat, is the access town to Flathead National Forest and the southern gateway to Glacier National Park, which straddles the Great Divide all the way up to the Canadian border. With an inland water area of 143.2 square miles, including Hungry Horse Reservoir, Whitefish Lake, and Flathead Lake, and nearly 2.5 million acres of public lands, Kalispell earns 3,750 points in the Outdoor Assets category, the highest score among the retirement places.

Kalispell and surrounding Flathead County also score well in the Common Denominators category, particularly when the hundreds of thousands of summer visitors disappear after Labor Day. While the collection of books in its single public library earns only a C rating, the rustic Montana resort earns four AA ratings—the highest possible—for per capita access to good restaurants, public golf courses, bowling centers, and movie theaters.

The Performing Arts category is quite another story. Kalispell has one artist series, the Flathead Community Concert Association, and one resident ensemble, the Glacier Orchestra and Chorale. The combined 14 dates scheduled by these institutions are good for just 140 points.

Hanover, New Hampshire (#22)

Where Kalispell's strength lies in its outdoor assets and San Diego's in its performing arts, Hanover's advantage lies in its balance between the outdoors, the performing arts, and common denominators.

You'll search town directories in vain for tenpin bowling anywhere in Hanover and surrounding Grafton County. But the place earns three AA ratings for public golf courses, movie theaters, and public libraries, and an A rating for good restaurants. Per capita access to these amenities earns Hanover 1,500 points.

Outdoors, Grafton County's low mountain topography embraces nearly 370,000 acres of public land, including a national forest, a stretch of the Appalachian National Scenic Trail, and 23 state forests and parks. Those lands, plus more than 30 square miles of natural lakes and ponds, earn the Yankee Belt retirement place 1,766 points for outdoor assets.

Indoors, 54 of the performing arts bookings take place "Under the Big Hop" at Dartmouth College's Hopkins Center. Plymouth State College to the east schedules another 8 performances during the academic year. These dates add 620 points to Hanover's leisure-living score.

RANKINGS: Leisure Living

Eleven criteria are used to derive the score for a retirement place's supply of leisure-living assets: (1) good restaurants, (2) holes of public golf courses, (3) certified lanes for tenpin bowling, (4) movie theaters, (5) public-library resources, (6) campus and civic auditorium bookings, (7) resident opera companies and symphony orchestras, (8) miles of ocean or Great Lakes coastlines, (9) inland water area, (10) national parks, forests, and wildlife refuges, and (11) state recreation areas.

Places that receive tie scores are given the same rank and listed alphabetically.

Retirement Places from First to Last

Rank	Score	Rank	Score	Rank	Score
1. Miami–Hialeah, FL	6,513	11. Eagle River, WI	4,450	21. Ann Arbor, MI	3,923
2. San Diego, CA	5,697	12. Medford–Ashland, OR	4,428	22. Hanover, NH	3,886
3. Kalispell, MT	5,590	13. Salinas–Seaside–		23. Bend, OR	3,863
4. Phoenix, AZ	5,566	Monterey, CA	4,410	24. Sarasota, FL	3,769
5. Hamilton–		14. Eugene–Springfield, OR	4,384	25. Maui, HI	3,718
Bitterroot Valley, MT	5,263	15. Virginia Beach–		26. Ocean City–	
6. Bellingham, WA	5,207	Norfolk, VA	4,360	Assateague Island, MD	3,560
7. Port Angeles–Strait of		16. Fort Collins–Loveland, CO	4,270	27. Charleston, SC	3,535
Juan de Fuca, WA	5,176	17. Naples, FL	4,262	27. Fort Lauderdale–	
8. Twain Harte–Yosemite, CA	4,892	18. Friday Harbor–San Juan		Hollywood–Pompano Beach,	
9. St. Petersburg–		Islands, WA	4,256	FL	3,535
Clearwater, FL	4,834	19. Fort Myers–Cape Coral, FL	4,141	29. St. George–Zion, UT	3,497
10. Cape Cod, MA	4,547	20. Missoula, MT	3,924	30. Coeur d'Alene, ID	3,415

Rank	Score		Rank	Score		Rank	Score
31. Flagstaff, AZ	3,345		63. Brownsville–Harlingen, TX	2,540		96. Lake Havasu City– Kingman, AZ	1,650
32. Newport–Lincoln City, OR	3,324		64. San Luis Obispo, CA	2,521		97. Iowa City, IA	1,646
33. Melbourne–Titusville– Palm Bay, FL	3,288		65. Brunswick– Golden Isles, GA	2,507		98. Chico–Paradise, CA	1,639
34. Santa Fe, NM	3,283					99. Yuma, AZ	1,606
35. Camden–Penobscot Bay, ME	3,242		66. Petoskey–Straits of Mackinac, MI	2,484		100. New Paltz– Ulster County, NY	1,601
36. Oscoda–Huron Shore, MI	3,233		67. Hendersonville– Brevard, NC	2,471			
37. Burlington, VT	3,162		68. Colorado Springs, CO	2,444		101. Monticello–Liberty, NY	1,594
38. Bennington, VT	3,135		69. Carson City–Minden, NV	2,435		102. Litchfield County, CT	1,583
39. Hot Springs– Lake Ouachita, AR	3,123		70. Tucson, AZ	2,425		103. Fort Walton Beach, FL	1,575
40. Clayton–Clarkesville, GA	3,122					104. Charlottesville, VA	1,526
			71. Biloxi–Gulfport, MS	2,396		105. Springfield, MO	1,507
41. North Conway– White Mountains, NH	3,100		72. Laconia– Lake Winnipesaukee, NH	2,388		106. Keene, NH	1,505
42. Easton–Chesapeake Bay, MD	3,078		73. Ocala, FL	2,357		107. Las Cruces, NM	1,468
43. Bar Harbor– Frenchman Bay, ME	3,076		74. Ocean County, NJ	2,346		108. Asheville, NC	1,462
43. Door County, WI	3,076		75. Front Royal, VA	2,344		109. Columbia County, NY	1,456
45. Las Vegas, NV	3,069		76. Cape May, NJ	2,322		110. Lancaster, PA	1,442
46. Daytona Beach, FL	3,047		76. Panama City, FL	2,322		111. Winchester, VA	1,436
47. Traverse City– Grand Traverse Bay, MI	3,045		78. Branson–Cassville– Table Rock Lake, MO	2,260		112. Blacksburg, VA	1,408
48. Albuquerque, NM	3,029		79. Austin, TX	2,208		113. Kerrville, TX	1,404
49. Prescott, AZ	2,991		80. Amherst–Northampton, MA	2,185		114. Bradenton, FL	1,342
50. West Palm Beach– Boca Raton– Delray Beach, FL	2,981		81. Mountain Home– Bull Shoals, AR	2,172		115. Roswell, NM	1,332
			82. Myrtle Beach, SC	2,162		116. Portsmouth– Dover–Durham, NH	1,309
51. Orlando, FL	2,950		83. Lexington, KY	2,103		117. Fairhope–Gulf Shores, AL	1,281
52. Redding, CA	2,897		84. Rehoboth Bay–Indian River Bay, DE	2,088		118. Burnet– Marble Falls–Llano, TX	1,254
53. Bloomington– Brown County, IN	2,814		85. Lakeland–Winter Haven, FL	2,085		119. Boise, ID	1,238
54. Kauai, HI	2,785		86. Red Bluff– Sacramento Valley, CA	2,058		120. Fredericksburg, TX	1,204
55. San Antonio, TX	2,764		87. Reno, NV	2,008		121. Athens, GA	1,190
56. Madison, WI	2,745		88. Olympia, WA	1,999		122. Chapel Hill, NC	1,099
57. Rhinelander, WI	2,740		89. Santa Rosa–Petaluma, CA	1,975		123. Gainesville– Lake Lanier, GA	1,067
58. Grand Junction, CO	2,729		90. Houghton Lake, MI	1,967		124. Southport, NC	1,047
59. Hilton Head–Beaufort, SC	2,645		91. Fayetteville, AR	1,772		125. Crossville, TN	962
60. Grass Valley–Truckee, CA	2,634		92. Canandaigua, NY	1,707		126. Paris–Big Sandy, TN	893
61. Oak Harbor– Whidbey Island, WA	2,568		93. Murray–Kentucky Lake, KY	1,690		127. Deming, NM	801
62. Clear Lake, CA	2,553		94. Grand Lake– Lake Tenkiller, OK	1,668		128. Franklin County, TN	725
			95. State College, PA	1,658		129. McAllen–Edinburg– Mission, TX	719
						130. Athens–Cedar Creek Lake, TX	631
						131. Canton–Lake Tawakoni, TX	527

Retirement Places Listed Alphabetically

Retirement Place	Rank		Retirement Place	Rank		Retirement Place	Rank
Albuquerque, NM	48		Brownsville–Harlingen, TX	63		Columbia County, NY	109
Amherst–Northampton, MA	80		Brunswick–Golden Isles, GA	65		Crossville, TN	125
Ann Arbor, MI	21		Burlington, VT	37		Daytona Beach, FL	46
Asheville, NC	108					Deming, NM	127
Athens, GA	121		Burnet–Marble Falls– Llano, TX	118		Door County, WI	43
Athens–Cedar Creek Lake, TX	130		Camden–Penobscot Bay, ME	35		Eagle River, WI	11
Austin, TX	79		Canandaigua, NY	92		Easton–Chesapeake Bay, MD	42
Bar Harbor–Frenchman Bay, ME	43		Canton–Lake Tawakoni, TX	131		Eugene–Springfield, OR	14
Bellingham, WA	6		Cape Cod, MA	10		Fairhope–Gulf Shores, AL	117
Bend, OR	23		Cape May, NJ	76		Fayetteville, AR	91
Bennington, VT	38		Carson City–Minden, NV	69		Flagstaff, AZ	31
Biloxi–Gulfport, MS	71		Chapel Hill, NC	122		Fort Collins–Loveland, CO	16
Blacksburg, VA	112		Charleston, SC	27		Fort Lauderdale–Hollywood– Pompano Beach, FL	27
Bloomington– Brown County, IN	53		Charlottesville, VA	104		Fort Myers–Cape Coral, FL	19
Boise, ID	119		Chico–Paradise, CA	98		Fort Walton Beach, FL	103
Bradenton, FL	114		Clayton–Clarkesville, GA	40		Franklin County, TN	128
Branson–Cassville– Table Rock Lake, MO	78		Clear Lake, CA	62		Fredericksburg, TX	120
			Coeur d'Alene, ID	30			
			Colorado Springs, CO	68			

Retirement Place	Rank	Retirement Place	Rank	Retirement Place	Rank
Friday Harbor–San Juan Islands, WA	18	Medford–Ashland, OR	12	Prescott, AZ	49
Front Royal, VA	75	Melbourne–Titusville– Palm Bay, FL	33	Red Bluff–Sacramento Valley, CA	86
Gainesville–Lake Lanier, GA	123	Miami–Hialeah, FL	1	Redding, CA	52
		Missoula, MT	20	Rehoboth Bay–Indian River Bay, DE	84
Grand Junction, CO	58	Monticello–Liberty, NY	101		
Grand Lake–Lake Tenkiller, OK	94			Reno, NV	87
Grass Valley–Truckee, CA	60	Mountain Home–Bull Shoals, AR	81	Rhinelander, WI	57
Hamilton–Bitterroot Valley, MT	5	Murray–Kentucky Lake, KY	93	Roswell, NM	115
Hanover, NH	22	Myrtle Beach, SC	82	St. George–Zion, UT	29
		Naples, FL	17	St. Petersburg–Clearwater, FL	9
Hendersonville–Brevard, NC	67				
Hilton Head–Beaufort, SC	59	New Paltz–Ulster County, NY	100	Salinas–Seaside–Monterey, CA	13
Hot Springs–Lake Ouachita, AR	39	Newport–Lincoln City, OR	32	San Antonio, TX	55
Houghton Lake, MI	90	North Conway– White Mountains, NH	41	San Diego, CA	2
Iowa City, IA	97	Oak Harbor–Whidbey Island, WA	61	San Luis Obispo, CA	64
		Ocala, FL	73	Santa Fe, NM	34
Kalispell, MT	3				
Kauai, HI	54	Ocean City– Assateague Island, MD	26	Santa Rosa–Petaluma, CA	89
Keene, NH	106	Ocean County, NJ	74	Sarasota, FL	24
Kerrville, TX	113	Olympia, WA	88	Southport, NC	124
Laconia–Lake Winnipesaukee, NH	72	Orlando, FL	51	Springfield, MO	105
		Oscoda–Huron Shore, MI	36	State College, PA	95
Lake Havasu City–Kingman, AZ	96				
Lakeland–Winter Haven, FL	85	Panama City, FL	76	Traverse City–Grand Traverse Bay, MI	47
Lancaster, PA	110	Paris–Big Sandy, TN	126	Tucson, AZ	70
Las Cruces, NM	107	Petoskey–Straits of Mackinac, MI	66	Twain Harte–Yosemite, CA	8
Las Vegas, NV	45	Phoenix, AZ	4	Virginia Beach–Norfolk, VA	15
		Port Angeles–Strait of Juan de Fuca, WA	7	West Palm Beach–Boca Raton– Delray Beach, FL	50
Lexington, KY	83				
Litchfield County, CT	102			Winchester, VA	111
Madison, WI	56	Portsmouth–Dover–Durham, NH	116	Yuma, AZ	99
Maui, HI	25				
McAllen–Edinburg–Mission, TX	129				

PLACE PROFILES: Leisure Living

The following profiles catalog leisure-living features in each retirement place.

The profiles begin with Common Denominators—selected everyday options that ought to be available everywhere. Each item's access rating is shown in the right-hand column. (AA indicates the best access and C the worst.)

The second category, Performing Arts Calendar, counts the annual number of dates booked by local campus and civic auditoriums for touring fine arts groups as reported by *Musical America*'s latest survey. The dates of resident ensembles—opera companies that are members of Opera America and orchestras belonging to the American Symphony Orchestra League—are also counted.

The third category, Outdoor Assets, counts each place's miles of ocean or Great Lakes coastline, its square miles of inland water, and the public acreage for all state parks and national forests, national parks, and wildlife refuges located there. The figures for inland water count ponds and lakes if their surface areas are 40 acres or more; streams, canals, and rivers are also counted if their width is one-eighth mile or

more. The water area along irregular Great Lakes and ocean coastlines is counted, too, if the bays, inlets, and estuaries are between 1 and 10 miles in width. Lengths of ocean and Great Lakes coastlines are estimated from state totals measured by the National Oceanic and Atmospheric Administration. A selected list of units of the National Park System, national forests, and national wildlife refuges is included. The following abbreviations are used in this section:

NF	National forest	NP	National park
NHP	National historic park	NRA	National recreation area
NHS	National historic site	NS	National seashore
NM	National monument	NWR	National wildlife refuge

The figure in parentheses beside each major heading is the number of points awarded the place for assets in that category. A star preceding a place's name highlights it as one of the top 15 places for leisure living.

Information comes from these sources: ABC Leisure Magazines, *Musical America: 1986 International Directory of the Performing Arts*, 1986; American Bowling Congress, unpublished zip code data, 1986; American Symphony Orchestra League, *Orchestra and Business*

Directory, 1986; R. R. Bowker Co., *American Library Directory*, 1985; National Golf Foundation, unpublished administrative records, 1986; Opera America, *Profile*, 1986; Places Rated partnership, 1986 survey of state library associations and state parks and recreation departments; Rand McNally & Company, *Mobil Travel Guide* (7 volumes), 1986; U.S. Department of Agriculture, *Land Areas of the National Forest System*, 1986; U.S. Department of Commerce, Bureau of the Census, *1982*

Census of Selected Service Establishments, 1985, and unpublished land and water area measurements, 1985; U.S. Department of Commerce, National Oceanic and Atmospheric Administration, *The Coastline of the United States*, 1975; U.S. Department of the Interior, Fish and Wildlife Service, unpublished master deed listing, 1986; and National Park Service, *Index to the National Park System and Related Areas*, 1986, and unpublished master deed listing, 1986.

Albuquerque, NM

Rating

Common Denominators (1,000 points)
Good restaurants: 3 *, 7 **, 4 ***   **B**
Golf courses: 7 private (135 holes); 1 daily fee (27 holes);
    4 municipal (81 holes)   **C**
Bowling centers: 10 (288 lanes)   **A**
Movie theaters: 18   **A**
Public libraries: 9 (496,117 volumes)   **C**
Performing Arts Calendar (1,360 points)
Campus and civic auditorium bookings: 29 dates
Resident ensembles:
    Albuquerque Civic Light Opera (40 dates)
    Albuquerque Opera Theatre (15 dates)
    Chamber Orchestra of Albuquerque (20 dates)
    New Mexico Symphony Orchestra (32 dates)
Outdoor Assets (669 points)
National forests, parks, wildlife refuges:
    Bitter Lake NWR (23,350 acres)
    Cibola NF (76,482 acres)
State recreation areas: 1 (170 acres)

Score: 3,029
Rank: 48

Amherst–Northampton, MA

Common Denominators (1,400 points)
Good restaurants: 1 *, 4 **, 3 ***   **A**
Golf courses: 3 private (36 holes); 7 daily fee (90 holes)   **B**
Bowling centers: 1 (32 lanes)   **C**
Movie theaters: 7   **AA**
Public libraries: 18 (721,317 volumes)   **AA**
Performing Arts Calendar (520 points)
Campus and civic auditorium bookings: 40 dates
Resident ensembles:
    Five College Symphony Orchestra (8 dates)
    Project Opera (4 dates)
Outdoor Assets (265 points)
Inland water area: 17.1 square miles
    Knightville Reservoir
    Quabbin Reservoir
State recreation areas: 8 (7,573 acres)

Score: 2,185
Rank: 80

Ann Arbor, MI

Common Denominators (1,400 points)
Good restaurants: 2 *, 8 **, 3 ***   **B**
Golf courses: 8 private (117 holes); 11 daily fee (171
    holes); 3 municipal (54 holes)   **A**
Bowling centers: 11 (232 lanes)   **AA**
Movie theaters: 9   **B**
Public libraries: 9 (497,098 volumes)   **A**
Performing Arts Calendar (2,320 points)
Campus and civic auditorium bookings: 86 dates
Resident ensembles:
    Ann Arbor Chamber Orchestra (67 dates)
    Ann Arbor Symphony Orchestra (5 dates)
    Ars Musica Symphony Orchestra (50 dates)
    Comic Light Opera Guild (6 dates)
    Eastern Michigan University Symphony Orchestra
        (9 dates)
    University of Michigan Symphony Orchestra (9 dates)

Outdoor Assets (203 points)

Rating

Inland water area: 12.5 square miles
State recreation areas: 2 (10,799 acres)

Score: 3,923
Rank: 21

Asheville, NC

Common Denominators (700 points)
Good restaurants: 1 *, 1 **, 1 ***   **C**
Golf courses: 5 private (90 holes); 2 daily fee (27 holes);
    2 municipal (36 holes)   **C**
Bowling centers: 2 (48 lanes)   **C**
Movie theaters: 5   **B**
Public libraries: 10 (253,530 volumes)   **B**
Performing Arts Calendar (320 points)
Campus and civic auditorium bookings: 20 dates
Resident ensembles:
    Asheville Symphony Orchestra (12 dates)
Outdoor Assets (442 points)
Inland water area: 0.8 square miles
National forests, parks, wildlife refuges:
    Blue Ridge Parkway (5,411 acres)
    Pisgah NF (31,464 acres)

Score: 1,462
Rank: 108

Athens, GA

Common Denominators (1,100 points)
Good restaurants: 1 *   **C**
Golf courses: 1 private (27 holes); 2 daily fee (27 holes)   **C**
Bowling centers: 1 (24 lanes)   **C**
Movie theaters: 5   **AA**
Public libraries: 3 (203,799 volumes)   **AA**
Performing Arts Calendar (90 points)
Campus and civic auditorium bookings: 9 dates

Score: 1,190
Rank: 121

Athens–Cedar Creek Lake, TX

Common Denominators (300 points)
Golf courses: 1 private (9 holes); 1 daily fee (9 holes)   **C**
Public libraries: 2 (61,696 volumes)   **B**
Outdoor Assets (331 points)
Inland water area: 60.3 square miles
    Cedar Creek Lake
State recreation areas: 1 (1,582 acres)

Score: 631
Rank: 130

Austin, TX

Common Denominators (700 points)
Good restaurants: 3 *, 4 **, 2 ***   **C**
Golf courses: 15 private (324 holes); 10 daily fee (126
    holes); 5 municipal (81 holes)   **C**
Bowling centers: 11 (262 lanes)   **C**
Movie theaters: 21   **B**
Public libraries: 11 (923,420 volumes)   **B**
Performing Arts Calendar (1,430 points)
Campus and civic auditorium bookings: 99 dates

Rating

Resident ensembles:
    Austin Symphony Orchestra (28 dates)
    Austin Civic Orchestra (16 dates)
Outdoor Assets (78 points)
Inland water area: 35.6 square miles
    Tom Miller Dam
State recreation areas: 1 (632 acres)

Score: 2,208
Rank: 79

Bar Harbor–Frenchman Bay, ME

Common Denominators (1,600 points)

	Rating
Good restaurants: 4 *, 9 **, 1 ***	AA
Golf courses: 3 private (27 holes); 8 daily fee (90 holes)	AA
Bowling centers: 1 (4 lanes)	C
Movie theaters: 2	A
Public libraries: 2 (139,602)	AA

Outdoor Assets (1,476 points)
Atlantic coastline: 30 miles
Inland water area: 392.8 square miles
    Frenchman Bay
National forests, parks, wildlife refuges:
    Acadia NP (36,386 acres)
    Franklin Island NWR (12 acres)
    Seal Island NWR (65 acres)
State recreation areas: 7 (2,682 acres)

Score: 3,076
Rank: 43

★ Bellingham, WA

Common Denominators (1,600 points)

	Rating
Good restaurants: 2 **, 1 ***	B
Golf courses: 2 private (36 holes); 7 daily fee (81 holes); 2 municipal (27 holes)	A
Bowling centers: 4 (76 lanes)	A
Movie theaters: 9	AA
Public libraries: 16 (317,687 volumes)	AA

Performing Arts Calendar (160 points)
Campus and civic auditorium bookings: 6 dates
Resident ensembles:
    Bellingham Western Symphony Orchestra (10 dates)
Outdoor Assets (3,447 points)
Puget Sound coastline: 30 miles
Inland water area: 54.1 square miles
    Baker Lake
    Ross Lake
    Lake Whatcom
National forests, parks, wildlife refuges:
    Mt. Baker NF (452,629 acres)
    North Cascades NP (281,413 acres)
    Ross Lake NRA (107,663 acres)
State recreation areas: 2 (1,205 acres)

Score: 5,207
Rank: 6

Bend, OR

Common Denominators (1,300 points)

	Rating
Good restaurants: 1 *, 1 **	C
Golf courses: 1 private (18 holes); 7 daily fee (135 holes); 1 municipal (18 holes)	AA
Bowling centers: 4 (42 lanes)	A
Movie theaters: 7	AA
Public libraries: 3 (59,335 volumes)	C

Outdoor Assets (2,563 points)
Inland water area: 29.3 square miles
    Crane Prairie Reservoir
    Wickiup Reservoir
National forests, parks, wildlife refuges:
    Deschutes NF (979,136 acres)
State recreation areas: 8 (4,096 acres)

Score: 3,863
Rank: 23

Bennington, VT

Common Denominators (1,700 points)

	Rating
Good restaurants: 2 *, 1 **	A
Golf courses: 3 private (45 holes); 3 daily fee (45 holes)	A
Bowling centers: 2 (28 lanes)	A
Movie theaters: 2	AA
Public libraries: 4 (101,345 volumes)	AA

Performing Arts Calendar (160 points)
Campus and civic auditorium bookings: 12 dates
Resident ensembles:
    Sage City Symphony (4 dates)
Outdoor Assets (1,275 points)
Inland water area: 0.8 square miles
National forests, parks, wildlife refuges:
    Appalachian Trail (375 acres)
    Green Mountain NF (108,696 acres)
State recreation areas: 3 (931 acres)

Score: 3,135
Rank: 38

Biloxi–Gulfport, MS

Common Denominators (1,100 points)

	Rating
Good restaurants: 2 *, 5 **, 2 ***	B
Golf courses: 4 private (189 holes); 7 daily fee (153 holes); 3 municipal (36 holes)	A
Bowling centers: 6 (112 lanes)	B
Movie theaters: 7	B
Public libraries: 12 (321,141 volumes)	B

Performing Arts Calendar (150 points)
Campus and civic auditorium bookings: 7 dates
Resident ensembles:
    Gulf Coast Opera Theatre (3 dates)
    Gulf Coast Symphony Orchestra (5 dates)
Outdoor Assets (1,146 points)
Gulf coastline: 45 miles
Inland water area: 22.7 square miles
    Biloxi Bay
    St. Louis Bay
National forests, parks, wildlife refuges:
    DeSoto NF (61,389 acres)
    Gulf Islands NS (19,997 acres)
State recreation areas: 2 (393 acres)

Score: 2,396
Rank: 71

Blacksburg, VA

Common Denominators (900 points)

	Rating
Good restaurants: 1 **, 1 ***	B
Golf courses: 2 private (27 holes); 1 daily fee (18 holes)	C
Bowling centers: 2 (40 lanes)	B
Movie theaters: 2	B
Public libraries: 1 (96,198 volumes)	B

Performing Arts Calendar (100 points)
Campus and civic auditorium bookings: 6 dates
Resident ensembles:
    New River Valley Symphony (4 dates)
Outdoor Assets (408 points)
Inland water area: 1.5 square miles
National forests, parks, wildlife refuges:
    Appalachian Trail (150 acres)
    Jefferson NF (19,231 acres)

Score: 1,408
Rank: 112

Bloomington–Brown County, IN

Common Denominators (1,200 points)

	Rating
Good restaurants: 3 **, 2 ***	B
Golf courses: 2 private (27 holes); 3 daily fee (54 holes); 1 municipal (18 holes)	B
Bowling centers: 2 (56 lanes)	B
Movie theaters: 5	A
Public libraries: 3 (192,100 volumes)	A

Rating

Performing Arts Calendar (850 points)
Campus and civic auditorium bookings: 50 dates
Resident ensembles:
    Bloomington Symphony Orchestra (5 dates)
    Indiana University Philharmonic Orchestra (30 dates)
Outdoor Assets (764 points)
Inland water area: 31.4 square miles
    Lake Lemon
    Monroe Lake
National forests, parks, wildlife refuges:
    Hoosier NF (35,552 acres)
State recreation areas: 1 (15,543 acres)

Score: 2,814
Rank: 53

Boise, ID
Common Denominators (900 points)
Good restaurants: 2 **   C
Golf courses: 4 private (72 holes); 3 daily fee (45 holes);
    1 municipal (9 holes)   C
Bowling centers: 5 (98 lanes)   B
Movie theaters: 8   A
Public libraries: 5 (293,958 volumes)   B
Performing Arts Calendar (260 points)
Campus and civic auditorium bookings: 6 dates
Resident ensembles:
    Boise Opera (3 dates)
    Boise Philharmonic (17 dates)
Outdoor Assets (78 points)
Inland water area: 8.6 square miles
    Lucky Peak Lake
National forests, parks, wildlife refuges:
    Boise NF (4,211 acres)
State recreation areas: 3 (826 acres)

Score: 1,238
Rank: 119

Bradenton, FL
Common Denominators (800 points)
Good restaurants: 1 *, 2 **   C
Golf courses: 6 private (90 holes); 7 daily fee (126 holes);
    1 municipal (18 holes)   A
Bowling centers: 2 (88 lanes)   B
Movie theaters: 3   C
Public libraries: 4 (163,207 volumes)   C
Outdoor Assets (542 points)
Gulf coastline: 20 miles
Inland water area: 52.2 square miles
National forests, parks, wildlife refuges:
    De Soto National Memorial (26 acres)
    Passage Key NWR (36 acres)
    Hobe Sound NWR (967 acres)
State recreation areas: 2 (573 acres)

Score: 1,342
Rank: 114

Branson–Cassville–
Table Rock Lake, MO
Common Denominators (1,400 points)
Good restaurants: 1 *, 5 **, 1 ***   A
Golf courses: 5 daily fee (45 holes); 1 municipal (9 holes) A
Bowling centers: 3 (32 lanes)   B
Movie theaters: 2   B
Public libraries: 2 (173,452 volumes)   AA
Outdoor Assets (860 points)
Inland water area: 120.5 square miles
    Bull Shoals Lake
    Table Rock Lake
    Lake Taneycomo
National forests, parks, wildlife refuges:
    Mark Twain NF (133,997 acres)

Rating

State recreation areas: 2 (3,732 acres)
Score: 2,260
Rank: 78

Brownsville–Harlingen, TX
Common Denominators (800 points)
Good restaurants: 3 *, 6 **, 1 ***   B
Golf courses: 3 private (63 holes); 2 daily fee (54 holes);
    1 municipal (27 holes)   C
Bowling centers: 3 (64 lanes)   C
Movie theaters: 10   A
Public libraries: 8 (249,037 volumes)   C
Outdoor Assets (1,740 points)
Gulf coastline: 31 miles
Inland water area: 262.9 square miles
    Laguna Atascosa
    Laguna Madre
National forests, parks, wildlife refuges:
    Laguna Atascosa NWR (44,922 acres)
    Lower Rio Grande Valley NWR (528 acres)
State recreation areas: 2 (217 acres)

Score: 2,540
Rank: 63

Brunswick–Golden Isles, GA
Common Denominators (1,800 points)
Good restaurants: 1 *, 6 **   AA
Golf courses: 2 private (27 holes); 3 daily fee (81 holes);
    1 municipal (36 holes)   AA
Bowling centers: 1 (24 lanes)   B
Movie theaters: 3   AA
Public libraries: 1 (200,472 volumes)   AA
Outdoor Assets (707 points)
Atlantic coastline: 21 miles
Inland water area: 45.1 square miles
    St. Simons Sound
National forests, parks, wildlife refuges:
    Fort Frederica NM (216 acres)

Score: 2,507
Rank: 65

Burlington, VT
Common Denominators (1,500 points)
Good restaurants: 1 *, 6 **, 3 ***   A
Golf courses: 1 private (18 holes); 8 daily fee (117 holes) A
Bowling centers: 6 (114 lanes)   AA
Movie theaters: 6   A
Public libraries: 8 (181,200 volumes)   B
Performing Arts Calendar (840 points)
Campus and civic auditorium bookings: 55 dates
Resident ensembles:
    Vermont Symphony Orchestra (20 dates)
    Vermont Youth Orchestra (9 dates)
Outdoor Assets (822 points)
Inland water area: 81.1 square miles
    Lake Champlain
State recreation areas: 5 (13,414 acres)

Score: 3,162
Rank: 37

Burnet–Marble Falls–Llano, TX
Common Denominators (1,100 points)
Golf courses: 1 private (18 holes); 5 daily fee (99 holes) AA
Movie theaters: 2   AA
Public libraries: 2 (79,226 volumes)   A
Outdoor Assets (154 points)
Inland water area: 53.9 square miles
    Lake Buchanan
    Lake Lyndon B. Johnson
State recreation areas: 2 (4,549 acres)

Score: 1,254
Rank: 118

Rating

Camden–Penobscot Bay, ME
Common Denominators (1,600 points)
Good restaurants: 1 *, 4 **, 2 ***   AA
Golf courses: 1 private (9 holes); 5 daily fee (63 holes)   AA
Movie theaters: 2   AA
Public libraries: 10 (153,260 volumes)   AA
Outdoor Assets (1,642 points)
Atlantic coastline: 45 miles
Inland water area: 103 square miles
    Penobscot Bay
National forests, parks, wildlife refuges:
    Acadia NP (3,130 acres)
State recreation areas: 6 (3,091 acres)

Score: 3,242
Rank: 35

Canandaigua, NY
Common Denominators (1,400 points)
Good restaurants: 2 *, 2 **, 2 ***   A
Golf courses: 4 private (45 holes); 7 daily fee (108 holes)   A
Bowling centers: 5 (160 lanes)   AA
Movie theaters: 2   C
Public libraries: 11 (185,046 volumes)   A
Performing Arts Calendar (160 points)
Campus and civic auditorium bookings: 16 dates
Outdoor Assets (147 points)
Inland water area: 18.2 square miles
    Canandaigua Lake
State recreation areas: 5 (841 acres)

Score: 1,707
Rank: 92

Canton–Lake Tawakoni, TX
Common Denominators (500 points)
Golf courses: 1 private (18 holes)
Movie theaters: 3   AA
Public libraries: 2 (39,287 volumes)   C
Outdoor Assets (27 points)
Inland water area: 4.6 square miles
    Lake Tawakoni

Score: 527
Rank: 131

★ Cape Cod, MA
Common Denominators (1,500 points)
Good restaurants: 11 *, 23 **, 7 ***, 1 ****   AA
Golf courses: 8 private (153 holes); 18 daily fee (252 holes); 5 municipal (81 holes)   AA
Bowling centers: 3 (36 lanes)   C
Movie theaters: 14   AA
Public libraries: 9 (219,953 volumes)   B
Performing Arts Calendar (770 points)
Campus and civic auditorium bookings: 3 dates
Resident ensembles:
    Cape Cod Symphony Orchestra (20 dates)
    College Light Opera Company (54 dates)
Outdoor Assets (2,277 points)
Atlantic coastline: 80 miles
Inland water area: 56.9 square miles
    Cape Cod Bay
    Wellfleet Harbor
National forests, parks, wildlife refuges:
    Cape Cod NS (41,897 acres)
    Monomoy NWR (2,657 acres)
State recreation areas: 5 (5,488 acres)

Score: 4,547
Rank: 10

Cape May, NJ
Common Denominators (1,500 points)
Good restaurants: 1 *, 7 **, 2 ***   AA

Rating

Golf courses: 1 private (18 holes); 3 daily fee (45 holes); 1 municipal (9 holes)   B
Bowling centers: 1 (32 lanes)   C
Movie theaters: 11   AA
Public libraries: 3 (380,634 volumes)   AA
Outdoor Assets (822 points)
Atlantic coastline: 40 miles
Inland water area: 23.3 square miles
    Cape May Harbor
State recreation areas: 2 (531 acres)

Score: 2,322
Rank: 76

Carson City–Minden, NV
Common Denominators (1,600 points)
Good restaurants: 2 *, 5 **, 1 ***   AA
Golf courses: 3 daily fee (45 holes); 1 municipal (18 holes)   A
Bowling centers: 1 (44 lanes)   A
Movie theaters: 4   AA
Public libraries: 1 (71,486 volumes)   B
Outdoor Assets (835 points)
Inland water area: 39.3 square miles
    Lake Tahoe
National forests, parks, wildlife refuges:
    Eldorado NF (53 acres)
    Toiyabe NF (70,287 acres)
State recreation areas: 1 (2 acres)

Score: 2,435
Rank: 69

Chapel Hill, NC
Common Denominators (800 points)
Good restaurants: 1 *, 1 **, 2 ***   A
Golf courses: 2 private (36 holes); 4 daily fee (54 holes)   B
Bowling centers: 1 (12 lanes)   C
Movie theaters: 2   C
Public libraries: 2 (89,049 volumes)   C
Performing Arts Calendar (290 points)
Campus and civic auditorium bookings: 25 dates
Resident ensembles:
    University of North Carolina Symphony Orchestra
    (4 dates)
Outdoor Assets (9 points)
Inland water area: 0.7 square miles

Score: 1,099
Rank: 122

Charleston, SC
Common Denominators (900 points)
Good restaurants: 1 *, 3 **, 4 ***   B
Golf courses: 8 private (162 holes); 6 daily fee (108 holes); 1 municipal (18 holes)   C
Bowling centers: 6 (164 lanes)   B
Movie theaters: 8   B
Public libraries: 10 (349,779 volumes)   B
Performing Arts Calendar (660 points)
Campus and civic auditorium bookings: 12 dates
Resident ensembles:
    Charleston Opera Company (14 dates)
    Charleston Symphony Orchestra (40 dates)
Outdoor Assets (1,975 points)
Atlantic coastline: 75 miles
Inland water area: 108.2 square miles
    Bulls Bay
    Intracoastal Waterway
National forests, parks, wildlife refuges:
    Cape Romain NWR (3,440 acres)
    Fort Sumter NM (189 acres)
    Francis Marion NF (58,914 acres)
State recreation areas: 3 (1,536 acres)

Score: 3,535
Rank: 27

Rating

Charlottesville, VA
Common Denominators (1,100 points)
Good restaurants: 2 **, 2 ***   B
Golf courses: 4 private (90 holes); 2 daily fee (36 holes);
   4 municipal (54 holes)   A
Bowling centers: 1 (40 lanes)   C
Movie theaters: 4   B
Public libraries: 2 (243,308 volumes)   A
Performing Arts Calendar (220 points)
Campus and civic auditorium bookings: 12 dates
Resident ensembles:
   University and Community Symphony (10 dates)
Outdoor Assets (206 points)
Inland water area: 0.1 square miles
National forests, parks, wildlife refuges:
   Appalachian Trail (689 acres)
   Shenandoah NP (29,800 acres)

Score: 1,526
Rank: 104

Chico–Paradise, CA
Common Denominators (700 points)
Good restaurants: 1 **   C
Golf courses: 1 private (18 holes); 4 daily fee (36 holes);
   2 municipal (36 holes)   C
Bowling centers: 2 (58 lanes)   C
Movie theaters: 5   B
Public libraries: 1 (246,845 volumes)   B
Performing Arts Calendar (180 points)
Campus and civic auditorium bookings: 9 dates
Resident ensembles:
   Chico Symphony Orchestra (4 dates)
   Paradise Symphony Orchestra (5 dates)
Outdoor Assets (759 points)
Inland water area: 30.1 square miles
   Lake Oroville
National forests, parks, wildlife refuges:
   Lassen NF (49,237 acres)
   Plumas NF (81,992 acres)
State recreation areas: 4 (12,474 acres)

Score: 1,639
Rank: 98

Clayton–Clarkesville, GA
Common Denominators (800 points)
Good restaurants: 1 **   B
Golf courses: 2 private (36 holes); 1 daily fee (9 holes); 1
   municipal (9 holes)   B
Public libraries: 3 (141,763 volumes)   AA
Outdoor Assets (2,322 points)
Inland water area: 7.4 square miles
   Lake Burton
   Lake Rabun
National forests, parks, wildlife refuges:
   Appalachian Trail (190 acres)
   Chattahoochee NF (188,666 acres)
State recreation areas: 2 (1,402 acres)

Score: 3,122
Rank: 40

Clear Lake, CA
Common Denominators (800 points)
Good restaurants: 1 **   C
Golf courses: 5 daily fee (54 holes)   A
Bowling centers: 2 (22 lanes)   B
Movie theaters: 1   C
Public libraries: 1 (53,000 volumes)   C
Outdoor Assets (1,753 points)
Inland water area: 67.1 square miles
   Clear Lake
   Indian Valley Reservoir
National forests, parks, wildlife refuges:
   Mendocino NF (253,874 acres)

Rating

State recreation areas: 2 (1,433 acres)

Score: 2,553
Rank: 62

Coeur d'Alene, ID
Common Denominators (1,500 points)
Good restaurants: 1 **, 2 ***   A
Golf courses: 4 private (72 holes); 3 daily fee (45 holes);
   1 municipal (9 holes)   A
Bowling centers: 4 (68 lanes)   AA
Movie theaters: 3   A
Public libraries: 5 (100,987 volumes)   B
Performing Arts Calendar (110 points)
Campus and civic auditorium bookings: 5 dates
Resident ensembles:
   North Idaho Symphony Orchestra (6 dates)
Outdoor Assets (1,805 points)
Inland water area: 70 square miles
   Coeur d'Alene Lake
   Hayden Lake
   Spirit Lake
National forests, parks, wildlife refuges:
   Coeur d'Alene NF (241,484 acres)
   Kaniksu NF (3,602 acres)
State recreation areas: 3 (12,710 acres)

Score: 3,415
Rank: 30

Colorado Springs, CO
Common Denominators (1,100 points)
Good restaurants: 2 *, 9 **, 3 ***   B
Golf courses: 8 private (198 holes); 2 daily fee (27 holes);
   2 municipal (45 holes)   C
Bowling centers: 13 (310 lanes)   AA
Movie theaters: 14   A
Public libraries: 11 (237,354 volumes)   C
Performing Arts Calendar (970 points)
Campus and civic auditorium bookings: 29 dates
Resident ensembles:
   Colorado Opera Festival (3 dates)
   Colorado Springs Symphony Orchestra (65 dates)
Outdoor Assets (374 points)
Inland water area: 2.1 square miles
National forests, parks, wildlife refuges:
   Pike NF (100,728 acres)

Score: 2,444
Rank: 68

Columbia County, NY
Common Denominators (1,300 points)
Good restaurants: 1 ***, 1 ****   A
Golf courses: 3 private (54 holes); 1 daily fee (9 holes)   C
Bowling centers: 4 (66 lanes)   AA
Movie theaters: 1   C
Public libraries: 11 (146,571 volumes)   AA
Outdoor Assets (156 points)
Inland water area: 9.6 square miles
   Copake Lake
State recreation areas: 4 (6,808 acres)

Score: 1,456
Rank: 109

Crossville, TN
Common Denominators (900 points)
Good restaurants: 1 ***   B
Golf courses: 2 private (36 holes); 3 daily fee (45 holes)   AA
Bowling centers: 1 (16 lanes)   B
Public libraries: 1 (13,805 volumes)   C
Outdoor Assets (62 points)
Inland water area: 2.1 square miles
State recreation areas: 1 (1,720 acres)

Score: 962
Rank: 125

Rating

Daytona Beach, FL
Common Denominators (1,300 points)
Good restaurants: 4 *, 8 **, 3 ***, 1 ****   A
Golf courses: 5 private (99 holes); 13 daily fee (234
holes); 2 municipal (54 holes)   A
Bowling centers: 7 (226 lanes)   A
Movie theaters: 11   B
Public libraries: 13 (479,045 volumes)   B
Performing Arts Calendar (350 points)
Campus and civic auditorium bookings: 28 dates
Resident ensembles:
Stetson University Orchestra (7 dates)
Outdoor Assets (1,397 points)
Atlantic coastline: 49 miles
Inland water area: 151.9 square miles
Intracoastal Waterway
Lake Dexter
National forests, parks, wildlife refuges:
Canaveral NS (28,148 acres)
Lake Woodruff NWR (18,225 acres)
State recreation areas: 3 (3,194 acres)

Score: 3,047
Rank: 46

Deming, NM
Common Denominators (800 points)
Golf courses: 1 daily fee (9 holes)   B
Bowling centers: 1 (8 lanes)   B
Public libraries: 1 (47,169 volumes)   AA
Outdoor Assets (1 point)
State recreation areas: 2 (313 acres)

Score: 801
Rank: 127

Door County, WI
Common Denominators (1,800 points)
Good restaurants: 6 *, 6 **   AA
Golf courses: 6 daily fee (99 holes); 1 municipal (18
holes)   AA
Bowling centers: 4 (34 lanes)   AA
Movie theaters: 1   B
Public libraries: 1 (132,060 volumes)   AA
Outdoor Assets (1,276 points)
Great Lakes coastline: 100 miles
Inland water area: 20.5 square miles
Sturgeon Bay
National forests, parks, wildlife refuges:
Gravel Island NWR (27 acres)
Green Bay NWR (2 acres)
State recreation areas: 4 (4,959 acres)

Score: 3,076
Rank: 43

★ Eagle River, WI
Common Denominators (2,000 points)
Good restaurants: 3 *, 5 **, 1 ***   AA
Golf courses: 2 private (27 holes); 4 daily fee (45 holes);
1 municipal (9 holes)   AA
Bowling centers: 2 (18 lanes)   AA
Movie theaters: 1   AA
Public libraries: 7 (48,578 volumes)   AA
Outdoor Assets (2,450 points)
Inland water area: 150.5 square miles
Plum Lake
Trout Lake
Yellow Birch Lake
National forests, parks, wildlife refuges:
Chequamegon NF (6,457 acres)
Nicolet NF (47,759 acres)
State recreation areas: 1 (68,472 acres)

Score: 4,450
Rank: 11

Rating

Easton–Chesapeake Bay, MD
Common Denominators (1,600 points)
Good restaurants: 1 ***   A
Golf courses: 2 private (36 holes); 1 municipal (27 holes)   A
Bowling centers: 1 (24 lanes)   AA
Movie theaters: 1   B
Public libraries: 1 (95,521 volumes)   AA
Performing Arts Calendar (40 points)
Campus and civic auditorium bookings: 4 dates
Outdoor Assets (1,438 points)
Chesapeake coastline: 40 miles
Inland water area: 67.7 square miles
Chesapeake Bay
State recreation areas: 1 (29 acres)

Score: 3,078
Rank: 42

★ Eugene–Springfield, OR
Common Denominators (1,100 points)
Good restaurants: 2 *, 4 **, 3 ***   B
Golf courses: 3 private (45 holes); 9 daily fee (126 holes);
1 municipal (9 holes)   B
Bowling centers: 10 (150 lanes)   B
Movie theaters: 12   A
Public libraries: 4 (325,904 volumes)   B
Performing Arts Calendar (480 points)
Campus and civic auditorium bookings: 12 dates
Resident ensembles:
Eugene Opera (7 dates)
Eugene Symphony Orchestra (23 dates)
University of Oregon Symphony Orchestra (6 dates)
Outdoor Assets (2,804 points)
Pacific coastline: 30 miles
Inland water area: 58.2 square miles
Fall Creek Lake
Fern Ridge Lake
Lookout Point Lake
National forests, parks, wildlife refuges:
Oregon Islands NWR (542 acres)
Siuslaw NF (242,747 acres)
Umpqua NF (151,588 acres)
Willamette NF (1,021,784 acres)
State recreation areas: 19 (4,850 acres)

Score: 4,384
Rank: 14

Fairhope–Gulf Shores, AL
Common Denominators (700 points)
Good restaurants: 2 *, 1 **   C
Golf courses: 3 private (63 holes); 1 daily fee (18 holes);
1 municipal (18 holes)   C
Bowling centers: 3 (40 lanes)   B
Movie theaters: 2   C
Public libraries: 7 (121,496 volumes)   B
Outdoor Assets (581 points)
Gulf coastline: 27 miles
Inland water area: 91.1 square miles
Bon Secour Bay
National forests, parks, wildlife refuges:
Bon Secour NWR (2,499 acres)
State recreation areas: 1 (6,000 acres)

Score: 1,281
Rank: 117

Fayetteville, AR
Common Denominators (1,200 points)
Good restaurants: 2 **, 2 ***   B
Golf courses: 1 private (18 holes); 3 daily fee (36 holes)   C
Bowling centers: 2 (68 lanes)   A
Movie theaters: 4   A
Public libraries: 1 (215,000 volumes)   A
Performing Arts Calendar (340 points)
Campus and civic auditorium bookings: 14 dates

Rating

Resident ensembles:
   North Arkansas Symphony Orchestra (20 dates)
Outdoor Assets (232 points)
Inland water area: 5.3 square miles
National forests, parks, wildlife refuges:
   Ozark NF (23,242 acres)
State recreation areas: 1 (1,699 acres)

Score: 1,772
Rank: 91

Flagstaff, AZ

Common Denominators (1,400 points)
Good restaurants: 1 *, 3 **, 3 ***, 1 ****   AA
Golf courses: 4 private (72 holes); 3 daily fee (54 holes);
   1 municipal (9 holes)   A
Bowling centers: 6 (60 lanes)   A
Movie theaters: 2   C
Public libraries: 7 (190,735 volumes)   A
Performing Arts Calendar (210 points)
Campus and civic auditorium bookings: 6 dates
Resident ensembles:
   Flagstaff Symphony Orchestra (15 dates)
Outdoor Assets (1,735 points)
Inland water area: 58.9 square miles
   Mormon Lake
National forests, parks, wildlife refuges:
   Apache-Sitgreaves NF (284,125 acres)
   Coconino NF (1,409,611 acres)
   Glen Canyon NRA (47,545 acres)
   Grand Canyon NP (673,497 acres)
   Kaibab NF (126,038 acres)
   Lake Mead NRA (83,166 acres)
   Navajo NM (40 acres)
   Prescott NF (43,695 acres)
   Sunset Crater NM (3,040 acres)
   Walnut Canyon NM (2,012 acres)
   Wupatki NM (35,253 acres)
State recreation areas: 1 (10 acres)

Score: 3,345
Rank: 31

Fort Collins–Loveland, CO

Common Denominators (1,200 points)
Good restaurants: 2 *, 2 **, 2 ***   B
Golf courses: 3 private (45 holes); 2 daily fee (27 holes);
   5 municipal (72 holes)   B
Bowling centers: 7 (108 lanes)   A
Movie theaters: 8   A
Public libraries: 3 (240,806 volumes)   B
Performing Arts Calendar (720 points)
Campus and civic auditorium bookings: 51 dates
Resident ensembles:
   Colorado State University Symphony Orchestra
      (6 dates)
   Fort Collins Symphony Orchestra (15 dates)
Outdoor Assets (2,350 points)
Inland water area: 29 square miles
   Horsetooth Reservoir
National forests, parks, wildlife refuges:
   Rocky Mountain NP (143,582 acres)
   Roosevelt NF (624,988 acres)
State recreation areas: 2 (4,916 acres)

Score: 4,270
Rank: 16

Fort Lauderdale–Hollywood–
Pompano Beach, FL

Common Denominators (1,000 points)
Good restaurants: 2 *, 12 **, 21 ***, 2 ****   B
Golf courses: 23 private (495 holes); 30 daily fee (666
   holes); 5 municipal (108 holes)   B
Bowling centers: 19 (544 lanes)   B
Movie theaters: 44   A
Public libraries: 26 (1,228,619 volumes)   C

Rating

Performing Arts Calendar (2,240 points)
Campus and civic auditorium bookings: 84 dates
Resident ensembles:
   Broward Community College Symphony Orchestra
      (19 dates)
   Florida Pops Orchestra (5 dates)
   Gold Coast Opera (9 dates)
   The Opera Guild (4 dates)
   Philharmonic Orchestra of Florida (70 dates)
   South Florida Symphony Orchestra (30 dates)
   Telemann Society Orchestra (3 dates)
Outdoor Assets (295 points)
Atlantic coastline: 25 miles
Inland water area: 10.2 square miles
State recreation areas: 2 (431 acres)

Score: 3,535
Rank: 27

Fort Myers–Cape Coral, FL

Common Denominators (1,400 points)
Good restaurants: 8 *, 11 **, 4 ***   A
Golf courses: 14 private (261 holes); 20 daily fee (360
   holes); 2 municipal (36 holes)   AA
Bowling centers: 8 (166 lanes)   A
Movie theaters: 10   B
Public libraries: 7 (354,370 volumes)   B
Performing Arts Calendar (1,160 points)
Campus and civic auditorium bookings: 99 dates
Resident ensembles:
   Southwest Florida Symphony Orchestra (17 dates)
Outdoor Assets (1,581 points)
Gulf coastline: 38 miles
Inland water area: 238 square miles
   Caloosahatchee River Estuary
   Pine Island Sound
   San Carlos Bay
National forests, parks, wildlife refuges:
   Caloosahatchee NWR (40 acres)
   J. N. "Ding" Darling NWR (4,960 acres)
   Matlacha Pass NWR (231 acres)
   Pine Island NWR (404 acres)
State recreation areas: 4 (2,063 acres)

Score: 4,141
Rank: 19

Fort Walton Beach, FL

Common Denominators (1,000 points)
Good restaurants: 4 **, 1 ***   B
Golf courses: 3 private (54 holes); 7 daily fee (117 holes);
   1 municipal (27 holes)   A
Bowling centers: 4 (80 lanes)   A
Movie theaters: 2   C
Public libraries: 3 (79,485 volumes)   C
Outdoor Assets (575 points)
Gulf coastline: 24 miles
Inland water area: 59.6 square miles
   Choctawhatchee Bay
National forests, parks, wildlife refuges:
   Choctawhatchee NF (675 acres)
   Gulf Islands NS (3,485 acres)
   State recreation areas: 1 (357 acres)

Score: 1,575
Rank: 103

Franklin County, TN

Common Denominators (400 points)
Golf courses: 2 private (18 holes); 1 daily fee (9 holes)   C
Movie theaters: 1   B
Public libraries: 1 (21,653 volumes)   C
Performing Arts Calendar (110 points)
Campus and civic auditorium bookings: 5 dates
Resident ensembles:
   Sewanee Summer Music Center Orchestra (6 dates)

	Rating

Outdoor Assets (215 points)
Inland water area: 23.7 square miles
    Lake Woods
    Tims Ford Lake
State recreation areas: 1 (413 acres)
Score: 725
Rank: 128

Fredericksburg, TX
Common Denominators (1,200 points)
Golf courses: 1 municipal (9 holes) — B
Bowling centers: 1 (10 lanes) — A
Movie theaters: 1 — AA
Public libraries: 1 (35,784 volumes) — A
Outdoor Assets (4 points)
National forests, parks, wildlife refuges:
    Lyndon B. Johnson NHP (197 acres)
State recreation areas: 1 (354 acres)
Score: 1,204
Rank: 120

Friday Harbor–
San Juan Islands, WA
Common Denominators (1,200 points)
Golf courses: 2 daily fee (18 holes) — AA
Movie theaters: 1 — AA
Public libraries: 3 (38,384 volumes) — AA
Outdoor Assets (3,056 points)
Puget Sound coastline: 115 miles
Inland water area: 89.3 square miles
National forests, parks, wildlife refuges:
    San Juan Island NHP (1,752 acres)
    San Juan Islands NWR (379 acres)
State recreation areas: 14 (6,255 acres)
Score: 4,256
Rank: 18

Front Royal, VA
Common Denominators (1,600 points)
Good restaurants: 1 *, 1 ** — A
Golf courses: 3 daily fee (54 holes) — AA
Bowling centers: 1 (18 lanes) — A
Movie theaters: 1 — A
Public libraries: 1 (37,791 volumes) — A
Outdoor Assets (744 points)
National forests, parks, wildlife refuges:
    Appalachian Trail (816 acres)
    George Washington NF (6,177 acres)
    Shenandoah NP (13,692 acres)
Score: 2,344
Rank: 75

Gainesville–Lake Lanier, GA
Common Denominators (500 points)
Golf courses: 1 daily fee (18 holes); 1 municipal (18 holes) — B
Bowling centers: 1 (24 lanes) — C
Movie theaters: 1 — C
Public libraries: 1 (87,969 volumes) — C
Outdoor Assets (567 points)
Inland water area: 48.5 square miles
    Lake Sidney Lanier
Score: 1,067
Rank: 123

Grand Junction, CO
Common Denominators (1,200 points)
Good restaurants: 1 *, 1 **, 1 *** — B
Golf courses: 1 private (18 holes); 1 daily fee (18 holes); 2 municipal (27 holes) — C
Bowling centers: 3 (92 lanes) — AA
Movie theaters: 3 — B
Public libraries: 6 (210,000 volumes) — A
Performing Arts Calendar (150 points)
Campus and civic auditorium bookings: 4 dates
Resident ensembles:
    Grand Junction Symphony Orchestra (11 dates)
Outdoor Assets (1,379 points)
Inland water area: 32.9 square miles
National forests, parks, wildlife refuges:
    Colorado NM (20,454 acres)
    Grand Mesa NF (252,648 acres)
    Manti Lasal NF (4,542 acres)
    Uncompahgre NF (207,256 acres)
    White River NF (81,289 acres)
State recreation areas: 3 (2,456 acres)
Score: 2,729
Rank: 58

Grand Lake–Lake Tenkiller, OK
Common Denominators (1,300 points)
Good restaurants: 2 **, 3 ***, 1 **** — AA
Golf courses: 1 private (9 holes); 2 daily fee (18 holes); 2 municipal (27 holes) — A
Bowling centers: 3 (30 lanes) — B
Movie theaters: 3 — A
Public libraries: 3 (32,500 volumes) — C
Performing Arts Calendar (40 points)
Campus and civic auditorium bookings: 4 dates
Outdoor Assets (328 points)
Inland water area: 100.2 square miles
    Lake O' The Cherokees
    Tenkiller Ferry Lake
State recreation areas: 8 (1,811 acres)
Score: 1,668
Rank: 94

Grass Valley–Truckee, CA
Common Denominators (1,200 points)
Good restaurants: 3 **, 3 ***, 1 **** — AA
Golf courses: 3 private (54 holes); 4 daily fee (54 holes) — A
Bowling centers: 2 (22 lanes) — C
Movie theaters: 3 — A
Public libraries: 1 (74,420 volumes) — C
Outdoor Assets (1,434 points)
Inland water area: 14.3 square miles
    Englebright Lake
    Prosser Creek Reservoir
National forests, parks, wildlife refuges:
    Tahoe NF (162,043 acres)
    Toiyabe NF (2,574 acres)
State recreation areas: 4 (5,057 acres)
Score: 2,634
Rank: 60

★ Hamilton–
Bitterroot Valley, MT
Common Denominators (1,600 points)
Good restaurants: 1 *** — A
Golf courses: 1 private (9 holes); 1 municipal (18 holes) — A
Bowling centers: 3 (28 lanes) — AA
Movie theaters: 1 — A
Public libraries: 3 (42,563 volumes) — A
Outdoor Assets (3,663 points)
Inland water area: 6.5 square miles
National forests, parks, wildlife refuges:
    Bitterroot NF (1,105,918 acres)
    Lee Metcalf NWR (2,696 acres)
    Lolo NF (8,131 acres)
State recreation areas: 3 (13,458 acres)
Score: 5,263
Rank: 5

Rating

Hanover, NH
Common Denominators (1,500 points)
Good restaurants: 1 *, 4 **, 1 ***   A
Golf courses: 2 private (18 holes); 10 daily fee (117
  holes); 1 municipal (18 holes)   AA
Movie theaters: 5   AA
Public libraries: 10 (173,676 volumes)   AA
Performing Arts Calendar (620 points)
Campus and civic auditorium bookings: 62 dates
Outdoor Assets (1,766 points)
Inland water area: 30.3 square miles
  Mascoma Lake
  Newfound Lake
National forests, parks, wildlife refuges:
  Appalachian Trail (5,760 acres)
  White Mountain NF (340,887 acres)
State recreation areas: 23 (22,618 acres)

Score: 3,886
Rank: 22

Hendersonville–Brevard, NC
Common Denominators (1,000 points)
Good restaurants: 1 **   C
Golf courses: 4 private (54 holes); 10 daily fee (153 holes) AA
Bowling centers: 2 (50 lanes)   B
Movie theaters: 1   C
Public libraries: 4 (137,678 volumes)   B
Performing Arts Calendar (360 points)
Campus and civic auditorium bookings: 25 dates
Resident ensembles:
  Brevard Opera Workshop (6 dates)
  Hendersonville Symphony Orchestra (5 dates)
Outdoor Assets (1,111 points)
Inland water area: 2.3 square miles
National forests, parks, wildlife refuges:
  Blue Ridge Parkway (1,553 acres)
  Carl Sandburg Home NHS (263 acres)
  Nantahala NF (4,082 acres)
  Pisgah NF (100,008 acres)

Score: 2,471
Rank: 67

Hilton Head–Beaufort, SC
Common Denominators (1,400 points)
Good restaurants: 1 *, 5 **, 5 ***   AA
Golf courses: 14 private (279 holes); 10 daily fee (207
  holes)   AA
Bowling centers: 1 (24 lanes)   C
Movie theaters: 4   A
Public libraries: 2 (91,842 volumes)   B
Outdoor Assets (1,245 points)
  Atlantic coastline: 36 miles
Inland water area: 112.5 square miles
  Port Royal Sound
  National forests, parks, wildlife refuges:
  Pinckney Island NWR (1,325 acres)
State recreation areas: 1 (5,000 acres)

Score: 2,645
Rank: 59

Hot Springs–Lake Ouachita, AR
Common Denominators (1,400 points)
Good restaurants: 6 **, 1 ***   A
Golf courses: 3 private (54 holes); 4 daily fee (81 holes)   A
Bowling centers: 2 (48 lanes)   A
Movie theaters: 2   B
Public libraries: 1 (134,099 volumes)   A
Outdoor Assets (1,723 points)
Inland water area: 77.5 square miles
  Lake Ouachita
National forests, parks, wildlife refuges:
  Hot Springs NP (5,135 acres)

Ouachita NF (106,824 acres)
State recreation areas: 1 (370 acres)

Score: 3,123
Rank: 39

Houghton Lake, MI
Common Denominators (1,500 points)
Good restaurants: 1 *, 1 **   A
Golf courses: 5 daily fee (63 holes)   AA
Bowling centers: 2 (20 lanes)   AA
Public libraries: 2 (56,444 volumes)   AA
Outdoor Assets (467 points)
Inland water area: 52 square miles
  Higgins Lake
  Houghton Lake
  Lake St. Helen
National forests, parks, wildlife refuges:
  Huron NF (40 acres)
State recreation areas: 2 (1,390 acres)

Score: 1,967
Rank: 90

Iowa City, IA
Common Denominators (1,300 points)
Good restaurants: 3 **   B
Golf courses: 1 private (9 holes); 3 daily fee (27 holes); 1
  municipal (18 holes)   B
Bowling centers: 2 (48 lanes)   B
Movie theaters: 5   AA
Public libraries: 4 (190,638 volumes)   A
Performing Arts Calendar (260 points)
Campus and civic auditorium bookings: 20 dates
Resident ensembles:
  University of Iowa Symphony Orchestra (6 dates)
Outdoor Assets (86 points)
Inland water area: 9.1 square miles
  Coralville Reservoir
  Lake Macbride
State recreation areas: 1 (1,073 acres)

Score: 1,646
Rank: 97

★ Kalispell, MT
Common Denominators (1,700 points)
Good restaurants: 4 *, 8 **   AA
Golf courses: 3 daily fee (63 holes); 1 municipal (18
  holes)   AA
Bowling centers: 6 (58 lanes)   AA
Movie theaters: 3   AA
Public libraries: 1 (14,426 volumes)   C
Performing Arts Calendar (140 points)
Campus and civic auditorium bookings: 6 dates
Resident ensembles:
  Glacier Orchestra and Chorale (8 dates)
Outdoor Assets (3,750 points)
Inland water area: 143.2 square miles
  Flathead Lake
  Hungry Horse Reservoir
  Whitefish Lake
National forests, parks, wildlife refuges:
  Flathead NF (1,715,680 acres)
  Glacier NP (643,137 acres)
  Kootenai NF (53,453 acres)
  Lolo NF (18,907 acres)
State recreation areas: 5 (9,780 acres)

Score: 5,590
Rank: 3

Kauai, HI
Common Denominators (1,100 points)
Golf courses: 4 daily fee (63 holes); 1 municipal (18
  holes)   AA

	Rating
Movie theaters: 2	A
Public libraries: 5 (141,952 volumes)	AA

Performing Arts Calendar (50 points)
Campus and civic auditorium bookings: 5 dates
Outdoor Assets (1,635 points)
Pacific coastline: 137 miles
Inland water area: 10 square miles
National forests, parks, wildlife refuges:
   Huleia NWR (238 acres)
   Hanalei NWR (917 acres)
State recreation areas: 11 (13,794 acres)

Score: 2,785
Rank: 54

Keene, NH
Common Denominators (1,000 points)

	Rating
Good restaurants: 2 **	B
Golf courses: 2 private (18 holes); 5 daily fee (63 holes)	A
Movie theaters: 1	C
Public libraries: 21 (316,301 volumes)	AA

Performing Arts Calendar (190 points)
Campus and civic auditorium bookings: 19 dates
Outdoor Assets (315 points)
Inland water area: 19 square miles
   Spofford Lake
   Silver Lake
State recreation areas: 17 (17,277 acres)

Score: 1,505
Rank: 106

Kerrville, TX
Common Denominators (1,400 points)

	Rating
Good restaurants: 1 *, 1 **, 1 ***	A
Golf courses: 1 private (18 holes); 1 municipal (36 holes)	A
Bowling centers: 1 (16 lanes)	B
Movie theaters: 2	AA
Public libraries: 1 (57,540 volumes)	B

Outdoor Assets (4 points)
State recreation areas: 1 (497 acres)

Score: 1,404
Rank: 113

Laconia–Lake Winnipesaukee, NH
Common Denominators (1,600 points)

	Rating
Good restaurants: 1 *, 2 **, 1 ***	A
Golf courses: 1 private (9 holes); 9 daily fee (99 holes)	AA
Bowling centers: 1 (24 lanes)	B
Movie theaters: 2	A
Public libraries: 10 (191,790 volumes)	AA

Outdoor Assets (788 points)
Inland water area: 66.9 square miles
   Lake Winnipesaukee
State recreation areas: 18 (4,688 acres)

Score: 2,388
Rank: 72

Lake Havasu City–Kingman, AZ
Common Denominators (800 points)

	Rating
Good restaurants: 1 *, 1 **	C
Golf courses: 4 daily fee (81 holes); 1 municipal (9 holes)	A
Bowling centers: 2 (36 lanes)	B
Movie theaters: 1	C
Public libraries: 5 (71,846 volumes)	C

Outdoor Assets (850 points)
Inland water area: 186 square miles
   Lake Havasu
   Lake Mead
National forests, parks, wildlife refuges:
   Grand Canyon NP (517,223 acres)
   Havasu NWR (11,908 acres)
   Kaibab NF (5,468 acres)
   Lake Mead NRA (799,213 acres)
   Pipe Spring NM (40 acres)

State recreation areas: 1 (13,000 acres)

Score: 1,650
Rank: 96

Lakeland–Winter Haven, FL
Common Denominators (1,100 points)

	Rating
Good restaurants: 7 **, 9 ***, 2 ****	A
Golf courses: 8 private (144 holes); 6 daily fee (126 holes); 5 municipal (99 holes)	B
Bowling centers: 7 (240 lanes)	A
Movie theaters: 9	B
Public libraries: 7 (262,707 volumes)	C

Performing Arts Calendar (500 points)
Campus and civic auditorium bookings: 45 dates
Resident ensembles:
   Lakeland Symphony Orchestra (5 dates)
Outdoor Assets (485 points)
Inland water area: 187.2 square miles
   Lake Pierce
   Lake Rosalie
   Lake Weohyakapka
State recreation areas: 1 (5,030 acres)

Score: 2,085
Rank: 85

Lancaster, PA
Common Denominators (800 points)

	Rating
Good restaurants: 6 **, 2 ***	C
Golf courses: 5 private (90 holes); 9 daily fee (171 holes)	C
Bowling centers: 12 (282 lanes)	A
Movie theaters: 5	C
Public libraries: 8 (502,394 volumes)	B

Performing Arts Calendar (480 points)
Campus and civic auditorium bookings: 28 dates
Resident ensembles:
   Lancaster Opera Workshop (20 dates)
Outdoor Assets (162 points)
Inland water area: 31.5 square miles
   Muddy Run Reservoir
State recreation areas: 1 (224 acres)

Score: 1,442
Rank: 110

Las Cruces, NM
Common Denominators (1,000 points)

	Rating
Good restaurants: 2 **, 1 ***	B
Golf courses: 5 private (90 holes); 2 daily fee (36 holes)	C
Bowling centers: 1 (32 lanes)	C
Movie theaters: 5	A
Public libraries: 2 (216,197 volumes)	A

Performing Arts Calendar (360 points)
Campus and civic auditorium bookings: 30 dates
Resident ensembles:
   Las Cruces Symphony (6 dates)
Outdoor Assets (108 points)
National forests, parks, wildlife refuges:
   San Andres NWR (2 acres)
   White Sands NM (52,778 acres)
State recreation areas: 1 (140 acres)

Score: 1,468
Rank: 107

Las Vegas, NV
Common Denominators (900 points)

	Rating
Good restaurants: 3 *, 14 **, 27 ***, 1 ****	A
Golf courses: 3 private (54 holes); 7 daily fee (117 holes); 4 municipal (54 holes)	C
Bowling centers: 10 (388 lanes)	A
Movie theaters: 14	C
Public libraries: 17 (625,863 volumes)	C

Performing Arts Calendar (550 points)
Campus and civic auditorium bookings: 32 dates

Rating

Resident ensembles:
    Las Vegas Chamber Symphony Orchestra (6 dates)
    Las Vegas Civic Symphony (6 dates)
    Las Vegas Opera Company (11 dates)
Outdoor Assets (1,619 points)
Inland water area: 209.8 square miles
    Lake Mead
National forests, parks, wildlife refuges:
    Desert NWR (828,755 acres)
    Lake Mead NRA (589,105 acres)
    Moapa Valley NWR (32 acres)
    Toiyabe NF (58,040 acres)
State recreation areas: 3 (66,160 acres)

Score: 3,069
Rank: 45

Lexington, KY
Common Denominators (900 points)
Good restaurants: 4 **, 3 ***, 2 ****   B
Golf courses: 10 private (153 holes); 7 daily fee (117
    holes); 3 municipal (54 holes)   B
Bowling centers: 6 (156 lanes)   B
Movie theaters: 8   C
Public libraries: 8 (439,871 volumes)   B
Performing Arts Calendar (1,200 points)
Campus and civic auditorium bookings: 101 dates
Resident ensembles:
    Central Kentucky Youth Orchestra (7 dates)
    Lexington Philharmonic Orchestra (12 dates)
Outdoor Assets (3 points)
Inland water area: 0.9 square miles
State recreation areas: 1 (10 acres)

Score: 2,103
Rank: 83

Litchfield County, CT
Common Denominators (1,400 points)
Good restaurants: 3 *, 3 **, 1 ***   B
Golf courses: 8 private (90 holes); 6 daily fee (63 holes);
    1 municipal (18 holes)   B
Bowling centers: 3 (100 lanes)   A
Movie theaters: 6   A
Public libraries: 21 (578,732 volumes)   AA
Outdoor Assets (183 points)
Inland water area: 23.5 square miles
    Bantam Lake
    Lake Winchester
National forests, parks, wildlife refuges:
    Appalachian Trail (4,943 acres)
State recreation areas: 19 (2,186 acres)

Score: 1,583
Rank: 102

Madison, WI
Common Denominators (1,400 points)
Good restaurants: 3 *, 5 **   C
Golf courses: 5 private (81 holes); 7 daily fee (117 holes);
    4 municipal (72 holes)   B
Bowling centers: 23 (386 lanes)   AA
Movie theaters: 13   A
Public libraries: 18 (904,207 volumes)   AA
Performing Arts Calendar (1,200 points)
Campus and civic auditorium bookings: 70 dates
Resident ensembles:
    Madison Opera (4 dates)
    Madison Symphony Orchestra (9 dates)
    University of Wisconsin Symphony (7 dates)
    Wisconsin Chamber Orchestra (30 dates)
Outdoor Assets (145 points)
Inland water area: 34.7 square miles
    Lake Mendota
    Lake Monona

Rating

State recreation areas: 2 (765 acres)
Score: 2,745
Rank: 56

Maui, HI
Common Denominators (1,000 points)
Golf courses: 2 private (18 holes); 6 daily fee (162 holes);
    1 municipal (18 holes)   AA
Bowling centers: 2 (30 lanes)   C
Movie theaters: 3   B
Public libraries: 7 (198,734 volumes)   A
Performing Arts Calendar (320 points)
Campus and civic auditorium bookings: 10 dates
Resident ensembles:
    Maui Philharmonic Society (10 dates)
    Maui Symphony Orchestra (12 dates)
Outdoor Assets (2,398 points)
Pacific coastline: 210 miles
Inland water area: 9.4 square miles
National forests, parks, wildlife refuges:
    Haleakala NP (27,621 acres)
    Kakahaia NWR (45 acres)
    Kalaupapa NHP (10,752 acres)
State recreation areas: 11 (285 acres)

Score: 3,718
Rank: 25

McAllen–Edinburg–Mission, TX
Common Denominators (600 points)
Good restaurants: 2 *, 3 **   C
Golf courses: 5 private (72 holes); 4 daily fee (54 holes);
    3 municipal (54 holes)   C
Bowling centers: 4 (66 lanes)   C
Movie theaters: 12   B
Public libraries: 10 (324,820 volumes)   C
Performing Arts Calendar (50 points)
Resident ensembles:
    Valley Symphony Orchestra (5 dates)
Outdoor Assets (69 points)
Inland water area: 12.4 square miles
National forests, parks, wildlife refuges:
    Lower Rio Grande Valley NWR (2,476 acres)
    Santa Ana NWR (2,901 acres)
State recreation areas: 1 (587 acres)

Score: 719
Rank: 129

★ Medford–Ashland, OR
Common Denominators (800 points)
Good restaurants: 3 **, 1 ***   B
Golf courses: 2 private (36 holes); 4 daily fee (36 holes);
    1 municipal (9 holes)   C
Bowling centers: 3 (74 lanes)   B
Movie theaters: 5   B
Public libraries: 12 (154,516 volumes)   C
Performing Arts Calendar (80 points)
Campus and civic auditorium bookings: 8 dates
Outdoor Assets (3,548 points)
Inland water area: 14.4 square miles
    Emigrant Reservoir
    Howard Prairie Reservoir
    Hyatt Reservoir
National forests, parks, wildlife refuges:
    Crater Lake NP (947 acres)
    Klamath NF (26,334 acres)
    Rogue River NF (411,704 acres)
    Umpqua NF (822,585 acres)
State recreation areas: 7 (1,386 acres)

Score: 4,428
Rank: 12

Rating

Melbourne–Titusville–Palm Bay, FL
Common Denominators (900 points)
Good restaurants: 1 *, 5 **, 1 ***   C
Golf courses: 4 private (81 holes); 6 daily fee (99 holes);
    4 municipal (72 holes)   B
Bowling centers: 5 (104 lanes)   C
Movie theaters: 14   A
Public libraries: 7 (472,823 volumes)   B
Performing Arts Calendar (300 points)
Campus and civic auditorium bookings: 12 dates
Resident ensembles:
    Brevard Symphony Orchestra (18 dates)
Outdoor Assets (2,088 points)
Atlantic coastline: 72 miles
Inland water area: 299 square miles
    Banana River
    Indian River
    Lake Washington
National forests, parks, wildlife refuges:
    Canaveral NS (29,479 acres)
    St. Johns NWR (5,264 acres)
State recreation areas: 1 (578 acres)

Score: 3,288
Rank: 33

★ Miami–Hialeah, FL
Common Denominators (800 points)
Good restaurants: 9 *, 16 **, 21 ***, 1 ****, 1 *****   B
Golf courses: 14 private (333 holes); 8 daily fee (252
    holes); 12 municipal (171 holes)   C
Bowling centers: 12 (454 lanes)   C
Movie theaters: 64   B
Public libraries: 26 (2,479,720 volumes)   B
Performing Arts Calendar (2,660 points)
Campus and civic auditorium bookings: 71 dates
Resident ensembles:
    Florida International University Orchestra (10 dates)
    Greater Miami Opera Association (126 dates)
    Miami Chamber Society (14 dates)
    South Florida Symphony Orchestra (45 dates)
Outdoor Assets (3,053 points)
Atlantic coastline: 50 miles
Inland water area: 64.2 square miles
    Biscayne Bay
National forests, parks, wildlife refuges:
    Big Cypress National Preserve (19,516 acres)
    Biscayne NP (171,369 acres)
    Everglades NP (415,952 acres)
State recreation areas: 4 (1,906 acres)

Score: 6,513
Rank: 1

Missoula, MT
Common Denominators (1,600 points)
Good restaurants: 7 **, 1 ***   AA
Golf courses: 1 private (18 holes); 1 daily fee (9 holes); 2
    municipal (27 holes)   B
Bowling centers: 2 (60 lanes)   A
Movie theaters: 6   AA
Public libraries: 1 (160,819 volumes)   A
Performing Arts Calendar (180 points)
Campus and civic auditorium bookings: 12 dates
Resident ensembles:
    Missoula Symphony Orchestra (6 dates)
Outdoor Assets (2,144 points)
Inland water area: 36 square miles
    Salmon Lake
    Seeley Lake
National forests, parks, wildlife refuges:
    Bitterroot NF (7,920 acres)
    Flathead NF (168,070 acres)

Rating

    Lolo NF (519,620 acres)
Score: 3,924
Rank: 20

Monticello–Liberty, NY
Common Denominators (1,400 points)
Golf courses: 1 private (9 holes); 11 daily fee (171 holes);
    2 municipal (36 holes)   AA
Bowling centers: 5 (50 lanes)   A
Movie theaters: 6   AA
Public libraries: 8 (102,394 volumes)   A
Performing Arts Calendar (80 points)
Campus and civic auditorium bookings: 8 dates
Outdoor Assets (114 points)
Inland water area: 20.6 square miles
    Neversink Reservoir
    Swinging Bridge Reservoir
State recreation areas: 1 (1,409 acres)

Score: 1,594
Rank: 101

Mountain Home–Bull Shoals, AR
Common Denominators (1,200 points)
Good restaurants: 2 *, 1 **, 1 ***   A
Golf courses: 1 daily fee (18 holes)   C
Bowling centers: 3 (46 lanes)   AA
Movie theaters: 2   A
Public libraries: 2 (48,500 volumes)   C
Outdoor Assets (972 points)
Inland water area: 94.1 square miles
    Bull Shoals Lake
    Norfork Lake
National forests, parks, wildlife refuges:
    Buffalo National River (26,921 acres)
    Ozark NF (64,798 acres)
State recreation areas: 1 (663 acres)

Score: 2,172
Rank: 81

Murray–Kentucky Lake, KY
Common Denominators (1,200 points)
Good restaurants: 1 **   C
Golf courses: 3 private (45 holes); 5 daily fee (72 holes)   A
Bowling centers: 3 (42 lanes)   A
Movie theaters: 2   B
Public libraries: 4 (129,500 volumes)   A
Performing Arts Calendar (50 points)
Campus and civic auditorium bookings: 5 dates
Outdoor Assets (440 points)
Inland water area: 61.2 square miles
    Kentucky Lake
State recreation areas: 2 (3,144 acres)

Score: 1,690
Rank: 93

Myrtle Beach, SC
Common Denominators (1,400 points)
Good restaurants: 10 **, 2 ***   AA
Golf courses: 1 private (9 holes); 29 daily fee (612 holes)   AA
Bowling centers: 2 (38 lanes)   C
Movie theaters: 9   AA
Public libraries: 4 (138,384 volumes)   C
Outdoor Assets (762 points)
Atlantic coastline: 75 miles
Inland water area: 2.3 square miles
State recreation areas: 1 (312 acres)

Score: 2,162
Rank: 82

Naples, FL
Common Denominators (1,600 points)
Good restaurants: 6 **, 4 ***, 1 ****   AA

Rating

Golf courses: 15 private (333 holes); 13 daily fee (234 holes) **AA**
Bowling centers: 5 (114 lanes) **AA**
Movie theaters: 5 **A**
Public libraries: 5 (111,585 volumes) **C**
Performing Arts Calendar (100 points)
Campus and civic auditorium bookings: 10 dates
Outdoor Assets (2,562 points)
Gulf coastline: 40 miles
Inland water area: 112.8 square miles
  Lake Trafford
National forests, parks, wildlife refuges:
  Big Cypress National Preserve (413,979 acres)
  Everglades NP (39,262 acres)
State recreation areas: 3 (57,641 acres)
Score: 4,262
Rank: 17

New Paltz–Ulster County, NY
Common Denominators (1,100 points)
Good restaurants: 1 *, 5 ** **B**
Golf courses: 3 private (36 holes); 14 daily fee (153 holes) **A**
Bowling centers: 3 (64 lanes) **C**
Movie theaters: 6 **B**
Public libraries: 16 (312,240 volumes) **A**
Performing Arts Calendar (300 points)
Campus and civic auditorium bookings: 30 dates
Outdoor Assets (201 points)
Inland water area: 30.4 square miles
  Ashokan Reservoir
State recreation areas: 2 (10,489 acres)
Score: 1,601
Rank: 100

Newport–Lincoln City, OR
Common Denominators (1,400 points)
Good restaurants: 5 **, 1 ***, 1 **** **AA**
Golf courses: 5 daily fee (54 holes) **AA**
Bowling centers: 2 (20 lanes) **B**
Movie theaters: 1 **B**
Public libraries: 3 (49,029 volumes) **B**
Outdoor Assets (1,924 points)
Pacific coastline: 50 miles
Inland water area: 11.8 square miles
  Alsea Bay
  Devils Lake
  Yaquina Bay
National forests, parks, wildlife refuges:
  Oregon Islands NWR (38 acres)
  Siuslaw NF (171,161 acres)
State recreation areas: 29 (2,027 acres)
Score: 3,324
Rank: 32

North Conway– White Mountains, NH
Common Denominators (1,600 points)
Good restaurants: 5 **, 4 *** **AA**
Golf courses: 1 private (18 holes); 9 daily fee (117 holes) **AA**
Movie theaters: 2 **AA**
Public libraries: 12 (145,269 volumes) **AA**
Outdoor Assets (1,500 points)
Inland water area: 57.7 square miles
  Lake Winnipesaukee
  Ossipee Lake
  Silver Lake
National forests, parks, wildlife refuges:
  White Mountain NF (145,005 acres)
State recreation areas: 14 (8,133 acres)
Score: 3,100
Rank: 41

Rating

Oak Harbor–Whidbey Island, WA
Common Denominators (1,600 points)
Good restaurants: 1 * **C**
Golf courses: 2 private (27 holes); 3 daily fee (36 holes) **A**
Bowling centers: 3 (56 lanes) **AA**
Movie theaters: 4 **AA**
Public libraries: 1 (438,433 volumes) **AA**
Outdoor Assets (968 points)
Puget Sound coastline: 60 miles
Inland water area: 11 square miles
  Saratoga Passage
  Skagit Bay
National forests, parks, wildlife refuges:
  San Juan Islands NWR (65 acres)
State recreation areas: 9 (3,379 acres)
Score: 2,568
Rank: 61

Ocala, FL
Common Denominators (700 points)
Good restaurants: 2 **, 1 *** **C**
Golf courses: 4 private (54 holes); 3 daily fee (54 holes); **C**
  2 municipal (27 holes)
Bowling centers: 3 (112 lanes) **A**
Movie theaters: 3 **C**
Public libraries: 14 (173,000 volumes) **C**
Performing Arts Calendar (160 points)
Resident ensembles:
  Central Florida Community College Aeolian Players
    (4 dates)
  Marion Chamber Music Society (4 dates)
  Ocala Festival Orchestra (8 dates)
Outdoor Assets (1,497 points)
Inland water area: 52.5 square miles
  Lake Bryant
  Lake Kerr
  Lake Weir
National forests, parks, wildlife refuges:
  Ocala NF (274,783 acres)
Score: 2,357
Rank: 73

Ocean City– Assateague Island, MD
Common Denominators (1,800 points)
Good restaurants: 4 **, 1 *** **AA**
Golf courses: 2 private (36 holes); 2 daily fee (45 holes);
  1 municipal (9 holes) **AA**
Bowling centers: 2 (28 lanes) **AA**
Movie theaters: 1 **B**
Public libraries: 1 (85,961 volumes) **AA**
Outdoor Assets (1,760 points)
Atlantic coastline: 31 miles
Inland water area: 110 square miles
  Chincoteague Bay
  Isle of Wight Bay
  Sinepuxent Bay
National forests, parks, wildlife refuges:
  Assateague Island NS (23,227 acres)
  Chincoteague NWR (910 acres)
State recreation areas: 2 (14,032 acres)
Score: 3,560
Rank: 26

Ocean County, NJ
Common Denominators (800 points)
Good restaurants: 3 ** **C**
Golf courses: 5 private (63 holes); 4 daily fee (54 holes);
  2 municipal (36 holes) **C**
Bowling centers: 7 (192 lanes) **B**
Movie theaters: 9 **C**
Public libraries: 3 (611,080 volumes) **A**
Performing Arts Calendar (130 points)
Campus and civic auditorium bookings: 9 dates

Rating   Rating

Resident ensembles:
   Garden State Philharmonic (4 dates)
Outdoor Assets (1,416 points)
Atlantic coastline: 50 miles
Inland water area: 113.8 square miles
   Barnegat Bay
National forests, parks, wildlife refuges:
   Edwin B. Forsythe NWR (8,189 acres)
State recreation areas: 5 (7,519 acres)

Score: 2,346
Rank: 74

Olympia, WA
Common Denominators (1,200 points)
Good restaurants: 1 *, 1 **   C
Golf courses: 1 private (18 holes); 6 daily fee (99 holes)   B
Bowling centers: 5 (80 lanes)   B
Movie theaters: 6   A
Public libraries: 1 (607,000 volumes)   AA
Performing Arts Calendar (360 points)
Campus and civic auditorium bookings: 30 dates
Resident ensembles:
   Olympia Symphony Orchestra (6 dates)
Outdoor Assets (439 points)
Puget Sound coastline: 10 miles
Inland water area: 47 square miles
   Budd Inlet
   Case Inlet
National forests, parks, wildlife refuges:
   Nisqually NWR (1,985 acres)
   Olympic NF (10 acres)
   Snoqualmie NF (612 acres)
State recreation areas: 1 (840 acres)

Score: 1,999
Rank: 88

Orlando, FL
Common Denominators (700 points)
Good restaurants: 2 *, 9 **, 5 ***   C
Golf courses: 11 private (216 holes); 31 daily fee (504
   holes); 1 municipal (18 holes)   B
Bowling centers: 19 (518 lanes)   B
Movie theaters: 21   C
Public libraries: 13 (445,793 volumes)   C
Performing Arts Calendar (1,690 points)
Campus and civic auditorium bookings: 38 dates
Resident ensembles:
   Festival Chamber Orchestra (3 dates)
   Florida Symphony Orchestra (107 dates)
   Florida Symphony Youth Orchestra (9 dates)
   Orlando Opera Company, Inc. (6 dates)
   University of Central Florida Orchestra (6 dates)
Outdoor Assets (560 points)
Inland water area: 297.1 square miles
   Lake Apopka
   Lake Kissimmee
   Lake Tohopekaliga
State recreation areas: 2 (14,399 acres)

Score: 2,950
Rank: 51

Oscoda–Huron Shore, MI
Common Denominators (1,200 points)
Golf courses: 4 daily fee (63 holes)   AA
Bowling centers: 2 (20 lanes)   A
Movie theaters: 2   AA
Public libraries: 3 (18,000 volumes)   C
Outdoor Assets (2,033 points)
Great Lakes coastline: 40 miles
Inland water area: 19.4 square miles
   Tawas Lake
National forests, parks, wildlife refuges:
   Huron NF (105,606 acres)

State recreation areas: 1 (175 acres)

Score: 3,233
Rank: 36

Panama City, FL
Common Denominators (900 points)
Good restaurants: 1 *, 4 **   B
Golf courses: 4 private (81 holes); 4 daily fee (54 holes)   B
Bowling centers: 3 (56 lanes)   B
Movie theaters: 4   B
Public libraries: 12 (83,421 volumes)   C
Performing Arts Calendar (270 points)
Campus and civic auditorium bookings: 27 dates
Outdoor Assets (1,152 points)
Gulf coastline: 44 miles
Inland water area: 123.8 square miles
   St. Andrew Bay
   West Bay
State recreation areas: 1 (1,082 acres)

Score: 2,322
Rank: 76

Paris–Big Sandy, TN
Common Denominators (500 points)
Good restaurants: 1 **   C
Golf courses: 3 private (27 holes); 1 municipal (18 holes)   C
Bowling centers: 1 (12 lanes)   C
Movie theaters: 1   C
Public libraries: 2 (31,000 volumes)   C
Outdoor Assets (393 points)
Inland water area: 77.4 square miles
   Kentucky Lake
State recreation areas: 2 (2,289 acres)

Score: 893
Rank: 126

Petoskey–Straits of
Mackinac, MI
Common Denominators (1,800 points)
Good restaurants: 4 *, 8 **   AA
Golf courses: 5 private (81 holes); 3 daily fee (72 holes)   AA
Bowling centers: 1 (24 lanes)   AA
Movie theaters: 1   A
Public libraries: 2 (56,000 volumes)   A
Outdoor Assets (684 points)
Great Lakes coastline: 50 miles
Inland water area: 16.5 square miles
   Little Traverse Bay
   Walloon Lake
State recreation areas: 2 (867 acres)

Score: 2,484
Rank: 66

★ Phoenix, AZ
Common Denominators (800 points)
Good restaurants: 9 *, 19 **, 15 ***, 4 ****   B
Golf courses: 38 private (774 holes); 39 daily fee (630
   holes); 12 municipal (189 holes)   C
Bowling centers: 28 (790 lanes)   B
Movie theaters: 35   C
Public libraries: 27 (2,713,448 volumes)   B
Performing Arts Calendar (4,150 points)
Campus and civic auditorium bookings: 256 dates
Resident ensembles:
   Arizona Opera Company (6 dates)
   Arizona State University Symphony Orchestra
     (15 dates)
   Mesa Symphony Orchestra (12 dates)
   Metropolitan Pops Orchestra (5 dates)
   Phoenix Chamber Music Society (13 dates)
   Phoenix Symphony Orchestra (93 dates)
   Scottsdale Symphony Orchestra (10 dates)
   Sun City Symphony Orchestra (5 dates)
Outdoor Assets (616 points)
Inland water area: 97.9 square miles

Rating   Rating

Apache Lake
Bartlett Reservoir
Canyon Lake
Cave Creek Dam
National forests, parks, wildlife refuges:
  Tonto NF (658,683 acres)
State recreation areas: 3 (6,260 acres)

Score: 5,566
Rank: 4

★ Port Angeles–Strait of Juan de Fuca, WA

Common Denominators (1,800 points)
Good restaurants: 3 **   A
Golf courses: 1 private (18 holes); 2 daily fee (36 holes)   A
Bowling centers: 5 (50 lanes)   AA
Movie theaters: 3   AA
Public libraries: 1 (139,459 volumes)   AA
Performing Arts Calendar (60 points)
Resident ensembles:
  Port Angeles Symphony Orchestra (6 dates)
Outdoor Assets (3,316 points)
Puget Sound coastline: 90 miles
Inland water area: 36 square miles
  Lake Crescent
  Ozette Lake
National forests, parks, wildlife refuges:
  Dungeness NWR (285 acres)
  Flattery Rocks NWR (125 acres)
  Olympic NF (200,095 acres)
  Olympic NP (329,185 acres)
  Quillayute Needles NWR (104 acres)
State recreation areas: 2 (211 acres)

Score: 5,176
Rank: 7

Portsmouth–Dover–Durham, NH

Common Denominators (700 points)
Good restaurants: 1 *, 7 **, 2 ***   B
Golf courses: 5 private (99 holes); 11 daily fee (126 holes)   C
Bowling centers: 2 (34 lanes)   C
Movie theaters: 7   C
Public libraries: 11 (487,442 volumes)   B
Performing Arts Calendar (100 points)
Campus and civic auditorium bookings: 10 dates
Outdoor Assets (509 points)
Atlantic coastline: 26 miles
Inland water area: 40.3 square miles
  Bow Lake
  Great Bay
  Portsmouth Harbor
State recreation areas: 24 (9,610 acres)

Score: 1,309
Rank: 116

Prescott, AZ

Common Denominators (900 points)
Good restaurants: 1 **   C
Golf courses: 1 private (18 holes); 2 daily fee (27 holes);
  1 municipal (18 holes)   B
Bowling centers: 2 (26 lanes)   C
Movie theaters: 4   A
Public libraries: 12 (144,408 volumes)   B
Performing Arts Calendar (200 points)
Campus and civic auditorium bookings: 20 dates
Outdoor Assets (1,891 points)
Inland water area: 4.2 square miles
  Pleasant Lake
National forests, parks, wildlife refuges:
  Coconino NF (426,621 acres)
  Kaibab NF (25,119 acres)
  Montezuma Castle NM (841 acres)
  Prescott NF (1,193,876 acres)

Tonto NF (316,917 acres)
Tuzigoot NM (58 acres)
State recreation areas: 3 (720 acres)

Score: 2,991
Rank: 49

Red Bluff–Sacramento Valley, CA

Common Denominators (1,000 points)
Good restaurants: 1 **   C
Golf courses: 1 private (18 holes); 1 daily fee (9 holes)   C
Bowling centers: 2 (26 lanes)   B
Movie theaters: 2   A
Public libraries: 1 (73,592 volumes)   A
Outdoor Assets (1,058 points)
Inland water area: 3.1 square miles
  Black Butte Lake
National forests, parks, wildlife refuges:
  Lassen NF (188,903 acres)
  Lassen Volcanic NP (4,200 acres)
  Mendocino NF (127,766 acres)
  Trinity NF (76,947 acres)
State recreation areas: 2 (431 acres)

Score: 2,058
Rank: 86

Redding, CA

Common Denominators (1,100 points)
Good restaurants: 1 *, 2 **, 1 ***   B
Golf courses: 3 private (45 holes); 6 daily fee (63 holes)   B
Bowling centers: 5 (72 lanes)   B
Movie theaters: 4   B
Public libraries: 1 (251,320 volumes)   A
Performing Arts Calendar (70 points)
Resident ensembles:
  Shasta Symphony (7 dates)
Outdoor Assets (1,727 points)
Inland water area: 67.8 square miles
  Shasta Lake
  Whiskeytown Lake
National forests, parks, wildlife refuges:
  Lassen NF (249,223 acres)
  Lassen Volcanic NP (66,862 acres)
  Shasta NF (436,665 acres)
  Whiskeytown–Shasta–Trinity NRA (42,488 acres)
State recreation areas: 4 (12,889 acres)

Score: 2,897
Rank: 52

Rehoboth Bay–Indian River Bay, DE

Common Denominators (1,200 points)
Good restaurants: 1 *, 4 **   B
Golf courses: 5 private (63 holes); 2 daily fee (27 holes)   C
Bowling centers: 4 (100 lanes)   AA
Movie theaters: 3   B
Public libraries: 14 (232,734 volumes)   A
Performing Arts Calendar (60 points)
Campus and civic auditorium bookings: 6 dates
Outdoor Assets (828 points)
Atlantic coastline: 52 miles
Inland water area: 37.1 square miles
  Indian River Bay
  Rehoboth Bay
National forests, parks, wildlife refuges:
  Prime Hook NWR (8,817 acres)
State recreation areas: 5 (6,093 acres)

Score: 2,088
Rank: 84

Reno, NV

Common Denominators (1,300 points)
Good restaurants: 8 *, 13 **, 5 ***, 2 ****   AA

Rating

	Rating
Golf courses: 1 private (18 holes); 2 daily fee (45 holes); 4 municipal (81 holes)	B
Bowling centers: 5 (150 lanes)	A
Movie theaters: 6	B
Public libraries: 7 (354,042 volumes)	B

Performing Arts Calendar (210 points)
Campus and civic auditorium bookings: 6 dates
Resident ensembles:
   Nevada Opera Association (9 dates)
   Reno Philharmonic Association (6 dates)
Outdoor Assets (498 points)
Inland water area: 232.9 square miles
   Lake Tahoe
National forests, parks, wildlife refuges:
   Anaho Island NWR (248 acres)
   Sheldon NWR (187,200 acres)
   Toiyabe NF (65,315 acres)
State recreation areas: 2 (15,684 acres)

Score: 2,008
Rank: 87

Rhinelander, WI

Common Denominators (1,900 points)	
Good restaurants: 2 *, 3 **	AA
Golf courses: 3 private (36 holes); 3 daily fee (36 holes)	A
Bowling centers: 4 (42 lanes)	AA
Movie theaters: 2	AA
Public libraries: 4 (119,747 volumes)	AA

Outdoor Assets (840 points)
Inland water area: 106.4 square miles
   Tomahawk Lake
   Pelican Lake
   Willow Reservoir
National forests, parks, wildlife refuges:
   Nicolet NF (11,273 acres)
State recreation areas: 1 (53,544 acres)

Score: 2,740
Rank: 57

Roswell, NM

Common Denominators (1,100 points)	
Good restaurants: 2 **	B
Golf courses: 1 private (9 holes); 2 municipal (36 holes)	B
Bowling centers: 2 (40 lanes)	A
Movie theaters: 3	A
Public libraries: 1 (64,867 volumes)	C

Performing Arts Calendar (170 points)
Campus and civic auditorium bookings: 4 dates
Resident ensembles:
   Roswell Symphony Orchestra (13 dates)
Outdoor Assets (62 points)
Inland water area: 10.4 square miles
   Two Rivers Reservoir
National forests, parks, wildlife refuges:
   Lincoln NF (40,332 acres)
State recreation areas: 1 (1,611 acres)

Score: 1,332
Rank: 115

St. George–Zion, UT

Common Denominators (1,600 points)	
Good restaurants: 3 **, 1 ***	AA
Golf courses: 1 private (18 holes); 3 daily fee (36 holes); 2 municipal (27 holes)	AA
Bowling centers: 2 (24 lanes)	A
Movie theaters: 3	AA
Public libraries: 1 (40,000 volumes)	C

Performing Arts Calendar (170 points)
Campus and civic auditorium bookings: 12 dates
Resident ensembles:
   Southwest Symphony Orchestra (5 dates)
Outdoor Assets (1,727 points)
Inland water area: 1.1 square miles

National forests, parks, wildlife refuges:
   Dixie NF (394,393 acres)
   Zion NP (130,602 acres)
State recreation areas: 4 (9,966 acres)

Score: 3,497
Rank: 29

★ St. Petersburg– Clearwater, FL

Common Denominators (800 points)	
Good restaurants: 13 *, 21 **, 9 ***, 1 ****	A
Golf courses: 12 private (297 holes); 24 daily fee (432 holes); 4 municipal (72 holes)	B
Bowling centers: 8 (232 lanes)	C
Movie theaters: 15	C
Public libraries: 7 (925,603 volumes)	C

Performing Arts Calendar (2,510 points)
Campus and civic auditorium bookings: 156 dates
Resident ensembles:
   Florida Lyric Opera Association (20 dates)
   The Florida Opera (9 dates)
   Matinee Opera Theatre (60 dates)
   Tampa Bay Community Symphony (6 dates)
Outdoor Assets (1,524 points)
Gulf coastline: 40 miles
Inland water area: 70.8 square miles
   Old Tampa Bay
   Lake Tarpon
National forests, parks, wildlife refuges:
   Pinellas NWR (15 acres)
State recreation areas: 3 (5,171 acres)

Score: 4,834
Rank: 9

★ Salinas–Seaside– Monterey, CA

Common Denominators (1,600 points)	
Good restaurants: 7 *, 14 **, 11 ***, 1 ****	AA
Golf courses: 9 private (189 holes); 8 daily fee (171 holes); 3 municipal (45 holes)	A
Bowling centers: 5 (78 lanes)	C
Movie theaters: 18	AA
Public libraries: 18 (812,243 volumes)	AA

Performing Arts Calendar (1,170 points)
Campus and civic auditorium bookings: 4 dates
Resident ensembles:
   Monterey Peninsula Chamber Music Society (7 dates)
   Hidden Valley Opera Ensemble (60 dates)
   Monterey Bay Symphony Orchestra (18 dates)
   Monterey County Symphony Orchestra (24 dates)
   Sunset Center Lively Arts Series (4 dates)
Outdoor Assets (1,640 points)
Pacific coastline: 85 miles
Inland water area: 24 square miles
National forests, parks, wildlife refuges:
   Los Padres NF (304,578 acres)
   Pinnacles NM (1,283 acres)
State recreation areas: 15 (14,691 acres)

Score: 4,410
Rank: 13

San Antonio, TX

Common Denominators (600 points)	
Good restaurants: 9 *, 10 **, 9 ***	C
Golf courses: 17 private (333 holes); 6 daily fee (81 holes); 7 municipal (216 holes)	C
Bowling centers: 22 (586 lanes)	B
Movie theaters: 25	C
Public libraries: 6 (1,421,372 volumes)	C

Performing Arts Calendar (2,100 points)
Campus and civic auditorium bookings: 70 dates
Resident ensembles:
   Mid Texas Symphony Orchestra (6 dates)
   San Antonio Symphony Orchestra (134 dates)

Rating

Outdoor Assets (64 points)
Inland water area: 31.4 square miles
  Canyon Lake
  Colaveras Lake
National forests, parks, wildlife refuges:
  San Antonio Missions NHP (345 acres)
State recreation areas: 4 (518 acres)

Score: 2,764
Rank: 55

★ **San Diego, CA**
Common Denominators (600 points)
Good restaurants: 9 *, 25 **, 15 ***   C
Golf courses: 23 private (414 holes); 42 daily fee (828
  holes); 5 municipal (117 holes)   C
Bowling centers: 26 (856 lanes)   C
Movie theaters: 55   B
Public libraries: 37 (1,192,804 volumes)   C
Performing Arts Calendar (3,870 points)
Campus and civic auditorium bookings: 76 dates
Resident ensembles:
  Jewish Community Center Symphony Orchestra
    (14 dates)
  La Jolla Chamber Music Society (35 dates)
  La Jolla Civic Orchestra (6 dates)
  San Diego Chamber Orchestra (15 dates)
  San Diego Civic Light Opera Association (50 dates)
  San Diego Opera (21 dates)
  San Diego State University Symphony Orchestra
    (8 dates)
  San Diego Symphony Orchestra (152 dates)
  San Diego Youth Symphony (10 dates)
Outdoor Assets (1,227 points)
Pacific coastline: 55 miles
Inland water area: 52.5 square miles
  Cuyamaca Reservoir
  El Capitan Lake
  Lake Henshaw
  Lake Hodges
National forests, parks, wildlife refuges:
  Cabrillo NM (144 acres)
  Cleveland NF (288,124 acres)
  Tijuana Slough NWR (407 acres)
State recreation areas: 16 (46,971 acres)

Score: 5,697
Rank: 2

San Luis Obispo, CA
Common Denominators (1,000 points)
Good restaurants: 2 *, 5 **, 4 ***   A
Golf courses: 2 private (36 holes); 5 daily fee (63 holes);
  2 municipal (36 holes)   B
Bowling centers: 4 (56 lanes)   C
Movie theaters: 5   B
Public libraries: 15 (246,706 volumes)   B
Performing Arts Calendar (410 points)
Campus and civic auditorium bookings: 37 dates
Resident ensembles:
  San Luis Obispo County Symphony (4 dates)
Outdoor Assets (1,111 points)
Pacific coastline: 60 miles
Inland water area: 22.1 square miles
  Nacimiento Reservoir
National forests, parks, wildlife refuges:
  Los Padres NF (188,908 acres)
State recreation areas: 12 (14,788 acres)

Score: 2,521
Rank: 64

Santa Fe, NM
Common Denominators (1,500 points)
Good restaurants: 1 *, 9 **, 9 ***, 2 ****   AA
Golf courses: 1 daily fee (18 holes)   C

Rating

Bowling centers: 2 (56 lanes)   A
Movie theaters: 6   AA
Public libraries: 4 (217,774 volumes)   A
Performing Arts Calendar (790 points)
Campus and civic auditorium bookings: 37 dates
Resident ensembles:
  Orchestra of Santa Fe (7 dates)
  Santa Fe Opera (35 dates)
Outdoor Assets (993 points)
Inland water area: 6.8 square miles
  Cochiti Reservoir
National forests, parks, wildlife refuges:
  Bandelier NM (7,309 acres)
  Santa Fe NF (245,023 acres)
State recreation areas: 2 (355 acres)

Score: 3,283
Rank: 34

Santa Rosa–Petaluma, CA
Common Denominators (1,100 points)
Good restaurants: 2 *, 6 **, 2 ***   B
Golf courses: 2 private (27 holes); 13 daily fee (171
  holes); 3 municipal (63 holes)   B
Bowling centers: 9 (164 lanes)   B
Movie theaters: 9   B
Public libraries: 12 (647,114 volumes)   A
Performing Arts Calendar (340 points)
Campus and civic auditorium bookings: 12 dates
Resident ensembles:
  Santa Rosa Symphony (16 dates)
  Sonoma County Junior Symphony (6 dates)
Outdoor Assets (535 points)
Pacific coastline: 35 miles
Inland water area: 10.2 square miles
National forests, parks, wildlife refuges:
  San Pablo Bay NWR (249 acres)
State recreation areas: 15 (31,363 acres)

Score: 1,975
Rank: 89

Sarasota, FL
Common Denominators (1,300 points)
Good restaurants: 2 *, 6 **, 5 ***   A
Golf courses: 8 private (180 holes); 20 daily fee (369
  holes); 3 municipal (90 holes)   AA
Bowling centers: 7 (192 lanes)   A
Movie theaters: 7   B
Public libraries: 3 (178,020 volumes)   C
Performing Arts Calendar (1,480 points)
Campus and civic auditorium bookings: 96 dates
Resident ensembles:
  Florida West Coast Symphony Orchestra (24 dates)
  Florida West Coast Youth Orchestra (6 dates)
  Sarasota Community Orchestra (7 dates)
  Sarasota Opera Association (15 dates)
Outdoor Assets (989 points)
Gulf coastline: 35 miles
Inland water area: 31.9 square miles
State recreation areas: 2 (29,040 acres)

Score: 3,769
Rank: 24

Southport, NC
Common Denominators (500 points)
Golf courses: 7 daily fee (126 holes)   AA
Public libraries: 3 (46,502 volumes)   C
Outdoor Assets (547 points)
Atlantic coastline: 35 miles
Inland water area: 32.5 square miles
State recreation areas: 1 (1,773 acres)

Score: 1,047
Rank: 124

Rating

Rating

Springfield, MO
Common Denominators (1,000 points)
Good restaurants: 2 **, 3 ***   B
Golf courses: 4 private (63 holes); 1 daily fee (18 holes);
  3 municipal (45 holes)   C
Bowling centers: 6 (130 lanes)   A
Movie theaters: 5   C
Public libraries: 5 (353,998 volumes)   A
Performing Arts Calendar (490 points)
Campus and civic auditorium bookings: 18 dates
Resident ensembles:
  Springfield Regional Opera (10 dates)
  Springfield Symphony Orchestra (21 dates)
Outdoor Assets (17 points)
Inland water area: 0.4 square miles
National forests, parks, wildlife refuges:
  Wilson's Creek National Battlefield (1,184 acres)
Score: 1,507
Rank: 105

State College, PA
Common Denominators (1,000 points)
Good restaurants: 3 **   C
Golf courses: 4 private (54 holes); 2 daily fee (54 holes)   B
Bowling centers: 4 (55 lanes)   B
Movie theaters: 6   A
Public libraries: 2 (173,896 volumes)   B
Performing Arts Calendar (560 points)
Campus and civic auditorium bookings: 50 dates
Resident ensembles:
  Pennsylvania State University Symphony Orchestra
    (6 dates)
Outdoor Assets (98 points)
Inland water area: 6.1 square miles
State recreation areas: 6 (10,094 acres)
Score: 1,658
Rank: 95

Traverse City–Grand Traverse
Bay, MI
Common Denominators (1,500 points)
Good restaurants: 1 *, 2 **, 3 ***   AA
Golf courses: 1 private (18 holes); 6 daily fee (99 holes)   AA
Bowling centers: 2 (46 lanes)   A
Movie theaters: 2   B
Public libraries: 1 (68,000 volumes)   B
Performing Arts Calendar (510 points)
Campus and civic auditorium bookings: 11 dates
Resident ensembles:
  Interlochen Arts Academy Orchestra (15 dates)
  Traverse Symphony Orchestra (7 dates)
  World Youth Symphony Orchestra (18 dates)
Outdoor Assets (1,035 points)
Great Lakes coastline: 75 miles
Inland water area: 27.8 square miles
  Duck Lake
  Grand Traverse Bay
  Long Lake
National forests, parks, wildlife refuges:
  Manistee NF (2 acres)
State recreation areas: 2 (232 acres)
Score: 3,045
Rank: 47

Tucson, AZ
Common Denominators (900 points)
Good restaurants: 2 *, 5 **, 6 ***, 1 *****   B
Golf courses: 10 private (180 holes); 11 daily fee (180
  holes); 5 municipal (108 holes)   B
Bowling centers: 12 (324 lanes)   B
Movie theaters: 14   C
Public libraries: 2 (733,296 volumes)   B

Performing Arts Calendar (530 points)
Campus and civic auditorium bookings: 19 dates
Resident ensembles:
  Arizona Opera Company (6 dates)
  Civic Orchestra of Tucson (5 dates)
  Philharmonic Orchestra of Tucson (9 dates)
  Tucson Symphony Orchestra (14 dates)
Outdoor Assets (995 points)
Inland water area: 1.1 square miles
National forests, parks, wildlife refuges:
  Cabeza Prieta NWR (410,211 acres)
  Coronado NF (340,352 acres)
  Organ Pipe Cactus NM (330,519 acres)
  Saguaro NM (83,337 acres)
State recreation areas: 1 (5,511 acres)
Score: 2,425
Rank: 70

★ Twain Harte–Yosemite, CA
Common Denominators (1,200 points)
Good restaurants: 1 *, 2 **, 1 ***   A
Golf courses: 4 daily fee (45 holes)   A
Bowling centers: 1 (16 lanes)   C
Movie theaters: 2   A
Public libraries: 1 (47,827 volumes)   B
Outdoor Assets (3,692 points)
Inland water area: 42.7 square miles
  Beardley Lake
  Cherry Lake
  Don Pedro Reservoir
National forests, parks, wildlife refuges:
  Calaveras Bigtree NF (380 acres)
  Stanislaus NF (611,611 acres)
  Yosemite NP (430,099 acres)
State recreation areas: 3 (6,288 acres)
Score: 4,892
Rank: 8

★ Virginia Beach–Norfolk, VA
Common Denominators (900 points)
Good restaurants: 1 *, 9 **, 7 ***   C
Golf courses: 10 private (171 holes); 5 daily fee (90
  holes); 5 municipal (81 holes)   C
Bowling centers: 19 (508 lanes)   A
Movie theaters: 15   C
Public libraries: 29 (1,551,475 volumes)   A
Performing Arts Calendar (1,900 points)
Campus and civic auditorium bookings: 20 dates
Resident ensembles:
  Old Dominion University Symphony Orchestra (3 dates)
  Virginia Beach Pops (22 dates)
  The Virginia Opera (25 dates)
  Virginia Symphony/Virginia Pops (120 dates)
Outdoor Assets (1,560 points)
Chesapeake coastline: 55 miles
Inland water area: 118.7 square miles
  Lynnhaven Bay
National forests, parks, wildlife refuges:
  Great Dismal Swamp NWR (77,333 acres)
State recreation areas: 1 (2,770 acres)
Score: 4,360
Rank: 15

West Palm Beach–
Boca Raton–Delray Beach, FL
Common Denominators (900 points)
Good restaurants: 3 *, 11 **, 13 ***, 1 *****   B
Golf courses: 56 private, (1,359 holes); 30 daily fee (585
  holes); 10 municipal (180 holes)   A
Bowling centers: 9 (308 lanes)   C
Movie theaters: 24   B
Public libraries: 11 (488,774 volumes)   C
Performing Arts Calendar (1,070 points)
Campus and civic auditorium bookings: 52 dates

Rating

Resident ensembles:
    Boca Raton Symphonic Pops (30 dates)
    Greater Palm Beach Symphony (16 dates)
    Palm Beach Opera (9 dates)
Outdoor Assets (1,011 points)
Atlantic coastline: 47 miles
Inland water area: 235.9 square miles
    Lake Okeechobee
    Palm Beach Harbor
National forests, parks, wildlife refuges:
    Loxahatchee NWR (2,550 acres)
State recreation areas: 1 (842 acres)

Score: 2,981
Rank: 50

Winchester, VA

Common Denominators (1,300 points)
Good restaurants: 1 *, 1 **, 2 ***   A
Golf courses: 5 private (81 holes)
Bowling centers: 1 (40 lanes)   A
Movie theaters: 3   A
Public libraries: 2 (192,064 volumes)   AA
Performing Arts Calendar (40 points)
Campus and civic auditorium bookings: 4 dates
Outdoor Assets (96 points)
Inland water area: 0.5 square miles

Rating

National forests, parks, wildlife refuges:
    George Washington NF (4,873 acres)
Score: 1,436
Rank: 111

Yuma, AZ

Common Denominators (900 points)
Good restaurants: 1 *, 1 **   C
Golf courses: 1 private (18 holes); 2 daily fee (36 holes);
    2 municipal (27 holes)   B
Bowling centers: 3 (50 lanes)   B
Movie theaters: 2   C
Public libraries: 3 (167,558 volumes)   A
Performing Arts Calendar (280 points)
Campus and civic auditorium bookings: 20 dates
Resident ensembles:
    Yuma Community Orchestra (8 dates)
Outdoor Assets (426 points)
Inland water area: 37.3 square miles
    Imperial Reservoir
National forests, parks, wildlife refuges:
    Kofa NWR (523,041 acres)
State recreation areas: 1 (10 acres)

Score: 1,606
Rank: 99

 # ET CETERA: Leisure Living

ANOTHER BREAK AT 62 PLUS: GOLDEN AGE PASSPORTS

Since 1974, more than 3 million Golden Age Passports have been issued to U.S. citizens and permanent residents who are 62 or older. These are free permits to any national park, monument, or recreation area run by the federal government and are valid for the lifetime of the holder.

With a Golden Age Passport, friends who accompany you will also be admitted free as long as everyone arrives in the same private vehicle (a car, station wagon, pickup truck, motor home, or motorcycle; busloads don't qualify). If you walk in, the passport admits you, your spouse, and children.

It isn't necessary to obtain the passport before trucking off on a combined vacation and retirement-place inspection trip. You can get one at most federally operated recreation areas where they are used and at any National Park Service regional office, national forest supervisor's office, and most ranger station offices. They aren't available by mail, however; you have to obtain one in person. All you need is proof of age—a driver's license, birth certificate, or signed affidavit attesting to your age.

There are real savings involved if you plan on frequent visits to the national parks, forests, wildlife refuges, and Corps of Engineers waterways. Not only are entrance fees waived (they currently are $3 per person or $5 per vehicle), but the passport holder gets

an additional 50 percent discount on federal use fees, such as parking, overnight camping, and boat launching. With camping charges well over $10 a night, and with increased parking and boat-ramp fees, 50 percent discounts can add up to a real bargain.

RETIREMENT PLACES WITH THE BEST BASS FISHING

Black bass, the premier gamefish in North America, are found in lakes and rivers in every state but Alaska. They aren't abundant in all areas, and some regions do not have the large bass-holding waters that can withstand extensive public attention. *Field & Stream* recently named the 50 best fishing spots in the United States and Canada, and one or more of them are within 16 retirement places.

Amherst–Northampton, Massachusetts
Located in a wilderness setting just east of Amherst, the 25,000-acre Quabbin Reservoir is the largest body of water in Massachusetts and principal source of Boston's water supply. In addition to trout and salmon, it sports a good fishery for bass, particularly smallmouth, and is tightly managed for fishing and boating.

Branson–Cassville–Table Rock Lake, Missouri
Table Rock Lake, an impoundment of the White River

in southeastern Missouri, is surrounded by the Mark Twain National Forest. Its 43,100 acres are spread out in a meandering mazelike configuration of coves and creeks that amount to a plethora of bassy hideaways.

Burlington, Vermont

With the Green Mountains on the east and the Adirondack Mountains on the west, 120-mile-long Lake Champlain, a natural lake on the Vermont–New York border, is nestled in the midst of some outstanding country. The premier gamefish is smallmouth bass, especially in the northern sector. Largemouth bass are abundant, too, particularly in weedy bays. In addition, walleye, trout, salmon, and perch fishing is excellent.

Flagstaff, Arizona

At the northern edge of Coconino County, Lake Powell, a 186-mile-long impoundment straddling Utah and Arizona, is known as the ''Bass Capital of the

---

Most Popular National Park Units in the Retirement Places

National Park Unit	Annual Visitors	Retirement Place
Gulf Islands National Seashore	9,880,800	Biloxi–Gulfport, MS Fort Walton Beach, FL
Lake Mead National Recreation Area	6,952,100	Flagstaff, AZ Lake Havasu City–Kingman, AZ Las Vegas, NV
Cape Cod National Seashore	4,374,800	Cape Cod, MA
Acadia National Park	3,745,600	Bar Harbor–Frenchman Bay, ME Camden–Penobscot Bay, ME
Yosemite National Park	2,832,000	Twain Harte–Yosemite, CA
Grand Canyon National Park	2,711,500	Flagstaff, AZ Lake Havasu City–Kingman, AZ
Olympic National Park	2,532,100	Port Angeles–Strait of Juan de Fuca, WA
Assateague Island National Seashore	2,304,900	Ocean City–Assateague Island, MD
Rocky Mountain National Park	2,248,900	Fort Collins–Loveland, CO
Glen Canyon National Recreation Area	2,078,900	Flagstaff, AZ
Cabrillo National Monument	1,652,100	San Diego, CA
Glacier National Park	1,603,000	Kalispell, MT
Zion National Park	1,503,300	St. George–Zion, UT
Whiskeytown–Shasta–Trinity National Recreation Area	1,246,400	Redding, CA
Haleakala National Park	1,194,700	Maui, HI
Hot Springs National Park	1,112,800	Hot Springs–Lake Ouachita, AR

Source: National Park Service, *Statistical Abstract,* 1985.

RELOCATION RESOURCES

Not for nothing does this book count the acres in national parks, forests, and wildlife refuges. The 247 rural counties in the United States where more than one third of the land area is owned by the federal government are often retirement destinations, too, offering low-density living in the midst of spectacular scenery.

The federal agencies mentioned in this chapter have maps, listings, and descriptive brochures for recreation lands under their stewardship. For further information, send your specific requests to the following agencies. Tell them what part of the country you are interested in visiting and what kind of information you need. In some cases the agency may refer you to a district office in your area.

Department of Agriculture
National Forest Service
Publications Office
12th and Independence Ave., S.W.
Washington, DC 20090-6090

Department of the Interior
Fish and Wildlife Service
Publications Office
1717 H Street, N.W.
Washington, DC 20240

Department of the Interior
National Park Service
Office of Public Affairs
Public Inquiries
P.O. Box 37127
Washington, DC 20013-7127

West.'' Its 1,900 miles of shoreline nooks and crannies host largemouth bass.

Gainesville–Lake Lanier, Georgia

Lake Lanier is the most visited U.S. Army Corps of Engineers lake in the nation. Largemouth bass fishing among the 560 miles of shoreline, abundant coves and feeder creeks, and 38,000 acres of water supplied by the Chattahoochee and Chestatee rivers is excellent. Striped and white bass also draw anglers, but in the summer fishermen compete with weekend swimmers, water-skiers, and sailors and have to resort to weekday angling.

Hot Springs–Lake Ouachita, Arkansas

Lake Ouachita, a Corps of Engineers lake about 35 miles from Hot Springs, is part of the Ouachita National Forest and is known for a variety of good fishing. Largemouth and spotted (locally called ''Kentucky'') bass are plentiful here. Stripers, too, are abundant among the rotting timber left standing in this lake when it was flooded.

Laconia–Lake Winnipesaukee, New Hampshire

Squam Lake, location for the movie *On Golden Pond*, is noted for its smallmouth bass fishing. Its 44,000-acre neighbor, Lake Winnipesaukee, is the largest of New Hampshire's many lakes. Here, trout and landlocked salmon are the locally preferred fish, but many smallmouth and largemouth bass are caught as well.

Lake Havasu City–Kingman, Arizona

Lake Mohave, an impoundment on the Colorado River

downstream from Lake Mead (see **Las Vegas, Nevada**), is an excellent largemouth bass lake, providing good fishing on points, cliffs, brush, and other habitats that are typical of these weedless desert lakes. Cold water issuing from Hoover Dam makes the upper 15 miles more suitable for trout, but the rest of the 67-mile-long lake offers plenty of bass fishing opportunities.

Public Golf Holes: The States Ranked

State	Municipal Courses/Holes	Daily-Fee Courses/Holes	Total Public Courses/Holes
Michigan	73/1,161	446/6,813	519/7,974
Florida	67/1,224	356/6,525	423/7,749
California	145/2,547	328/5,004	473/7,551
Ohio	69/1,233	395/6,138	464/7,371
New York	101/1,854	371/5,076	472/6,930
Pennsylvania	36/612	331/5,202	367/5,814
Illinois	126/1,998	231/3,357	357/5,355
Texas	135/2,106	169/2,286	304/4,392
Wisconsin	58/864	238/3,168	296/4,032
Indiana	60/936	192/2,862	252/3,798
North Carolina	26/459	200/3,267	226/3,726
Minnesota	68/999	193/2,349	261/3,348
Massachusetts	36/567	174/2,340	210/2,907
New Jersey	41/747	88/1,494	129/2,241
Washington	42/666	108/1,404	150/2,070
South Carolina	6/90	115/1,971	121/2,061
Iowa	52/729	119/1,323	171/2,052
Arizona	30/441	86/1,359	116/1,800
Tennessee	40/648	75/999	115/1,647
Missouri	40/504	87/1,080	127/1,584
Colorado	57/918	48/621	105/1,539
Virginia	12/189	81/1,323	93/1,512
Kentucky	30/432	83/1,062	113/1,494
Georgia	34/540	63/936	97/1,476
Oregon	17/225	90/1,206	107/1,431
Oklahoma	49/720	53/639	102/1,359
Connecticut	33/567	53/738	86/1,305
Kansas	44/585	62/675	106/1,260
Maine	7/90	90/990	97/1,080
Nebraska	36/423	60/630	96/1,053
Alabama	33/477	39/549	72/1,026
New Hampshire	3/54	71/882	74/936
West Virginia	15/243	43/594	58/837
Idaho	24/315	38/441	62/756
Utah	35/477	24/279	59/756
North Dakota	43/423	28/261	71/684
Maryland	21/351	20/324	41/675
Louisiana	21/396	22/270	43/666
Hawaii	7/117	27/540	34/657
New Mexico	24/351	18/270	42/621
Arkansas	11/180	33/432	44/612
Vermont	—	45/612	45/612
South Dakota	24/279	32/306	56/585
Mississippi	13/171	22/342	35/513
Montana	17/216	24/297	41/513
Nevada	13/189	18/288	31/477
Rhode Island	3/45	28/369	31/414
Wyoming	14/189	20/216	34/405
Delaware	2/36	5/81	7/117
Alaska	1/9	1/18	2/27

Source: National Golf Foundation, unpublished data, 1986.

Lakeland–Winter Haven, Florida
The Florida Phosphate Pits, which are flooded, reclaimed phosphate-mining areas of varying size, possess an abundance of chunky largemouth bass, including plenty of trophy-size fish. There are lots of pits in the south-central mining country, and the newest publicly accessible ones are in the Tenoroc State Reserve outside of Lakeland.

Las Vegas, Nevada
Near Las Vegas and backed by the Hoover Dam, Lake Mead has lots of good bass cover, resulting in an abundance of 1- to 3-pound largemouth bass. Stripers, too, benefit from the expanded forage base and are popular on this lake, with small fish up to 10 pounds being plentiful.

Mountain Home–Bull Shoals, Arkansas
Bull Shoals is among the best largemouth bass waters in the Ozarks, has excellent spring and fall fishing, and provides good angling throughout the year for a variety of species, including white bass and crappies. Trout and smallmouth bass are also present.

Murray–Kentucky Lake, Kentucky
Kentucky Lake and Barkley Lake are magnets for warm-water anglers throughout the Midwest. Combined, they are the second-largest man-made water system in America, and their 3,500 miles of shoreline provide countless coves, bays, finders, and hideaways for bass. Largemouth and spotted (Kentucky) bass are plentiful, and smallmouth bass have become especially prominent in recent years.

Ocala, Florida
Good largemouth fishing can be had in many areas of Florida's lengthy and renowned St. Johns River, particularly Rodman Reservoir at the northern edge of the Ocala National Forest and Lake George, upriver yet south of Rodman Reservoir.

Orlando, Florida
There are a number of shallow, grassy lakes in Florida's Kissimmee River chain. Lake Kissimmee (the largest) and East and West Tohopekaliga are among the most prominent. West Toho is rated one of the best places for trophy bass, which is high praise in a state that has many trophy largemouth waters.

San Diego, California
San Diego's water supply lakes are small and intensively fished. Fifteen of these San Diego County Lakes are open to the public for fishing, and they have some of the best catch rates in California, including record-size Florida-strain largemouth bass.

West Palm Beach–Boca Raton–Delray Beach, Florida
Lake Okeechobee, at the western edge of this retirement place, is the most renowned of Florida's largemouth bass factories. It has over 200,000 acres of shallow, grass-filled water and is often the least affected Florida bass lake during late winter and early

spring, offering fantastic fishing when the weather is stable.

Source: Rand McNally, *Field & Stream 50 Great Bass Fishing Areas,* 1985.

HOW DOES YOUR GARDEN GROW?

If you are a dedicated gardener, then you're one of those hardy souls willing to deal with nature's varieties, from savage winters and sandy soils to slimy snails and slugs, to enjoy the splendor of June roses, vine-ripened tomatoes, and a blaze of petunias. You use the winter to read Katharine S. White's *Onward and Upward in the Garden* and the gardening catalogs, you put humus in the sandy soil, and you set out saucers of flat beer for the slugs. (No, it's not meant as a treat—they are attracted by the odor, climb in, get tipsy, and drown.)

You're also not alone if you love to garden. Of retired homeowners, 72 percent care for their lawns; 52 percent grow vegetables, with tomatoes, peppers, and cucumbers, in that order, the most popular crops. Impatiens, petunias, and marigolds are the front-runners in annuals among the 49 percent who grow flowers; roses are far and away the most popular perennials. Forty-eight percent grow shrubs, and 86 percent of those who grow vegetables also grow berries, with strawberries, red raspberries, and blueberries the favorites. Blackberries run a poor fourth. In the Midwest, 65 percent of households grow flowers as well as vegetables; in the East, 46 percent grow both. Nearly half of western households grow both vegetables and flowers, and a surprising 45 percent of western households also grow fruits and berries.

An acre or a pot, a treat for the eye or for the palate—no matter what your aim, gardening affords the delight of seemingly inexhaustible diversity. Years of growing both flowers and food reinforce your sense of change and renewal as well as your curiosity.

But what if you decide to move after retiring? Will the roses in your new garden bloom this year? Will the tomatoes thrive in the heat or the moisture, or the lack of both? Will the beloved tulips of the northern garden do well in the warm climate of the new home? (Probably, if you refrigerate the bulbs for a few months before planting.) Will the charming flowering dogwoods of the East prosper in the wintry blasts of the North Woods? (They won't prosper, but they will survive if placed in a sheltered spot.) You'll never know if the peonies of your last home will do well in the new location unless you try to transplant some of their fleshy roots. And if you try, maybe you can disprove the doomsayers who hold that oriental poppies can never be moved once planted (their long carrotlike root dislikes being transplanted). One old-timer claims you can't kill them.

As noted in an earlier chapter, the United States offers a dizzying number of variables in climate and terrain, many of which can either throw a sizable wrench into your gardening efforts or guarantee success. There are a few constraints, however, that you will find wherever you may decide to move.

Growing Seasons

The number of frost-free days ranges from a mere 8 in Barrow, Alaska, to 365 in Florida's Fort Lauderdale–Hollywood–Pompano Beach, Naples, and Miami–Hialeah, and in San Diego. The latter group would qualify as superior gardening areas from the standpoint of temperature, since killing frosts occur there less than one year in ten and plants can be grown year-round. Below are figures for some representative retirement places.

Growing Seasons and Killing Frosts

Retirement Place	Growing Season	Last Spring Frost	First Fall Frost
Albuquerque, NM	196 days	Apr. 16	Oct. 29
Asheville, NC	195	Apr. 12	Oct. 24
Bend, OR	62	June 17	Aug. 17
Boise, ID	171	Apr. 29	Oct. 16
Cape May, NJ	225	Apr. 4	Nov. 16
Kalispell, MT	135	May 12	Sept. 23
Lakeland–Winter Haven, FL	349	Jan. 10	Dec. 25
Las Vegas, NV	245	Mar. 13	Nov. 13
Lexington, KY	198	Apr. 13	Oct. 28
Medford–Ashland, OR	178	Apr. 25	Oct. 20
Miami–Hialeah, FL	365	—	—
Orlando, FL	319	Jan. 31	Dec. 17
Phoenix, AZ	317	Jan. 27	Dec. 11
Red Bluff–Sacramento Valley, CA	277	Feb. 25	Nov. 29
Reno, NV	141	May 14	Oct. 2
San Diego, CA	365	—	—
Springfield, MO	203	Apr. 10	Oct. 31
Tucson, AZ	261	Mar. 6	Nov. 23
Yuma, AZ	350	Jan. 11	Dec. 27

Source: National Oceanic and Atmospheric Administration, *Local Climatological Data,* 1986.

Soil

All soil is made up of varying amounts of clay particles, humus, and sand. The mix you have is dependent on where you live and on what others may have done to alter the natural state of the soil. Fortunately, the majority of plants are tolerant and will grow fairly well in most soils. Some can be grown most successfully in what is known as "acid soil." Other plants like sweet, or highly alkaline, soil. The acidity or alkalinity of soil is indicated by its pH number, a figure chemists use to measure the concentration of hydrogen ions (*pH* stands for "potential of hydrogen"). The midpoint in soil chemistry is 7, or neutral, on the pH scale. Less than 7 (down to 0) means acid; more than 7 (up to 14) means alkaline.

If you send a sample of soil to a testing laboratory, you may be told that it has a pH rating of 8.5, which would explain why the clematis looks so good, why you have the best onions and lettuce you've ever grown, and why your lilies and tomatoes are in bad shape. And now you know you'll have to put some alum or sulfur in the tomato patch.

You can test your soil yourself with litmus paper purchased at the drugstore. If the blue paper turns red when placed in moist soil, the soil is acid. If the red paper turns blue or purple, the soil is sweet. If there is no change, the soil is neutral. Or, you can take a representative slice of soil from the top down to about 6 inches, mix it, and send about half a cup to your county extension agent for testing.

A word of caution: if your soil is very acid or very sweet, take time to correct it, but change the pH by no more than a point per year.

Garden Pests

Unfortunately, pests are everywhere. If you leave the beetles and gypsy moths of the East for the gardens of California, chances are good that you will have to learn to do battle with snails and slugs, pests that were never a problem to you before. The cutworm that did damage only in the early part of the growing season in New England may reproduce several times a year in warm climates. One gardener who has lived in the East, on the Pacific Coast, and in the Midwest claims to have learned three distinct gardening rules, so pronounced are the variables of good gardening from area to area. And the ants, beetles, billbugs, borers, grubs, nematodes, and webworms are always with us.

So no matter where you live, you will have to have some kind of pest control. How much pesticide and what kind depends on the local pests, how perfect you want your crop to be, and what kind of growing season

you are coping with. Purists who abhor any kind of chemical spray will have to be extra diligent about the varieties of plants they buy, about keeping the gardening area free of any debris and weeds—both of which harbor insects and other pests—and about pruning assiduously.

Bowling Competition in the Retirement Places

For their size, Canandaigua, New York, (92 leagues, 2,517 players) and Door County, Wisconsin, (52 leagues, 1,091 players) see more bowling tournaments than larger retirement places. When it comes to the number of players, however, here are the top 20 associations.

Association	Leagues	Players
1. Greater Phoenix (AZ)	1,231	30,323
2. San Diego (CA)	774	16,642
3. Madison (WI)	602	16,181
4. Broward County (FL)	511	13,614
5. Orlando (FL)	555	12,837
6. Norfolk (VA)	370	11,607
7. Las Vegas (NV)	422	10,787
8. Miami (FL)	433	10,474
9. Ann Arbor (MI)	304	9,287
10. Colorado Springs (CO)	351	9,070
11. Albuquerque (NM)	312	8,882
12. Palm Beach County (FL)	307	8,792
13. St. Petersburg (FL)	293	7,197
14. Lancaster (PA)	330	7,108
15. Sarasota–Manatee (FL)	239	7,087
16. Charleston (SC)	257	5,799
17. Lexington (KY)	179	4,597
18. Ocean County (NJ)	173	4,517
19. Reno (NV)	196	4,349
20. Springfield (MO)	150	3,969

Source: American Bowling Congress, *Annual Report*, 1986.

Putting It All Together :

Retirement Regions and the Best All-Around Retirement Places

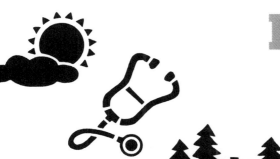
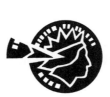
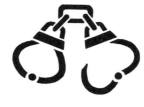

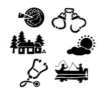

INTRODUCTION: Putting It All Together

Is there really an ideal place for retirement in America?

Various chambers of commerce, eager real estate promoters, and state tourism and economic development agencies may claim the title for their own particular locales. After all, with 21 million persons due to turn 65 during the 1980s, attracting footloose retired people to the Leisure Villages, Palm Shores, and Mountain Homes of this country is seen as a very promising growth industry.

By this book's criteria, the ideal place would have the climate of Maui, Hawaii, where the Pacific Ocean keeps the air temperature from ever dropping below 65 degrees or from topping 80 degrees much of the time. It would have to be a rural place if it were to match the low crime rate of Clayton–Clarkesville in the mountains of northeast Georgia, or the inexpensive housing of Branson–Cassville–Table Rock Lake in the Missouri Ozarks. Yet our ideal spot would also have to be a major metropolitan area to match San Diego's full range of health care facilities, public transportation, and continuing-education opportunities. For variety in recreation, you might choose a place like Miami–Hialeah, which not only has a busy calendar of symphony orchestra performances, opera productions, and guest artist dates but opportunities for outdoor activities as well. Finally, our ideal place should offer retired persons the low living costs of McAllen–Edinburg–Mission on the banks of the Rio Grande in southernmost Texas.

Obviously, this ideal retirement haven is a fiction. You can explore the geography long and hard, but you will never find the single retirement place that combines all of the ''bests'' according to *Retirement Places Rated*'s criteria. Moreover, because one person's retirement heaven can often be another's purgatory, and your rural retreat someone else's boondocks, one can argue that there really is no such thing as *the* ideal retirement place.

Because of better health care and increasing longevity, your retirement years can now amount to one quarter of your life span. Choosing where to spend these retirement years isn't an easy task. The best tactic is to focus on *your* own preferences and needs; the section ''Decisions, Decisions,'' at the front of the book, can help you identify what these preferences and needs might be. Having said as much, we can still try to discover which of the 131 places come closest to the ideal.

FINDING THE BEST ALL-AROUND RETIREMENT PLACES

Our method for determining America's best all-around retirement places is very simple: The ranks of every place for each of the six factors—money matters, climate, personal safety, services, housing, and leisure living—are added together for a cumulative score. Miami–Hialeah, for example, ranks 110th in money matters, 3rd in climate, 131st in personal safety, 13th in services, 105th in housing, and 1st in leisure living. The total of these ranks (110 + 3 + 131 + 13 + 105 + 1) equals 363, giving Miami–Hialeah a rank of 50 among the 131 retirement places. Because this rating system is based on ranks, the lower the cumulative score, the better the retirement place is judged to be all-around. The list that follows highlights the places that rise to the top as the better spots for retirement in America.

America's Top Retirement Places

Retirement Place	Cumulative Score
1. Murray–Kentucky Lake, KY	226
2. Clayton–Clarkesville, GA *	228
3. Hot Springs–Lake Ouachita, AR	237
4. Grand Lake–Lake Tenkiller, OK	253
5. Fayetteville, AR	263
6. St. George–Zion, UT	266
7. Brownsville–Harlingen, TX	267
8. Bloomington–Brown County, IN	268
9. San Antonio, TX *	279
10. Port Angeles–Strait of Juan de Fuca, WA	281
11. Mountain Home–Bull Shoals, AR *	295
12. Charleston, SC *	301
13. Bellingham, WA	302
14. Branson–Cassville–Table Rock Lake, MO *	307
14. Biloxi–Gulfport, MS	307
14. Athens–Cedar Creek Lake, TX *	307
17. Franklin County, TN *	312
18. Hamilton–Bitterroot Valley, MT *	315
18. Southport, NC *	315
20. Blacksburg, VA *	318
21. Daytona Beach, FL *	322
21. Asheville, NC *	322
23. Crossville, TN *	324
24. McAllen–Edinburg–Mission, TX *	325
25. Kalispell, MT *	332

* These places rank at the bottom—that is, 100th or lower—in one or more of the six factors.

In some respects, the list of the top 25 in this edition of *Retirement Places Rated* resembles that of the previous 1983 edition. Although their rankings have changed somewhat, 7 of the retirement places were in the top 25 before. Another 4 retirement places that were on the 1983 list appear again, but with slightly different geographic boundaries. Of the remaining retirement places on the list, 7 weren't featured at all in 1983; they are newcomers to this edition.

A Winning Place . . .

. . . is Murray–Kentucky Lake, an area composed of Calloway and Marshall counties in western Kentucky. Through a combination of factors, this Mid-South spot finishes at the top of the list of *Retirement Places Rated*'s 131 destinations.

In spite of statistics showing that 3 out of every 20 older adults in Murray–Kentucky Lake are newcomers, the place doesn't look at all like a standard resort-retirement destination with pockets of condominium development and adults-only housing.

Nor will Murray (population 14,248) strike the visitor as precious, even though the 1907 Louisville & Nashville freight depot has been moved to a big park on Arcadia Street to join the restored 1823 log cabin courthouse already there and though large and handsome 19th-century homes near the downtown square are being made over into bed-and-breakfast inns.

The area has been legally dry for as long as anyone can remember. Its Democratic congressman runs unopposed in general elections. This is where Briggs & Stratton makes small gasoline engines and Fisher-Price makes toys. The open country is a soybean, corn, and tobacco hinterland.

Why the area's top ranking as a retirement place? It has low health care and housing costs, excellent access to accredited hospitals, a high rating for personal safety, a good supply of physicians and medical specialists, an established public transit system, opportunities for continuing education at a mid-size state university, and a huge body of inland water along its entire eastern border.

But what about the things that can't be measured? What about those equally important day-to-day qualities like friendliness, volunteerism, and civic spirit?

Not for nothing did Murray compete successfully with major metropolitan areas for the new National Boy Scout Museum and its 54 original Norman Rockwell paintings, Baden-Powell memorabilia, multimedia theater, and research library. Location played a part. The city is smack in the center of 5 million Boy Scouts living within 500 miles. But the deciding factors were the community's widespread support and the local university's donation of land.

As in other college towns, the ebb and flow of community life is regulated by the academic calendar. Murray State University offers a rich variety of concerts, lectures, dramatic productions, art exhibits, and Ohio Valley Conference football and basketball games, all open to the public.

Outdoor recreation is ample and diverse. Just a few minutes from Murray, and joined to each other by a canal, are Kentucky Lake and Lake Barkley with nearly 3,500 miles of irregular shoreline. The lakes provide excellent fishing, sailing, swimming, and cruising. Land Between the Lakes, a 170,000-acre outdoor recreation area developed by the Tennessee Valley Authority, is a place to hike, ride, hunt, camp, or just lie on the beaches. Empire Farms, The Homeplace, and Woodlands Nature Center offer many demonstration and informational programs. The Buffalo Range, Silo Overlook, and Center Furnace are year-round sites.

The merchants in Murray stock a wide line of goods for everyday needs; a 45-minute trip to the large mall near Paducah or even a 2-hour jaunt down to Nashville, Tennessee, will put you in the midst of more specialized retail shops. Airports served by commercial airlines are also located in these two cities.

While Murray–Kentucky Lake scores no firsts in the elements *Retirement Places Rated* measures, neither does it make any errors. For some, this may simply mean the triumph of the average over the exceptional. For others, it is exceptional indeed that low living costs and crime rates, a high level of community services, a cosmopolitan university atmosphere, and extensive outdoor recreation can convene in one place. This authentic, small college town on the edge of the largest man-made body of water in the United States has those qualities in abundance.

Why have the rankings changed? For one thing, we have redefined the county components of several of the retirement places since 1983. For another, more recent data—particularly in the area of money matters—have caused some shifting in relative positions. But the main reason has to do with the scoring criteria. In some cases (state park acreage, for example, or health care costs) new factors have been adopted for scoring; in other cases, different weightings have been applied to old factors.

In reviewing the findings of this chapter (or any of the preceding chapters), be sure to note the close groupings of scores. With such close results, ranking retirement places from 1 to 131 may give the impression of greater differences between them than actually exist. Any ranking of 33 or higher, for example, puts a retirement place in the top quarter of retirement places featured in this book.

RANKINGS: Putting It All Together

The table below gives each retirement place's rank in each of *Retirement Places Rated*'s six chapters. On the table's right-hand side, the sum of these six ranks—the cumulative score—is also shown, as is the overall rank. For example, Cape Cod's cumulative score of 496 ranks it 114th overall among the 131 retirement places.

As in golf, the lower the cumulative score the better. The best possible score is 6, meaning a first-place rank in all six chapters.

The lowest possible rank a retirement place can receive is 131, so the worst possible cumulative score would be 786.

Retirement Place	Money Matters	Climate	Personal Safety	Services	Housing	Leisure Living	Cumulative Score	Overall Rank
Albuquerque, NM	81	71	124	29	55	48	408	79
Amherst–Northampton, MA	88	103	25	11	98	80	405	77
Ann Arbor, MI	126	98	110	7	118	21	480	107
Asheville, NC	40	62	48	35	29	108	322	21
Athens, GA	38	43	111	3	58	121	374	56
Athens–Cedar Creek Lake, TX	7	28	29	95	18	130	307	14
Austin, TX	99	26	102	19	89	79	414	82
Bar Harbor–Frenchman Bay, ME	55	111	21	70	72	43	372	55
Bellingham, WA	52	91	71	28	54	6	302	13
Bend, OR	51	110	44	48	86	23	362	48
Bennington, VT	103	109	33	56	108	38	447	97
Biloxi–Gulfport, MS	22	23	84	87	20	71	307	14
Blacksburg, VA	27	83	30	4	62	112	318	20
Bloomington–Brown County, IN	32	85	51	10	37	53	268	8
Boise, ID	90	94	78	42	48	119	471	106
Bradenton, FL	78	11	116	46	75	114	440	95
Branson–Cassville–Table Rock Lake, MO	25	68	3	124	9	78	307	14
Brownsville–Harlingen, TX	2	15	93	91	3	63	267	7
Brunswick–Golden Isles, GA	46	22	127	63	27	65	350	40
Burlington, VT	120	120	38	17	129	37	461	102
Burnet–Marble Falls–Llano, TX	73	35	12	121	33	118	392	69
Camden–Penobscot Bay, ME	43	111	23	60	73	35	345	36
Canandaigua, NY	111	105	22	74	104	92	508	120
Canton–Lake Tawakoni, TX	12	39	15	131	6	131	334	27
Cape Cod, MA	130	89	94	45	128	10	496	114
Cape May, NJ	113	65	104	51	123	76	532	126
Carson City–Minden, NV	114	100	58	61	111	69	513	122
Chapel Hill, NC	102	47	65	2	96	122	434	92

	Money Matters	Climate	Personal Safety	Services	Housing	Leisure Living	Cumulative Score	Overall Rank
Charleston, SC	49	29	126	30	40	27	301	12
Charlottesville, VA	98	57	70	9	93	104	431	88
Chico–Paradise, CA	53	45	85	21	67	98	369	53
Clayton–Clarkesville, GA	8	53	1	117	9	40	228	2
Clear Lake, CA	61	73	119	110	78	62	503	119
Coeur d'Alene, ID	34	107	72	53	38	30	334	27
Colorado Springs, CA	71	102	97	68	57	68	463	104
Columbia County, NY	74	108	46	85	100	109	522	124
Crossville, TN	4	76	9	103	7	125	324	23
Daytona Beach, FL	45	14	117	54	46	46	322	21
Deming, NM	6	67	87	129	4	127	420	86
Door County, WI	79	121	8	118	69	43	438	94
Eagle River, WI	19	130	19	127	71	11	377	59
Easton–Chesapeake Bay, MD	128	66	57	80	107	42	480	107
Eugene–Springfield, OR	67	79	82	24	90	14	356	45
Fairhope–Gulf Shores, AL	33	21	49	119	35	117	374	56
Fayetteville, AR	24	61	35	22	30	91	263	5
Flagstaff, AZ	23	114	96	27	44	31	335	29
Fort Collins–Loveland, CO	84	104	79	34	91	16	408	79
Fort Lauderdale–Hollywood–Pompano Beach, FL	129	4	122	50	116	27	448	98
Fort Myers–Cape Coral, FL	85	7	68	77	95	19	351	41
Fort Walton Beach, FL	47	20	41	114	59	103	384	63
Franklin County, TN	5	50	5	116	8	128	312	17
Fredericksburg, TX	68	27	4	111	45	120	375	58
Friday Harbor–San Juan Islands, WA	115	91	32	125	119	18	500	117
Front Royal, VA	28	75	39	111	41	75	369	53
Gainesville–Lake Lanier, GA	48	42	54	62	34	123	363	50
Grand Junction, CO	62	86	66	44	70	58	386	66
Grand Lake–Lake Tenkiller, OK	3	54	16	75	11	94	253	4
Grass Valley–Truckee, CA	63	87	53	82	117	60	462	103
Hamilton–Bitterroot Valley, MT	10	113	31	130	26	5	315	18
Hanover, NH	101	118	13	8	99	22	361	47
Hendersonville–Brevard, NC	58	52	14	98	50	67	339	32
Hilton Head–Beaufort, SC	70	25	125	86	88	59	453	99
Hot Springs–Lake Ouachita, AR	44	41	61	36	16	39	237	3
Houghton Lake, MI	13	128	95	97	12	90	435	93
Iowa City, IA	108	99	76	1	103	97	484	110
Kalispell, MT	37	129	56	83	24	3	332	25
Kauai, HI	96	2	67	69	127	54	415	83

	Money Matters	Climate	Personal Safety	Services	Housing	Leisure Living	Cumulative Score	Overall Rank
Keene, NH	95	124	18	52	102	106	497	115
Kerrville, TX	91	32	24	84	47	113	391	68
Laconia–Lake Winnipesaukee, NH	87	125	59	76	112	72	531	125
Lake Havasu City–Kingman, AZ	16	49	106	106	42	96	415	83
Lakeland–Winter Haven, FL	31	9	120	73	25	85	343	35
Lancaster, PA	105	80	20	72	114	110	501	118
Las Cruces, NM	14	72	108	40	13	107	354	43
Las Vegas, NV	100	46	128	78	84	45	481	109
Lexington, KY	89	70	91	23	77	83	433	90
Litchfield County, CT	127	96	10	102	130	102	567	130
Madison, WI	123	116	75	5	113	56	488	111
Maui, HI	117	1	92	93	131	25	459	100
McAllen–Edinburg–Mission, TX	1	17	69	107	2	129	325	24
Medford–Ashland, OR	56	81	60	37	87	12	333	26
Melbourne–Titusville–Palm Bay, FL	80	8	103	55	83	33	362	48
Miami–Hialeah, FL	110	3	131	13	105	1	363	50
Missoula, MT	57	127	64	12	74	20	354	43
Monticello–Liberty, NY	93	114	55	105	97	101	565	129
Mountain Home–Bull Shoals, AR	29	55	2	100	28	81	295	11
Murray–Kentucky Lake, KY	17	55	11	31	19	93	226	1
Myrtle Beach, SC	36	30	118	81	51	82	398	72
Naples, FL	124	6	89	103	126	17	465	105
New Paltz–Ulster County, NY	109	101	41	64	101	100	516	123
Newport–Lincoln City, OR	65	83	74	96	76	32	426	87
North Conway–White Mountains, NH	104	125	37	111	115	41	533	127
Oak Harbor–Whidbey Island, WA	66	90	6	125	85	61	433	90
Ocala, FL	21	16	115	120	32	73	377	59
Ocean City–Assateague Island, MD	64	59	121	91	43	26	404	76
Ocean County, NJ	112	78	62	109	124	74	559	128
Olympia, WA	72	88	50	39	63	88	400	74
Orlando, FL	83	10	123	67	65	51	399	73
Oscoda–Huron Shore, MI	18	117	41	108	22	36	342	34
Panama City, FL	35	19	109	101	23	76	363	50
Paris–Big Sandy, TN	20	58	16	121	5	126	346	38
Petoskey–Straits of Mackinac, MI	76	122	52	43	60	66	419	85
Phoenix, AZ	97	37	113	33	67	4	351	41
Port Angeles–Strait of Juan de Fuca, WA	60	95	47	16	56	7	281	10
Portsmouth–Dover–Durham, NH	121	118	27	99	121	116	602	131
Prescott, AZ	41	81	45	93	39	49	348	39

	Money Matters	Climate	Personal Safety	Services	Housing	Leisure Living	Cumulative Score	Overall Rank
Red Bluff–Sacramento Valley, CA	30	40	77	121	31	86	385	64
Redding, CA	59	38	83	41	64	52	337	31
Rehoboth Bay–Indian River Bay, DE	77	64	81	90	36	84	432	89
Reno, NV	116	106	107	15	81	87	512	121
Rhinelander, WI	50	130	34	58	49	57	378	62
Roswell, NM	26	63	101	89	1	115	395	70
St. George–Zion, UT	11	59	26	88	53	29	266	6
St. Petersburg–Clearwater, FL	107	11	99	49	61	9	336	30
Salinas–Seaside–Monterey, CA	122	51	98	56	120	13	460	101
San Antonio, TX	42	24	112	25	21	55	279	9
San Diego, CA	118	18	100	14	125	2	377	59
San Luis Obispo, CA	106	36	63	32	109	64	410	81
Santa Fe, NM	94	93	129	66	82	34	498	116
Santa Rosa–Petaluma, CA	125	48	73	38	122	89	495	113
Sarasota, FL	119	11	88	59	94	24	395	70
Southport, NC	9	30	7	128	17	124	315	18
Springfield, MO	54	68	80	20	14	105	341	33
State College, PA	69	97	28	6	110	95	405	77
Traverse City–Grand Traverse Bay, MI	86	122	40	26	80	47	401	75
Tucson, AZ	82	32	105	18	52	70	359	46
Twain Harte–Yosemite, CA	39	73	86	47	92	8	345	36
Virginia Beach–Norfolk, VA	92	44	90	65	79	15	385	64
West Palm Beach–Boca Raton–Delray Beach, FL	131	5	130	71	106	50	493	112
Winchester, VA	75	76	36	79	66	111	443	96
Yuma, AZ	15	32	114	115	15	99	390	67

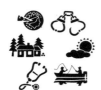

RETIREMENT REGIONS AND CHOICE PLACES

When it comes to finding your best place for retirement, you would do well to ignore the shopworn truisms about states and their track records in attracting retired persons. Considering Florida as a destination still means having to choose from thousands of cities, towns, and unincorporated places from Escambia County farm country in the northwest panhandle all the way down some 900 miles to Key West. People don't retire to states, they retire to specific places.

But viewing states as retirement destinations may not be a good idea for another reason. If your sights are set on the Desert Southwest, parts of five states make up that target. If you're tending toward mountain living, even more states fill the bill. Why not think of regions?

Here are 16 that look, feel, talk, and act differently from one another, yet the places within them share a number of characteristics. Few of their boundaries match the political borders you'll find in your road atlas; most of them embrace parts of more than one state and, conversely, some states are apportioned among more than one region. Southport, North Carolina, for example, is grouped with Fairhope–Gulf Shores, Alabama, and the other South Atlantic and Gulf Shore spots because it has more in common with them than Asheville in New Appalachia or Chapel Hill in the Mid-South.

On the following pages *Retirement Places Rated* describes the 16 regions into which the 131 retirement places seem to fall. Some have been resort country, on and off, for well over a century. Some have unsophisticated, small town manners. Others are relatively new and heavily promoted. One—Metropolitan South Florida—is nationally synonymous with retirement. Still others aren't associated with retirement by anyone but the savvy residents of nearby metropolitan areas. The North Woods country of Michigan and Wisconsin is such a place for Chicagoans, Milwaukeeans, and Detroiters. So are some of the Yankee Belt locations of coastal Maine and rural New Hampshire and Vermont to Bostonians and New Yorkers.

Each regional heading is accompanied by a list of the retirement places in the region, along with their overall ranks. Eleven of the regions include one or more of the 25 best all-around retirement places, and these are indicated with a star. For each of these choice locations, we offer a capsule description that we hope will pique your interest and also help you weigh the pros and cons in making plans for your retirement.

Whether you decide to move or end up staying right where you are, *Retirement Places Rated* hopes that your retirement years will rank among your best.

BIG TEN COUNTRY

Ann Arbor, MI (#107)
★ Bloomington–Brown County, IN (#8)
Iowa City, IA (#110)
Madison, WI (#111)

Heartland, Middle Earth, Breadbasket—the names sometimes given to the Central States evoke the change of seasons on featureless farmland, or an area mostly flown over by persons bound for either coast.

Though farming is important here, industry is more so in certain parts; though the land seems plain from the air, it is far from being homogeneous. To find what *Retirement Places Rated* calls Big Ten Country, take all the states that have a Lake Michigan frontage, add Minnesota and Iowa and Ohio, and home in on the locations of their well-known universities.

Four of these places (Columbus, Lansing–East Lansing, Madison, and Minneapolis–St. Paul) are also the home of state government. Two (Ann Arbor, Michigan, and Evanston, Illinois) are suburban parts of major metropolitan areas. Another four (Bloomington, Indiana; Champaign–Urbana, Illinois; Iowa City, Iowa; and West Lafayette, Indiana) are towns where the academic calendar dominates most of community life.

It isn't conjecture that Big Ten Country is a retirement region. The proportion of persons 65 and over tends to be greater in these college towns than it is in the nation as a whole. Big Ten universities here have huge alumni organizations, and many of these alums are returning for the benefits of the college town they knew years ago: past friendships, the cultural and recreational amenities, the youthful population, and the human services usually found only in large cities.

★ Bloomington–Brown County, Indiana (#8)

Bloomington represents the Monroe County college-town and high-technology side of this retirement place; the other side is Nashville's quaint Brown County covered bridge and its log cabins, antique shops, and art galleries. For the southern Indiana limestone quarry belt, this is a fortunate mix indeed.

When Kentuckians and Virginians first came here in the early 19th century, so the story goes, they found wildflower fields in full bloom. Indiana University was founded in 1820. Its tree-shaded campus, with neo-Gothic and modern university buildings (of limestone, naturally) is one of the most handsome in the country.

Pluses: Low health care and housing costs; excellent college-town amenities, including public transportation and an outstanding performing arts calendar.

Minuses: Continental climate with cold winters and hot summers may not be attractive to some; employment limited by competition from nearly 33,000 Indiana University students.

DESERT SOUTHWEST

Lake Havasu City–
  Kingman, AZ (#83)
Las Vegas, NV (#109)
Phoenix, AZ (#41)

Prescott, AZ (#39)
★ St. George–Zion, UT (#6)
Tucson, AZ (#46)
Yuma, AZ (#67)

The Desert Southwest, in the southern end of the Great Basin, lies between the country's two highest mountain ranges, the Rockies to the east and the Sierra Nevada to the west. These two mountain ranges not only add beauty, grandeur, and ruggedness to the region, they also block moist air coming from either the Pacific Ocean or the Gulf of Mexico. The entire region is high, mountainous, and dry, and valleys are dusty, with scant vegetation. The mountains and cliffsides, eroded by wind and sand, are jagged, angular, and knife-sharp.

If it's sun you're after, this is the place—Yuma is officially designated America's sunniest spot. Hot, sunny, cloudless days followed by cool, even chilly, nights are the rule here. This means you can enjoy outdoor activities in the daytime and still get a good night's rest . . . under a blanket or two.

Rapidly growing Arizona is the prototypical Sun Belt state. Tucson, a leading retirement area, has an excellent supply of health care and public transportation facilities. Metropolitan Phoenix is home to the largest retirement development in the world, Sun City. Many parts of the Desert Southwest, however, suffer from high crime rates and high housing costs (Las Vegas ranks 128th and 84th, respectively, in these categories), and the supply of health care facilities varies greatly from location to location.

Despite its rapid population growth (the seven retirement places profiled here grew an average of 25 percent since 1980, for example), this is thinly settled land. There is so much space here, with such great distances even between small towns, that people who have lived in thickly populated regions like the Great Lakes or the Northeast might find it difficult to adjust to the feeling of isolation.

★ St. George–Zion, Utah (#6)

One of the joys of living in southwestern Utah is experiencing the national park feeling 365 days a year, making it easy to enjoy a spontaneous picnic or a peaceful walk. Most likely the sun will be shining and you'll be comfortable in light clothing here in Utah's Dixie, where the summer is long and the winter is mild.

It wasn't always this relaxed and casual. The first hardy Mormon settlers lived in wagons in long rows on either side of an open ditch. The earliest homes were often only dugouts in the ground. Life was severely trying, but years of suffering and faith eventually brought results: orchards produced fruit, and corn, squash, and melons were raised on farms along the Virgin River. For a while cotton was grown, and in an attempt to produce silk, even mulberry trees were cultivated. Completed in 1877, the white Mormon Temple rises above green lawns and is visible for miles.

There is no rail service to St. George or Washington County, so it wasn't until the highway to Salt Lake City brought an outlet for crops, and later a steady stream of tourists, that the economy stabilized. Interstate Highway 15 is lightly traveled by national standards but provides a link to the bright lights and commerce of Las Vegas, the nearest major city, as well as reaching north to the Salt Lake Valley.

Among the 131 retirement places, the pace of home construction here is second only to Naples, Florida. A number of tiny towns stretch eastward from St. George following the Virgin River and its valley to the borders of Zion National Park. Clusters of cabins at Springdale denote the last village. Here, even though your home may be modest, the towering rock backdrop, in incredible shadings, adds a special dimension of grandeur.

Excellent outdoor recreation is offered at Zion National Park, Snow Canyon State Park, and Gunlock Lake State Beach. Shopping facilities at St. George are adequate for day-to-day needs. A medical center there will meet routine requirements, but specialized care must be sought elsewhere.

Pluses: Above-average access to public golf, good restaurants, and movie theaters; splendid natural setting; little criminal activity; low living costs; promising employment forecast.

Minuses: No public transportation; specialized health care may involve a long drive to Las Vegas; summers are hot and dry; Mormon tradition may be restrictive to some.

METROPOLITAN SOUTH FLORIDA

Bradenton, FL (#95)
★ Daytona Beach, FL (#21)
Fort Lauderdale–
  Hollywood–Pompano
  Beach, FL (#98)
Fort Myers–Cape Coral, FL
  (#41)
Lakeland–Winter Haven, FL
  (#35)
Melbourne–Titusville–
  Palm Bay, FL (#48)

Miami–Hialeah, FL (#50)
Naples, FL (#105)
Ocala, FL (#59)
Orlando, FL (#73)
St. Petersburg–
  Clearwater, FL (#30)
Sarasota, FL (#70)
West Palm Beach–Boca
  Raton–Delray Beach, FL
  (#112)

Perhaps because they so recently hailed from other places, few of Florida's residents are aware of the state's long and fascinating history. The land was first claimed by Spain in the 16th century, wrested away by the British, taken back by Spain, declared an independent republic by a group of Americans, and finally turned over by Spain to the United States in 1819. Very little happened in this remote, mosquito-infested outpost until the real estate boom of the 1920s. Then, dream cities sprouted up everywhere as the pitch of the real estate promoter was heard in the land. Property values increased from hour to hour, and thousands of persons bought unseen acres, many under salt water. It took three disasters—the hurricanes of 1926 and 1928 and the crash of 1929—to burst the bubble. But by then, the lure of Florida had been implanted in the American soul.

Today the Florida peninsula constitutes America's tropics. The state's first "tourist," Juan Ponce de Leon, didn't find his fountain of youth when he stepped ashore near St. Augustine in 1513, but modern-day retired persons, who are moving here at the rate of a thousand per week, are still trying. Whether beside a Fort Lauderdale condo swimming pool, on a Fort Myers beach, at a Miami jai alai fronton, or on a St. Petersburg park bench, they look for rejuvenation.

Florida, especially in the "frostproof" counties south of Gainesville and St. Augustine, has been elevated to its so-called "mega-state" niche by a migration unique in American history. In 1950, the state had 2 ½ million people; when the 1980 census figures were tallied, the total had climbed to nearly 10 million, nearly all of the increase coming from people moving from other states. By 1990, it is safe to predict, Florida will be the fourth most-populous state, behind only California, New York, and Texas.

★ Daytona Beach, Florida (#21)

One of the oldest of the Florida resorts, Daytona Beach with its triple waterfront—the Atlantic and both banks of the Halifax River—has developed into a major retirement community. One out of every four residents is over 65. The area is especially popular, too, with college students vacationing during their winter and spring breaks.

The 25-mile 500-foot-wide "World's Most Famous Beach" is rock hard. In 1903, Alexander Winton set the world's record for automobiles of 68 miles per hour here. Automobiles are still allowed on certain sections of the beach, but now the speed limit is 10 mph.

Among the 13 Metropolitan South Florida places profiled in this book, Daytona Beach and surrounding Volusia County are rated best due to a combination of leisure living, services, and cost-of-living factors. Health care costs here are typical of the U.S. average, but they are much less than the costs in three retirement places immediately to the south, West Palm Beach–Boca Raton–Delray Beach, Fort Lauderdale–Hollywood–Pompano Beach, and Miami–Hialeah.

Median housing prices resemble those of inland Ocala and Lakeland–Winter Haven rather than the higher prices on the coast. Types of homes here include condos, single-family homes, duplexes, and mobile homes. For single houses and condos, it is currently a buyer's market. Prices range from $45,000 to $150,000 on the mainland and $60,000 to $175,000 on the peninsula.

Outdoors, this resort area is blessed with a long coastline, many inland lakes, and numerous public golf courses. For a resort area, it also has an above-average number of dates for the performing arts.

Pluses: Generally low living costs; ocean setting at a southerly latitude; mild winters; abundant supply of good restaurants and public golf courses together with a fair set of performing arts bookings; established health care and public transportation services; opportunities for continuing education at local colleges.

Minuses: One of the worst crime rates among the retirement places; sluggish employment forecast.

MID-ATLANTIC METRO BELT

Canandaigua, NY (#120)
Cape May, NJ (#126)
Charlottesville, VA (#88)
Columbia County, NY (#124)
Easton–Chesapeake Bay, MD (#107)
Lancaster, PA (#118)
Monticello–Liberty, NY (#129)
New Paltz–Ulster County, NY (#123)
Ocean City–Assateague Island, MD (#76)
Ocean County, NJ (#128)
Rehoboth Bay–Indian River Bay, DE (#89)
State College, PA (#77)
Virginia Beach–Norfolk, VA (#64)

The area south from New York City to Washington and through the northern Virginia suburbs to Richmond is the most densely settled in America. Many metro areas in this region—notably Newark, Trenton, Philadelphia, Wilmington, and Baltimore—are saddled with the twin curses of sunset industries and long-term population losses.

In the midst of this stagnation, one can easily forget the pockets of retirement growth not visible from the Amtrak rails or Interstate Highway 95: the Atlantic beach counties, Chesapeake Bay, the Catskills, and smaller metro areas like civilized Lancaster, Pennsylvania; State College, in the Nittany Valley; and Charlottesville, Virginia, south of Washington and northwest of Richmond.

The 130 miles of New Jersey's sandy Atlantic coastline, particularly from the tip of Cape May north to Toms River, is rebounding after years of decline. One in five residents of Ocean County is over 65, compared with the U.S. average of one in nine. The retired newcomers among them didn't have to come far; they are often New Yorkers and Philadelphians, some returning after a disappointing stint in Florida. Many planned retirement communities have been built or are being developed here, though people who want less structure can find many small seaside towns, particularly south of Atlantic City (still seedy, in spite of casino gambling and new hotels) and west of the Garden State Parkway.

Farther south, you'll find retirement destinations within hailing distance of Washington and Baltimore on the Delmarva Peninsula and the shores of Chesapeake Bay. Many of the bigger summer resorts resemble Miami Beach rather than the charming, small seaside communities they once were before the opening of the Chesapeake Bay Bridge in 1952. Delaware's Rehoboth Beach, which has a winter population of 1,730 and a summer population of 50,000, calls itself the nation's summer capital because so many federal workers crowd its beaches. Ocean City, just over the border in Maryland, is also a popular resort among Washington and Baltimore residents.

MID-SOUTH

Athens, GA (#56)
Chapel Hill, NC (#92)
★ Crossville, TN (#23)
★ Franklin County, TN (#17)

Lexington, KY (#90)
★ Murray–Kentucky Lake, KY (#1)
Paris–Big Sandy, TN (#38)

This region is neither north nor too far south to be thoroughly Dixie. It's in the center of the country's eastern half. More precisely, it includes North Carolina's and Georgia's Piedmont (but not their mountains —they are part of New Appalachia) and most of Kentucky and Tennessee.

Middle Tennessee, hemmed in by the looping Tennessee River, is gently rolling bluegrass country: fertile, well-watered, and famous for its fine livestock. The heart of the state, it is rich in tradition and history, and its rural people cling to southern folkways.

Kentucky encompasses mountains in its sandstone area, deep gorges and caves in its limestone region, and swampy flats and oxbow lagoons in the far western part of the state. This end of Kentucky is called the Purchase, after the Jackson Purchase, which bought 8,500 square miles in Kentucky and Tennessee from the Chickasaw Indians.

Although Kentucky always had plenty of navigable rivers, it wasn't until the TVA projects of the 30s and 40s that it had a large number of lakes. These impoundments, created by dams on the Tennessee River and its tributaries, have transformed both Kentucky and Tennessee into front-runners for fishing and water recreation.

Why is the Mid-South such an attractive retirement region? For one thing, the region lies north of more established retirement areas of the Sun Belt. Recent demographic research shows that although the Sun Belt still remains a big drawing card for older adults, the "Retirement Belt" seems to be widening inexorably north. People are discovering the benefits of being closer to their former homes in the Midwest or Northeast, the desirability of mild, four-season climates as opposed to the monotony of the semitropical varieties, and the great advantages of low costs and low crime rates compared with many retirement areas farther south.

Furthermore, the gently rolling terrain with its pleasant scenery, the unhurried pace of life (far less manic than in many parts of Florida), and the outdoor

recreational options coupled with the weather to enjoy them fully make the Mid-South a winner. Like neighboring New Appalachia, this region has 3 retirement places that rank in the top 25.

★ Crossville, Tennessee (#23)

Crossville (population 6,394) is the seat of Tennessee's Cumberland County. It is also the site of Cumberland Mountain State Park, a protected wilderness area in the great Cumberland Plateau, the largest timbered plateau in America. The park contains cabin accommodations for visitors, a group lodge, a restaurant, and hundreds of camping and hiking sites. It covers 1,720 acres and has a 50-acre lake. Also nearby is the Obed Wild and Scenic River.

Crossville's elevation (1,881 feet) and southerly location are the principal reasons for its pleasant climate. Like the other places in the mountain South, Crossville enjoys long springs and falls, mild winters, and summers that are quite warm during the day but cool at night.

The cultural activities and special points of interest are limited, due to the county's small size (population 31,900). The Cumberland County Playhouse, Tennessee's largest professional theatre, offers five productions each season. For other live fine arts performances, it's only an hour's drive to the University of Tennessee in Knoxville. Crossville's country atmosphere has a calico-and-dulcimer tinge to it. Like places in the Ozarks and Ouachitas, and places in New Appalachia, too, 19th-century crafts are being relearned. The many small and rustic country and general stores add variety to this pretty rural setting.

Crossville's disadvantages are in three standard services: health care, public transportation, and continuing education. But its ratings for personal safety, housing, and money matters are impressive.

Pluses: Extremely low housing and health care costs; low personal taxes; high rating for personal safety; pleasant summer months; mountain vistas.

Minuses: No public transportation; few medical specialists; no local colleges for continuing-education opportunities; limited public recreation land.

★ Franklin County, Tennessee (#17)

What geologists call the Central Basin, some Tennesseans call the Heartland. It's a pocket of gently rolling hills and bluegrass meadows enclosed by the towering Highland Rim. It is also one of the richest tobacco and horse-farming areas in the state. Franklin County, down on the Alabama border, is the Heartland's southern extent.

The key to Franklin County's recent growth as a retirement destination isn't so much the topography's undeniable appeal as it is the construction of Tims Ford Dam and Reservoir by the Tennessee Valley Authority (TVA) in 1970. The 10,700-acre reservoir, on the headwaters of the Elk River, is one of the most picturesque of the TVA lakes and one of the top bass fishing and boating lakes in the Southeast. Year-round fishing can also find a substantial yield of rockfish, bluegill, catfish, and crappie for the angler's enjoyment.

Over the last 15 years, a good deal of low-density residential development has taken place along Tims Ford. Upriver along the shore of Woods Reservoir, researchers at University of Tennessee's Space Institute carry on exotic work on aeroacoustics and gas diagnostics. On a mountaintop farther east, the University of the South (locally called Sewanee) has a 10,000-acre campus with buildings reminiscent of a High Church English village.

Pluses: High rating for personal safety; extremely low housing and health care costs; low personal taxes; mild, four-season, continental climate.

Minuses: Few local medical specialists; no public transportation; limited performing arts attractions; limited opportunities for college-level continuing education.

★ Murray–Kentucky Lake, Kentucky (#1)

See page 199 for a detailed description of the number-one retirement place.

Pluses: Low health care and housing costs; excellent access to accredited hospitals; high rating for personal safety; good supply of physicians and medical specialists; established public transit system; opportunities for continuing education at a midsize state university.

Minuses: Limited fine arts calendar; hot summers; modest employment forecast.

NEW APPALACHIA

★ Asheville, NC (#21)
★ Blacksburg, VA (#20)
★ Clayton–Clarkesville, GA (#2)
Front Royal, VA (#53)

Gainesville–Lake Lanier, GA (#50)
Hendersonville–Brevard, NC (#32)
Winchester, VA (#96)

There's a 600-mile stretch of Appalachian Mountains from Frederick County in Virginia to Hall County, Georgia, that absorbed a good deal of antipoverty money during the 1960s and 1970s. Much of the area is still poor. Much of it, too, is as scenic as any place in the nation.

This is a land of peaks and ridges, rushing streams and thundering waterfalls. In the earliest spring days, the hillsides burst with flowering trees and shrubs: rhododendron, azalea, dogwood, and magnolia. The George Washington, Pisgah, and Chattahoochee national forests stand tall with black walnut, pine, beech, poplar, birch, and oak. The mountain vistas, especially along the Blue Ridge Parkway, show row after spectacular row of parallel mountain ridges. Distant parts of what you see from the road are so inaccessible that it's unlikely humans have regularly hiked more than 10 percent of the topography.

Because the area is bookended, so to speak, by Atlanta in the south and Washington in the north, it isn't at all unusual to encounter ex-urbanites from these major cities among the retired folks in places like Clayton in north Georgia, Asheville and Hendersonville in western North Carolina, and Blacksburg in the Virginia mountains. What is unusual are the new "Florida Clubs" formed by retired persons who settle here *after* a disappointing stint in the Sunshine State.

New Appalachia is becoming a major destination for retired persons, and many of the region's communities are virtually ideal for retirement living, offering a wide range of special services for older residents. The Appalachian counties generally combine low costs of living and housing, low crime rates, adequate health care facilities in most places, and some of the county's mildest four-season climates.

You're going to need a car to get around comfortably in much of this region, though. It is a rough wilderness area abundant in natural beauty, yet it is located within reach of major eastern population centers, which eliminates the feeling of isolation so often associated with wilderness areas.

★ Asheville, North Carolina (#21)

Asheville, seat of Buncombe County, serves the entire western tip of North Carolina—an area composed of about 20 counties—as headquarters for services, specialized shopping, and transportation. Despite its role as a commercial center, Asheville and the rest of the county conduct business at an easy, quiet pace. People always have time to "set a spell" and catch up on the latest local news and gossip.

One of Asheville's biggest assets is its mountain setting. Far, far off on every horizon are the spectacular ridges, rises, cliffs, domes, and peaks of the Blue Ridge. West of the city lie the Great Smoky Mountains, once the domain of the Cherokee Nation. Even though Asheville rests in a broad valley between two tall mountain ranges, the elevation of the city is still above 2,200 feet, which accounts for the year-round clear air and cool nights. You'll reach for a blanket nearly every night of the year in Asheville. Its springs and autumns, and especially its summers, are among the mildest in the nation.

But Buncombe County has many more attractions than just scenery and an eight-month stretch of pleasant weather. There's the Folk Arts Center on the Blue Ridge Parkway and Pisgah National Forest (composed of the remnants of George Vanderbilt's immense estate). Several outstanding ski areas. Wonderful and varied architecture. An extension of the University of North Carolina. Three country clubs. A new horse-show pavilion. A civic center and arena that book national acts and big-name entertainment. The Thomas Wolfe Auditorium, which provides symphonies, opera, and ballet. The Asheville Community Theatre. A minor league baseball team.

Asheville has a major shopping mall east of town, where all but the most specialized needs can be easily met. It also has four shopping centers. Additionally, the downtown area is full of boutiques, cafes, and gourmet food shops.

As lovely and special as Asheville is, it does have problems. There is some urban blight, and the effects of suburban growth and urban flight (many residents have moved to neighboring smaller towns, such as Hendersonville) are apparent in some sections. However, this retirement place remains strong on all counts.

Pluses: Spectacular southern mountain location; four-season climate characterized by cool nights and warm days from April through October; outstanding supply of physicians and accredited hospitals; moderate housing costs.

Minuses: Fewer cultural and entertainment amenities than larger metropolitan areas; lackluster employment growth forecast.

★ Blacksburg, Virginia (#20)

It might be argued that Virginia Tech (officially Virginia Polytechnic Institute and State University), one of the country's finest public universities, is all there is to mountainous Montgomery County. But hidden in the coves and on the mountainsides are a good many software engineers, artists, writers, and retired persons who can live anywhere they choose, and choose to live here. The Jefferson National Forest, off to the northwest, provides a backdrop of azaleas and flowering dogwood in spring, and brilliant hardwood foliage in fall.

Pluses: Low costs of living; large public transportation system for a community of its size; college town with artistic and cultural amenities and some opportunity for continuing education; crime rate less than one half the national average.

Minuses: Part-time employment limited by competition from over 23,000 Virginia Tech students; physician referrals may mean driving to Roanoke.

★ Clayton–Clarkesville, Georgia (#2)

Foxfire is both a lichen that glows in the dark and the name of a quarterly magazine and series of books that celebrates the folkways and commonsense abilities of northeastern Georgia's mountain people. Habersham and Rabun counties (the Clayton–Clarkesville retirement place) embrace part of their traditional home.

These counties are also in the midst of spectacular mountain recreation country. Rabun County borders the Appalachian Trail on the west. The Chattooga, a designated "wild scenic river" where the white-water sequences of *Deliverance* were filmed, is on the east. Just inside the county, Georgia's only ski slope operates on the north side of 4,760-foot Rabun Bald Mountain. To the south, the 1,000-foot Tallulah Gorge straddles the Rabun-Habersham county line. Overlying

both rural counties is a big chunk of Chattahoochee National Forest.

From all of the above, one might wonder whether this retirement place has bound up precious recreation land, leaving little to live on. Not true. While the prices of some private homes with long lake frontages resemble those of Lake Tahoe, reasonable prices can be found in and around the principal towns of Clarkesville, Clayton, Cornelia, and Demorest.

None of these towns will send the visitor into immediate ecstasy, although they are quiet, peaceful, and charming. The necessities of life are here to be sure, but for the exotic and the exciting, you must venture east to Greenville, South Carolina, or southwest to Atlanta to find the hustle and bustle, the specialty shopping, and that electric "buzz" that only bigger cities can give. Clayton–Clarkesville's strength lies in what it doesn't have (crime, high costs, rigorous weather, high taxes, congestion) rather than what it has. But what's wrong with that?

Pluses: Lowest crime rate of 131 retirement places; low health care and housing costs; spectacular mountain setting with ample outdoor recreation assets.

Minuses: No public transportation; limited facilities for health care; limited performing arts calendar.

NORTH WOODS

Door County, WI (#94)
Eagle River, WI (#59)
Houghton Lake, MI (#93)
Oscoda–Huron Shore, MI (#34)

Petoskey–Straits of Mackinac, MI (#85)
Rhinelander, WI (#62)
Traverse City–Grand Traverse Bay, MI (#75)

One region violating the "Law of Thermodemographics" (warm bodies eventually head south to the Sun Belt and stay there) has got to be that which includes the northern counties of Michigan's Lower Peninsula and several Wisconsin counties in Packer country near Green Bay. Winters here are long and cold. Spring, summer, and fall are lovely seasons but all too short.

During the 1970s, this area saw a population increase unequaled since waves of Finns, Germans, Czechs, and Poles arrived 80 years previously. On any summer weekend, campers, RVs, and boat-trailing cars crowd the northbound lanes of I-75 out of Detroit, I-94 out of Chicago, and I-43 out of Milwaukee. The traffic offers a clue to why the formerly depressed North Woods, forested with hemlock and Norway pine, have made a comeback.

The area's pull is strong for many vacationers from the big industrial cities of the Great Lakes. Many of these people decide to winterize their rural lakefront or flatwoods second home and retire for year-round residency.

This is recreation land with a rugged, Paul Bunyan flavor, not only in the summer months when the population doubles, but during the fall deer-hunting and winter skiing seasons, too. Most of Michigan's 11,000 and Wisconsin's 15,000 lakes are up here. "In some lakes," the *New York Times* reported in a recent profile of Eagle River and its environs, "the fishermen can see thirty feet down in waters forest green, or black, or blue, depending on the time of day or the perspective, and can retrieve dropped eyeglasses or snagged fishing lures."

In spite of high personal income and property taxes in these two North Woods states, the cost of living is still lower than in most other retirement regions. Except for small cities like Rhinelander and Sturgeon Bay in Wisconsin and Traverse City and Petoskey in Michigan, though, you won't find much in the way of structured retirement activities or a full range of health care facilities. Nor will you find expanding job prospects. Do expect to drive a good distance for retail shopping; this is rough, beautiful, but sparsely settled, country.

OZARKS AND OUACHITAS

★ Branson–Cassville–
  Table Rock Lake, MO (#14)

★ Fayetteville, AR (#5)

★ Grand Lake–Lake Tenkiller,
  OK (#4)

★ Hot Springs–Lake Ouachita,
  AR (#3)

★ Mountain Home–Bull Shoals,
  AR (#11)

Springfield, MO (#33)

Like New Appalachia, the Ozarks and Ouachitas of southern Missouri, northern and western Arkansas, and eastern Oklahoma are a kind of highland area with distinct folkways and geology and are undergoing rapid changes. In both areas, country craft galleries and bluegrass music festivals abound, and the mountain roads that wind through small towns also wind through some of the nation's prettiest countryside. (Here, as in New Appalachia, an automobile is a virtual necessity.) Many Ozark and Ouachita natives can trace their family names all the way back to Carolina and Virginia mountain roots.

Nearly 2 million people live in these hilly plateaus (the Ozarks) and ridge-valley mountains (the Ouachitas). Mention this region and you evoke an image of small-scale subsistence farming, chickens roosting in the hickory tree out back, shoeless springs and summers, moonshining, poverty, and isolation. Applied to the rural counties, the image was accurate until the 1960s. However, when the public utilities built hydroelectric dams, they produced a series of large impounded lakes in hardwood forests, which in turn produced resorts and a steady migration of retired people from Des Moines, Omaha, Tulsa, Oklahoma City, Memphis, Kansas City, St. Louis, and especially Chicago.

Some of the newcomers are what demographer Calvin Beale calls the new gentry—professional people with good incomes who can see themselves doing a bit of farming on a small section of land. Others he describes as the new peasantry, back-to-the-land types

interested in raising their own food, promoting conservation, maintaining rural values, and utilizing alternative fuel sources.

Lately, this region has been waking up to the problems that come with growth. Concerns about the loss of a special way of life are increasingly voiced; some locals say it may have already passed from the scene, never to be revived, despite local folk culture institutes and craft schools. The areas outside the biggest cities—Fayetteville and Fort Smith, Arkansas, and Springfield and Joplin, Missouri—aren't densely populated, yet some of the lakes are having pollution problems, and some of the better-known resorts are acquiring a tacky patina of liquor stores, fast-food outlets, tourist attractions, palmistry parlors, and diamond-appraisal shops.

★ Branson–Cassville–Table Rock Lake, Missouri (#14)

You could definitely do without a car much of the time in Cassville (population 2,091). The town map shows that the distance from the Sherwood Forest subdivision on the north side to City Hall on the south side can be walked in 20 minutes via Main Street. Each year, the Rotary Rodeo, the Old Soldiers' and Settlers' Reunion, the Fourth of July fireworks, and the Fall Foliage Festival are regular events.

This is one of many pleasant small towns in southwest Missouri. For one brief spell in the fall of 1861, it was the Confederate capital of the state, and the nearby steep terrain and canyonlike gorges became hideouts for Civil War guerrillas. Now it serves as the county seat and trading center of Barry County, one of Missouri's fast-growing Ozark recreation counties on the Arkansas border.

Branson (population 2,550), to the east, is a resort town and seat of Taney County. Nearby, Harold Bell Wright camped and wrote *The Shepherd of the Hills*, a novel quite famous around here. Nearby, too, is the School of the Ozarks campus, a liberal arts college where all students work in return for their room, board, and tuition.

The centerpiece of this small three-county area is 43,100-acre Table Rock Lake, a Corps of Engineers impoundment on the White River. According to *Sports Afield* magazine, it is the number-one bass lake in the United States.

Pluses: One of the safest retirement places and one of the least expensive; favorable part-time employment competition.

Minuses: No public transportation; no fine arts calendar; referral to medical specialists may mean traveling to Springfield; plateau climate with humid summers.

★ Fayetteville, Arkansas (#5)

Ever since the early 19th century when surveyors first staked out the land and promoters sold lots for settlement, Fayetteville has been the leading city in northwest Arkansas. During the Civil War, much of it burned to the ground as Union soldiers down from Missouri battled Confederate soldiers who had taken positions nearby on the Arkansas River.

When Washington County (of which Fayetteville is the seat) put up $100,000 for the Arkansas Industrial University in 1871, its future became more assured than that of other counties in that corner of the state. The school later became the University of Arkansas. The university is the home of the Razorbacks, and one wondered during the 1970s whether the city had any other bragging rights besides their Southwest Conference football team's winning record.

Fayetteville is eminently a college town. In autumn, with its brilliant maple and oak foliage and historic homes, it resembles New England. The university presence and nearness to the mountains has always attracted writers, artists, and professional persons. Now it is bringing back older alumni for retirement. One of the many benefits of living here is that, as long as there's room in the classroom and the student is over 60 years of age, the university will waive tuition fees for credit courses.

Pluses: Low crime rate; excellent supply of general physicians and accredited hospitals; opportunities for continuing education at a major state university; low living costs.

Minuses: Hot from June through September; lackluster job growth forecast; part-time employment limited by competition from nearly 15,000 students.

★ Grand Lake–Lake Tenkiller, Oklahoma (#4)

You won't get much argument from Sooners that the corner of their state where the Ozark Plateau spills over from Arkansas is the most beautiful part of Oklahoma. In autumn, the area is striking, with stands of oak, ash, and hickory changing colors over the hills and down the deep, narrow valleys. In the spring, dogwood, redbud, and wild plum blossoms splash the woods with color. Since the building of the Fort Gibson, Tenkiller Ferry, and Pensacola dams, the eastern and northeastern parts of the state rank near the top of the nation in total surface area of impounded water.

This region is also home to many Native Americans. Beginning in the 1830s, their ancestors were forcibly relocated here from the Southwest over the Trail of Tears. Until it was opened up to white settlement in 1889, this part of the state was Indian Territory; the county names—Cherokee, Choctaw, Creek, and Seminole—today recall some of the Five Civilized Tribes.

Lake O' The Cherokees (locals call it Grand Lake) is a huge man-made reservoir completed in 1941. It backs up the Neosho River for more than 60 miles, and along its 1,300 miles of shoreline (most of which is in Delaware County) are many resorts and fishing

camps. Jay (population 2,100) won the special county-seat election of 1908, beating Grove (population 3,378), now the largest town on the eastern shore. Both were trading centers for the local apple and berry farms during the Depression, but their businesses today cater to boaters and fishermen.

Lake Tenkiller, reaching up the Illinois River for 25 miles, is another huge impoundment started in 1947 and flooded in 1952. Tahlequah (population 9,708), the largest city in this retirement place, is historic on two counts: it has been the capital of the Cherokee Nation for nearly 150 years, and it is also the home of Northeastern State University, the second oldest university west of the Mississippi.

Pluses: Extremely low housing and health care costs; high rating for personal safety; continuing education available at a large state university; developed water recreation assets.

Minuses: No public transportation; specialized health care needs may mean traveling to Tulsa; short performing arts calendar; lackluster employment forecast.

★ Hot Springs–Lake Ouachita, Arkansas (#3)

If you're searching for a retirement place that will frequently draw visiting children and grandchildren, consider Hot Springs and the nearby lakes in Arkansas' Ouachita region. Its long history as a popular spa and resort gives the colorful town of Hot Springs (population 38,100) a wider array of entertainment facilities and a more cosmopolitan atmosphere than one might expect in a place of its size. Hot Springs surrounds portions of the 5,135-acre Hot Springs National Park. Each day, a million gallons of radioactive 143-degree water flow from 47 springs within the park. Since 1832, the springs have been administered by the federal government to prevent the inevitable charlatans and promoters from exploiting persons seeking hydrotherapy.

While the fact isn't generally known outside Arkansas, the city of Hot Springs faced big trouble in the 1981–82 recession. Historic buildings were deteriorating, the park service had closed many of the bathhouses, and other parts of Garland County were drawing off tourists. The city has since turned around. It has hired a full-time preservation manager, gotten the downtown designated the first National Register Historic District, and persuaded the park service to allow a private developer to rehabilitate and reopen the famous bathhouses.

If you are interested in structured retirement community living, you will find more options here than in any other place in the Ozark–Ouachita region. In addition, Hot Springs and surrounding Garland County offer a number of special services for older adults and several clubs for retired persons.

Pluses: Above-average supply of physicians and hospitals; extensive public transportation system; a balance of commercial leisure options and excellent natural recreation assets; favorable part-time employment prospects, particularly in services.

Minuses: Hot, humid summer months; limited performing arts attractions.

★ Mountain Home–Bull Shoals, Arkansas (#11)

Like other nearby towns, Bull Shoals and Mountain Home gain much of their revenue from one source, an aquatic creature called *Micropterus salmoides*, or the largemouth bass. The fish is as important to the local economy as automobiles are to Detroit or furniture to Grand Rapids.

A stroll down the main streets of Mountain Home (population 8,066), the largest town in Baxter County confirms this. Besides the usual retail establishments, there are taxidermy shops specializing in mounting your trophy bass. Enter almost any store and you can buy plastic worms in any and all colors of the rainbow —purple, gold, red, black, aqua, cream. They come in scents and flavors, too—licorice, strawberry, sassafras —to appeal, supposedly, to even the choosiest old bass. Also for sale are pork rinds, hula poppers, jitterbugs, flatfish, dive bombers, rubber frogs and crayfish, and hundreds of other kinds of artificial bait, plus rods, reels, tackle boxes, and bassboats.

On any given day, Norfork Lake, a huge (40 miles long) impoundment on the north fork of the White River, is dotted with skiffs as anglers try to hook and land a six-pounder. The reservoir is lined with marinas and boat docks. In the wooded hills and high meadows surrounding the lakes are many guest houses and cabins, trailer courts, and private homes.

Bull Shoals (population 1,312) also has a lovely natural setting and offers good facilities for fishing, hunting, and boating. More than 20 recreation areas and boating docks are located along Bull Shoals Lake, one of the White River group of lakes, which includes Beaver Lake in Arkansas and the Missouri lakes of Table Rock and Taneycomo. A dam completed in 1951 created the huge lake with a surface area of 45,000 acres, a shoreline of some 1,000 miles, and famous lunker largemouth bass fishing. Near Bull Shoals are Bull Shoals Caverns and Mountain Village 1890, a group of storefronts found in old towns in the area and carefully assembled in one place to preserve a genuine 19th-century Ozarks settlement.

Nights here can be warm in midsummer, but they are usually cool and comfortable the rest of the year, and the winters are mild. Between the two towns, U.S. Highway 62 winds around the higher hills and rides the tops of the lower ridges. Patches of hay and potatoes, and occasional strands of cotton alternate with corn and sorghum cane. Land that is too steep and rocky for cultivation is given over to pasture or woods.

Even if you're not an angler, Mountain Home–Bull Shoals offers great retirement living. One in four residents is over 65, compared with the national average of one in nine. Costs are low, the climate is mild yet variable, crime is practically nonexistent, and the pace of living is relaxed.

Pluses: Second lowest crime rate among the retirement places; expanding economy with favorable part-time job prospects; low health care and housing costs; popular water recreation area.

Minuses: No performing arts calendar; specialized health care needs may mean traveling to Fayetteville or Springfield.

PACIFIC BEACHES

Kauai, HI (#83)
Maui, HI (#100)
Salinas–Seaside–
  Monterey, CA (#101)

San Diego, CA (#59)
San Luis Obispo, CA (#81)
Santa Rosa–Petaluma, CA
  (#113)

A single word that most people associate with this region is *paradise*. It certainly isn't a distinct area, stretching as it does from the California coast to Hawaii. The retirement places here have only one thing in common: a shoreline on the Pacific Ocean.

Kauai and Maui are in the tropical climate zone, officially defined as anywhere temperatures never fall below 64 degrees Fahrenheit. Coastal California has a Mediterranean climate, typically described as mild and unchanging. Of the six retirement places in this region, all rank better than 51st for climatic mildness. With all this great weather, outdoor recreation options can be enjoyed year round.

Many California locations have been attracting older adults for years. San Diego is famed as a destination for retired Navy and Marine Corps personnel. Most of these spots provide a wide range of services for older adults and boast attractive retirement communities. Good health care facilities are available, as are transportation services for local and for intercity travel.

Nonetheless, because of the high cost of living, population growth in the Pacific retirement areas is expected to slow during the last years of this century. The living may be easy, but it is not cheap. Health care costs are among the highest in the United States. San Diego ranks 125th among the retirement places for affordable housing. Maui ranks 131st.

Pacific Beach retirement is great for those who can afford it, but despite the many recreational and cultural amenities and the terrific weather, the costs of living in paradise can run extremely high.

PACIFIC NORTHWEST CLOUD BELT

★ Bellingham, WA (#13)
Bend, OR (#48)
Eugene–Springfield, OR (#45)
Friday Harbor–San Juan
  Islands, WA (#117)
Medford–Ashland, OR (#26)

Newport–Lincoln City, OR
  (#87)
Oak Harbor–Whidbey Island,
  WA (#90)
Olympia, WA (#74)
★ Port Angeles–Strait of Juan
  de Fuca, WA (#10)

In the 1970s, no other state made so clear its desire to discourage immigration as did Oregon when its popular governor Tom McCall urged tourists to give the state a try. "But for heaven's sake," he quickly added, "don't come to live here." This awareness of the harm that rapid population growth can bring to beautiful, pristine land is commonly felt elsewhere in the Pacific Northwest.

Nevertheless, the near collapse of the lumber industry in Oregon and Washington in the early 1980s has caused local planners to behave like their counterparts in other states and to compete for industrial development and population growth.

Certain rural areas are being pitched as retirement havens—ironic, because older adults from the Great Lakes, the distant Northeast, and even sun-baked Southern California have been coming to this area for years to enjoy the clear air, quiet, and uncrowded space.

In the state of Washington, their destinations are most often the islands reachable by bridge or ferry from downtown Seattle, and places like Olympia, Port Angeles, Sequim, and Bellingham that front on Puget Sound.

The area, with the tall Cascades and Olympic Mountains in view, has a somewhat wet marine climate, low crime rates, and outstanding outdoor recreation endowments.

In Oregon, retired persons settle along the Pacific Coast and in the forested cities and towns along I-5 between Portland and the California border.

Calvin Beale, a well-known demographer who has followed American counties for decades as they grow, ebb, and grow again, observed not long ago that the popularity of the Pacific Northwest Cloud Belt just goes to show that "'Sun Belt' is a very imperfect synonym for population growth."

Between 1970 and 1980, for example, Bend and the surrounding forested environs in Deschutes County, Oregon, made up one of the fastest-growing places west of Florida.

Of more than 300 metropolitan areas in the United States, Olympia, Washington's groomed and parklike state capital, ranked in the top ten in rate of growth over the same period, along with the Florida metro areas of Ocala and Fort Myers–Cape Coral.

★ Bellingham, Washington (#13)

Whatcom County is Washington's northernmost coastal county. As much as any other location, it recalls the lumber and shipping heritage of the 19th-century Pacific Northwest. On its western edge are the deep waters of Georgia Strait; to the east are the Cascade Mountains, dominated by 10,778-foot Mt. Baker. Of the four incorporated places here, the largest by far is Bellingham (population 46,000).

Haven to counterculture types, young persons, and older adults as well, Bellingham is closer to Vancouver, British Columbia, than it is to Seattle. It is a growing city with many handsome turn-of-the-century homes. On Sehome Hill, overlooking the city and Bellingham Bay, sits Western Washington University. Lake Whatcom is at the eastern edge of town.

When the wet, clean salt air from the Pacific meets up with cold, clear mountain air, the result is precipitation. This is a constant fact of life in this retirement place. But the vistas are green, and the climate remarkably even all year round.

Pluses: Splendid outdoor recreation assets; above-average number of physicians; continuing education options available at both a two-year and a large state university.

Minuses: High health care costs; part-time employment limited by competition from students; cool, cloudy marine climate may not attract some.

★ Port Angeles–Strait of Juan de Fuca, Washington (#10)

On a mild winter afternoon on the Olympic Peninsula, there is nothing quite like taking your binoculars and driving out to the Coast Guard station at the end of Ediz Hook, a 4-mile sandbar curving out from the waterfront of Port Angeles, to watch the distant ship traffic arriving from all points in the Pacific bound for Puget Sound.

A Greek sailor nicknamed Juan de Fuca steered into this strait in 1592. Two hundred years later a Spanish mariner put into the impressive natural harbor on the south shore and named the Indian village he found there Port of Our Lady of the Angels. The name was shortened to Port Angeles by early settlers, then changed and rechanged until it stuck in 1890, when it became the seat of Clallam County.

Sitting atop the wild and beautiful Olympic Peninsula, Port Angeles and nearby Joyce and Sequim (locally pronounced "Skwim") have the Olympic Mountains behind them and the beaches along the Strait of Juan de Fuca at their front steps.

For such a small place (population 17,311), Port Angeles is truly a center of activity. There are several structured retirement communities in both Port Angeles and Sequim. The headquarters of the Olympic National Park is here. In summer, there is heavy ferry traffic to Vancouver Island and to Alaska.

Summer and fall, the hikers, berry pickers, clammers, crabbers, beachcombers, and fishermen are everywhere. During the winter, the Port Angeles Symphony puts on six concerts.

Pluses: Extensive public transportation system; spectacular natural setting; excellent supply of leisure-living amenities; low taxes; low crime rate.

Minuses: Cool, cloudy marine climate may not attract some; above-average health care costs; extremely limited performing arts options.

RIO GRANDE COUNTRY

Albuquerque, NM (#79)

★ Brownsville–
   Harlingen, TX (#7)

Deming, NM (#86)

Las Cruces, NM (#43)

★ McAllen–Edinburg–
   Mission, TX (#24)

Roswell, NM (#70)

Santa Fe, NM (#116)

The Rio Grande rises in the Rocky Mountains in southwestern Colorado, flows south through the center of New Mexico west of Santa Fe, through Albuquerque and Las Cruces, and serves as a 1,240-mile boundary between Texas and Mexico before emptying into the Gulf of Mexico some 60 miles downriver from Brownsville.

Like the Delta South, this area has a large ethnic population. Two of every five persons are Mexican-American, and one in ten is American Indian. Like the Delta South, too, Rio Grande Country is distinguished by low incomes, large families, poor housing, joblessness, low levels of education, and other social problems.

Along the river's southward progress are a few pockets of phenomenal retirement growth. Not only Albuquerque but also the cities of Roswell, Deming, and Las Cruces and the settled areas around them have all seen their number of residents over age 65 jump at three or more times the average national rate. This is also where several retirement subdivision promotions, notably Rio Rancho Estates and Cochiti Lake, went sour in the late 1970s.

Even with the well-publicized growth that most of arid and semiarid New Mexico has experienced, there are still fewer than eight persons per square mile. The desert-mesa vastness is imposing, the distances between towns great, and the loneliness outside city limits a little scary to retired persons hailing from large cities.

The lower valley in southmost Texas isn't lonely at all. Since 1980, Cameron County (Brownsville–Harlingen) and Hidalgo County (McAllen–Edinburg–Mission) have together gained 130,000 people, many of them retired midwesterners who found a climate as mild as Florida's and living costs nearly as low as Mexico's.

★ Brownsville–Harlingen, Texas (#7)

Onshore Gulf breezes make metropolitan Brownsville –Harlingen somewhat cooler than many inland Texas cities. Nonetheless, you know you're in the subtropics by the palms, royal poinciana, papaya, and banana trees that line the streets and are slowly recovering from the severe freeze of 1983. In August, you'll know it, too, by the visible heat waves rising from shimmering sand on South Padre Island. This retirement place, on the same latitude as Fort Lauderdale, is known to many as the "poor man's Florida."

Brownsville (population 96,300) is both an international seaport and a shrimp and deep-sea fishing

center. Harlingen (population 52,400) is more of a resort area with wide avenues and uncluttered thoroughfares. The Texas Highway Department ranks these two cities and all of surrounding Cameron County as the number one destination for long-term visitors. There are no smokestack industries, no skyscrapers to block the sun, or traffic snarls to fray your nerves. On the streets and in the shops of both cities, the language commonly spoken is Spanish. Culturally and economically, this area is more a part of Mexico than the United States.

Pluses: Established public transportation system; lowest composite cost-of-living index among 131 retirement places; Gulf coastline.

Minuses: Low ratings for personal safety; hot valley summers; limited performing arts attractions.

★ McAllen–Edinburg–Mission, Texas (#24)

Edinburg (population 24,075), McAllen (population 78,900), Mission (population 22,589), and Pharr (population 21,381) were centers for packing and marketing red grapefruit, oranges, limes, lemons, and winter vegetables grown in the lower Rio Grande valley until a freak freeze in 1983 ruined the citrus industry.

Even before that disaster, the devaluation of the Mexican peso shut down much of the business activity in Hidalgo County when thousands of customers from south of the border stopped crossing the bridge for daily retail shopping.

For all of that, plus the general recession in Texas, what possible explanation can there be for the lower valley's continued population growth? Part of the answer is immigration and part of it is retirement. Many of the citrus groves are being leveled into mobile-home parks. Valley bankers and businesspeople are welcoming "Winter Texans," who come down from states like Ohio, Wisconsin, Illinois, and Michigan, some for a few months stay, others for permanent residency.

Pluses: Lowest composite cost-of-living index among 131 retirement places; comprehensive health care system; continuing education opportunities at a large state university.

Minuses: Hot valley summers; middling ratings for personal safety; short performing arts calendar.

ROCKY MOUNTAINS

Boise, ID (#106)

Coeur d'Alene, ID (#27)

Colorado Springs, CO (#104)

Flagstaff, AZ (#29)

Fort Collins–Loveland, CO
   (#79)

Grand Junction, CO (#66)

★ Hamilton–Bitterroot Valley,
   MT (#18)

★ Kalispell, MT (#25)

Missoula, MT (#43)

What does green and rugged Coeur d'Alene in Idaho's panhandle have in common with sun-baked Deming in southwestern New Mexico? Very little. Yet the Census Bureau lumps them together in a region it labels Mountain. By better reasoning, Deming, with its desert and Hispanic flavors, more properly belongs in Rio Grande Country. When it comes to certain foothill-and-mountain counties in Arizona, Colorado, Idaho, and Montana, however, the feel is definitely high-country, definitely Rocky Mountains. In spite of the reservations many older adults have about high altitudes and cold winters, the Rockies are emerging from their vacation only status, becoming an area where older adults are moving for year-round living.

In Colorado, one can easily distinguish between the Eastern Slope and Western Slope areas. Large cities like Colorado Springs (in a setting that reminds many of Asheville in the North Carolina mountains) and Fort Collins are Eastern Slope. Grand Junction, near the Utah border, is the population center of the Western Slope. The two slopes have different political orientations and different growth rates.

In Idaho, where the population rose by a third in the 1970s, retired newcomers head for the city of Coeur d'Alene, within commuting distance of Spokane, Washington, or they settle near metropolitan Boise. In Montana, the spectacular but sparsely settled western counties—particularly Flathead, Lake, Missoula, and Ravalli—are the ones drawing older newcomers. In the Arizona high country, only cold weather and a low rating for personal safety (96th) kept Flagstaff from our list of 25 choice places; this locale made commendable showings in money matters (23rd), services (27th), and leisure assets (31st).

★ Hamilton–Bitterroot Valley, Montana (#18)

Bitterroot, Montana's state flower, has a small white rosette of 12 to 18 leaves. Flathead Indians who ate its root gave it a name that later stuck to the mountain range, river, and valley in Ravalli County where the flower is found most abundantly.

This valley has Montana's best orchards and some of its best land for truck gardens, but the growing season here is a limited one. Ravalli is one of 247 counties where more than a third of the land is national forest, park, or wilderness area. Hamilton, the county seat, is a small (population 2,661) trading center known for distinctive log-home kits that are shipped throughout the country. The town sits on U.S. route 93, one of the most spectacular routes in the United States; north is the college town of Missoula, and farther north is Kalispell and the Canadian border.

Pluses: Second highest rating for outdoor assets among 131 retirement places; low taxes; low housing costs; low crime rate.

Minuses: Long, rigorous winters; limited health care facilities; no public transportation or continuing-education options; no fine arts calendar.

★ Kalispell, Montana (#25)

Recognizing the economic realities of western Montana, this city has decided to call itself "Vacation City."

Each year, 3 million visitors come to see Glacier National Park, ski Big Mountain, and fish Flathead Lake, the biggest natural freshwater lake lying within a single state west of the Mississippi River.

Kalispell (a Pend d'Orielle Indian word for "prairie above the lake") started out when the Great Northern Railway arrived at the Flathead River in 1891. Most of the buildings on its broad, leafy streets are modern in design. Thanks to careful planning in the first three decades of this century, the city fits well into its spectacular setting.

While tourism plays the lead part in Flathead County's economy, art has a surprisingly strong supporting role. The Flathead River valley has some 30 professional artists who earn their living by painting, sculpting, carving, potting, and working with other mediums. It's a multimillion-dollar business here, strongly supported by Kalispell's Hockaday Center for the Arts, its annual Art Show and Auction.

Pluses: Low housing and health care costs; low taxes; highest score for outdoor assets among 131 retirement places.

Minuses: Long, cold winters; no public transportation; limited cultural attractions; lackluster job forecast.

SOUTH ATLANTIC AND GULF COAST SHORE

★ Biloxi–Gulfport, MS (#14)
Brunswick–Golden Isles, GA (#40)
★ Charleston, SC (#12)
Fairhope–Gulf Shores, AL (#56)
Fort Walton Beach, FL (#63)
Hilton Head–Beaufort, SC (#99)
Myrtle Beach, SC (#72)
Panama City, FL (#50)
Southport, NC (#18)

The retirement places in the South Atlantic and Gulf Coast Shore region have a special appeal and flavor. Although this coastline is dotted with many very old cities, such as Charleston and Galveston, it has enjoyed a boom growth only in recent years.

Most of these resort-retirement areas lie in low, marshy land either on the mainland itself or on nearby barrier islands. Palmetto palms, scrub oak, dune grass, and Spanish moss swaying in the sea breezes impart a languid, relaxed mood. Fishing shanties lie scattered near the piers and docks where shrimpers, crabbers, and trawlers moor. Stately planter-style cottages set back from the narrow street are almost hidden behind tall hedges and are surrounded by massive live oaks. Streets paved with old oyster and clam shells; small gift shops, boutiques, and shops offering seafood, gumbo, and chicory coffee; taverns and inns of all ages and sizes—these are what you'll find in every metro area, town, and village of the coastal islands.

The South Atlantic and Gulf Coast Shore resorts are less crowded and have lower living costs than most comparable places on the Florida peninsula. Furthermore, their summer months, while sometimes uncomfortable, are less rugged than those farther south. You are likely to find newer buildings and younger people here than in some older retirement havens.

On the minus side, crime rates are high. Of the nine retirement places in this region, only three—Southport, North Carolina; Fairhope–Gulf Shores, Alabama; Fort Walton Beach, Florida—have above-average ratings for personal safety. Health care facilities can be inadequate, and while housing costs are generally low for the region, some places (such as Hilton Head–Beaufort) are expensive. Finally, these low-lying oceanside locations are subject to damage from severe tropical storms.

★ Biloxi–Gulfport, Mississippi (#14)

Biloxi–Gulfport, which ranks 14th overall among the retirement places, is a metro area with a population over 200,000 encompassing two counties on Mississippi's Gulf shore.

Biloxi may be the oldest European town in the Mississippi Valley. Settled by the French in 1699, the city is confined to the low ridge of a narrow, fingerlike peninsula with 25 miles of coastline. It is not only a seaside resort, but a major fishing and shipbuilding center as well. The heaviest concentration of these industries is still to be found on the Point, or the eastern end of the peninsula. Here are the shrimp and oyster packing and canning plants, the fishing fleet, boatyards, and other maritime centers.

For those of you who think that Mardi Gras is celebrated only in New Orleans, make note that it is observed in Biloxi, too, although at a slightly more manageable level of insanity. There is also the annual shrimp festival, held the first Sunday in June, which includes the traditional Catholic blessing of the fleet.

Neighboring Gulfport has many of the attributes of Biloxi but lacks its colorful history and intimate charm. It's a bit more industrialized, with lumber, cotton, seafood canning, and shipbuilding as its major industries. However, it also has fine beaches, new housing developments of all types, and a reputation as an established resort area. Gulfport is a fisherman's paradise; the Mississippi Sound and a large number of lakes, rivers, bays, and bayous are within a few minutes' drive of downtown, and there are also excellent facilities for deep-sea fishing.

Like many metro areas, Biloxi–Gulfport has a soberingly high crime rate, ranking 84th out of 131 in this category. But it has low living costs: it ranks 22nd in money matters and 20th in homeowning costs.

Pluses: Low median housing values and extremely low property taxes; outstanding beach climate; abundant hospital facilities.

Minuses: Hurricane prone; no local colleges for continuing education; higher than average crime rate.

★ Charleston, South Carolina (#12)

If South Carolinians say that they are among the rare folk in the South who harbor no secret envy of Virginians, then native Charlestonians will probably say they envy no one at all.

This aristocratic and storied old American city is the survivor of floods, hurricanes, epidemics, and siege. Very fortunately, its homes, old churches, historic shrines, lovely gardens, winding streets, and intricate iron lace gateways have survived, too. And throughout nearly three centuries, it has carefully maintained its reputation for cultivated manners.

Located on a fine harbor on the Low Country coast where "the Ashley and Cooper rivers unite to form the Atlantic Ocean," Charleston traffics in waterborne international commerce. The bay, the tidal inlets, and the sea islands visible from the east battery, all provide recreation retreats.

After San Antonio, Charleston is the highest rated of any retirement place with more than 250,000 people. It isn't difficult to see why.

Pluses: Low living costs; excellent health care ratings; established public transit system; variety of colleges for continuing education; generally mild winter months; high marks for the performing arts; excellent outdoor recreation assets.

Minuses: Prone to hurricanes and tidal flooding; hot, humid summer months; a high level of criminal activity; modest economic outlook.

★ Southport, North Carolina (#18)

In the summer of 1986, Southport became Hazelhurst, Mississippi, when Hollywood production crews came in to film *Crimes of the Heart*. Located at the mouth of the Cape Fear River on North Carolina's southern Atlantic coast, the old town's collection of frame Victorian houses in its mile-square historic district lends a quaint flavor to what is mainly a beach resort. Unlike the Grand Strand immediately to the south in Myrtle Beach, South Carolina, however, the beaches here are relatively free of high rise condos and neon, stand-up eateries.

Until the late 1960s, Brunswick County (of which Southport is the seat) was dependent on pine plantations, turpentine distilleries, and fertilizer plants. The diversified economy today is based on agriculture, tourism, and commercial fishing. From the North Carolina Aquarium to the Dosher Hospital, older adults have a number of volunteer opportunities. Fishing and golf are possible almost all year. For specialized shopping and medical facilities, Wilmington, North Carolina's largest coastal city, is 35 miles up the Cape Fear River.

Pluses: Scenic, south Atlantic coastal setting; pleasant climate; low crime rate; low costs of living, particularly for housing.

Minuses: Limited health care facilities may require trips into Wilmington; no public transportation; limited performing arts calendar.

TAHOE BASIN AND THE OTHER CALIFORNIA

Carson City–Minden, NV (#122)

Chico–Paradise, CA (#53)

Clear Lake, CA (#119)

Grass Valley–Truckee, CA (#103)

Red Bluff–Sacramento Valley, CA (#64)

Redding, CA (#31)

Reno, NV (#121)

Twain Harte–Yosemite, CA (#36)

In California, three out of four residents live either in the Los Angeles basin or in metropolitan San Francisco–Oakland–San Jose. Everyone else lives in a part of the state the Beach Boys seem never to have sung about.

You might call it the Other California. Parts of it—the Mother Lode Country and the northern Sacramento Valley—are seeing a growing number of retired newcomers, most of whom are native Californians.

Mother Lode Country, the mountain-studded interior, with alpine meadows, blizzard-filled passes, clear lakes, trout streams, and magnificent scenery, was once a mining area and now is a tourist haven. Donner Lake, a popular summer beach resort, also doubles as a winter ski area. Even in midsummer, this high mountain lake tends to be on the chilly side. Tuolumne County, roughly a hundred miles to the south, contains spectacular Yosemite National Park, with all of the attendant opportunities for outstanding outdoor recreation. Although the gold rush is over, these areas continue to attract people with scenery, mountain climate, and open spaces. Places like Grass Valley, Nevada City, Truckee, and Twain Harte suffer from high living costs, especially those associated with owning a home.

Clear Lake, on the northwest fringe of the Great Interior Valley, is California's largest natural freshwater lake and centerpiece of Lake County's resort area. In addition to excellent fishing, Clear Lake (Bass Capital of the West) offers good boating facilities.

Water recreation is also available in nearby Tehama County at Red Bluff, where Diversion Dam spans the Sacramento River. Red Bluff has some splendid Victorian homes, as does Chico downriver. Both these areas have shown substantial growth in recent years, including a sizable increase due to in-migration of retired people from densely populated Southern California.

TEXAS INTERIOR

★ Athens–Cedar Creek Lake, TX (#14)

Austin, TX (#82)

Burnet–Marble Falls–Llano, TX (#69)

Canton–Lake Tawakoni, TX (#27)

Fredericksburg, TX (#58)

Kerrville, TX (#68)

★ San Antonio, TX (#9)

Of all the states, perhaps Texas occupies the most distinctive place in the American mind. To paraphrase a 50-year-old guidebook, Texas is so large that if it could be folded up and over, using its northernmost boundary as a hinge, McAllen would be plunked down in the middle of North Dakota; and if it were folded eastward, El Paso would lie just off the coast of Florida.

Out in the country, there are more internally sharp contrasts here than in any other state. Northeast Texas looks like Arkansas. East Texas is deeply southern, with small farms bringing in sugar cane, cotton, and rice. Southwest Texas is mainly lonely, open-range cattle country. Northwest Texas is dry and mountainous, looking like parts of New Mexico.

You'll find contrasting retirement regions, too. The lower Rio Grande valley is distinctly Hispanic and has winters as mild as Florida's. So do the Gulf Coast beaches, from South Padre Island up to just above Corpus Christi. Then there's an area in the middle of the state encompassing the lovely cedar-scented Hill Country along with metropolitan Austin and San Antonio.

According to certain visitors, Austin, state capital and home of the University of Texas, seems to have the same terrain and natural vegetation as New England. Metropolitan Austin is growing so quickly that its population is projected to double by the year 2000. Already, housing costs are breathtaking. It's a "books and bureaucrats" city, drawing a good many retired UT alumni from all over the nation along with retired Texas government employees.

San Antonio's appeal as a retirement destination, on the other hand, has four sources: Brooks, Kelly, Lackland, and Randolph. These are big Air Force bases. Many veterans who were posted to them during the 1940s have returned for the mild San Antonio winters, low living costs, and pleasant Hispanic atmosphere.

West of Austin and northwest of San Antonio, the Hill Country towns (Fredericksburg and Kerrville) have spic-and-span layouts in their old sections. These are towns settled by Germans who fled their homeland in the mid-19th century. So attractive is this area that much of it is experiencing second-home development by prosperous Texans and others from outside the state.

★ Athens–Cedar Creek Lake, Texas (#14)

The East Texas pine and post oak area southeast of Dallas, north of Houston, and west of Shreveport, Louisiana, has been attracting retired persons to its rolling terrain and lakes ever since the late 1960s. Athens, seat of Henderson County, is the largest town in a cluster of rural counties that surrounds Cedar Creek Lake, one of the most popular recreation areas in the state.

The Athens area, townspeople will tell you, is surrounded by so many lakes that it can almost qualify as an island. Aside from Cedar Creek Lake northwest of town, Lake Athens is just a ten-minute drive east on a county road; farther east, most of Henderson County's border lies along Lake Palestine.

Much of the place will feel like home to persons who grew up in smaller towns. There is a handsome courthouse square here, quiet neighborhoods, a country club district, and low-density residential developments around the lakes and in the midst of the agricultural hinterland. Like so many other small towns, long-time annual events offer a flavor: Black-Eyed Pea Jamboree, Texas Fiddlers' Reunion, the Henderson County Livestock Show, and the Athens Antique Fair.

Pluses: Mild winters, lovely springs and falls; extremely low living costs; crime rate less than half the national average.

Minuses: Health care needs may require a trip to Tyler or Dallas; no public transportation; few commercial recreation options.

★ San Antonio, Texas (#9)

This retirement place, which takes in three counties, has as its heart one of the handful of authentically different cities in America. In San Antonio, the South merges with the West, and North American culture blends with Latin. There is no better time to sample San Antonio's distinctive mix than during Fiesta Week each April. Originally staged as a memorial to the heroes of the Alamo, San Antonio's Fiesta has four parades, a multitude of ethnic dancers, food vendors, craft merchants, and art shows.

Winding through the heart of downtown is the San Antonio River, modest in size but used to the maximum. Dozens of bridges cross the river, which is lined with restaurants along a tree-shaded walkway. Shopping is offered in several regional malls as well as in downtown San Antonio. VIA Metropolitan Transit, the city public transportation agency, has one of the largest bus fleets in the country. A good network of freeways connects all parts of the city, and three interstate highways link the area to the rest of Texas.

Of retirement places with more than one-half million persons, San Antonio is rated the best in this book. What does this major metropolitan area offer retired persons besides atmosphere and charm? Obviously quite a bit, since even conservative estimates put the number of retired persons in Greater San Antonio at 15 percent of the population. With an established performing arts series and a full slate of outdoor entertainments, this retirement place doesn't suffer from too little to do. With 15 accredited hospitals, a medical school, and a VA medical center, the area's health care services are equally exceptional. Housing here is also affordable. San Antonio has a plentiful supply of homes for rent or purchase, condos, apartments, and retirement complexes.

Pluses: Mild winter months; low housing costs; low taxes; extensive public transportation system; impressive number of fine arts events.

Minuses: High crime rate; stressfully hot summers; high health care costs.

YANKEE BELT

Amherst–Northampton, MA (#77)

Bar Harbor–Frenchman Bay, ME (#55)

Bennington, VT (#97)

Burlington, VT (#102)

Camden–Penobscot Bay, ME (#36)

Cape Cod, MA (#114)

Hanover, NH (#47)

Keene, NH (#115)

Laconia–Lake Winnipesaukee, NH (#125)

Litchfield County, CT (#130)

North Conway–White Mountains, NH (#127)

Portsmouth–Dover–Durham, NH (#131)

In New England, the preferred retirement destinations aren't in heavily urbanized Connecticut, Massachusetts, or Rhode Island. One big exception is Massachusetts's Barnstable County (Cape Cod), where one in three residents since 1970 has been a newcomer and where one in five is now over age 65. Two future exceptions may be Hampshire County (Amherst–Northampton) in western Massachusetts and rural Litchfield County in Connecticut, an area discovered by upscale New Yorkers 15 years ago. To find the most popular retirement spots in the Yankee Belt, however, look in the countryside pockets of the north, in Maine, New Hampshire, and Vermont.

In the decade and a half since 1970, Maine's population has jumped 20 percent. By Sun Belt standards, such growth may seem paltry. For the Pine Tree State, though, it's been the fastest upsurge since the mid-19th century.

Most retired newcomers choose the rocky Atlantic coast over the hard-going farm areas and rough-cut paper- and lumber-mill towns in Maine's interior. Within the seascape counties—Hancock, Knox, Lincoln, and York—the places that draw retired people are the small lobster ports and summer resort towns off old U.S. Highway 1, places with names like Camden, Bar Harbor, Ellsworth, Wiscasset, and Rockland.

New Hampshire, too, is growing. Indeed, it is growing the most quickly of all the northeastern states —mainly at the expense of Massachusetts, its heavily taxed neighbor. You'll pay no income or sales taxes here (the only other state where this is still possible is Alaska). But you will pay handsomely for real estate along huge Lake Winnipesaukee's shoreline and around Hanover (home of Dartmouth College) and in the environs of North Conway, a resort town.

For all its attraction for disaffected New Yorkers and Pennsylvanians who come to live year round, Vermont remains the most rural state in America according to the Census Bureau. Two of every three residents here live beyond the built-up limits of cities. Much of the state unmistakably is a 19th-century Currier & Ives landscape of sugar maples, dairy farms, and steepled white Congregational churches that dominate every green town common. In early October, the brilliant fall foliage draws busloads of weekenders from Boston and New York. As a general rule, the southern counties (Bennington, for example) draw retired people, and the northern counties draw skiers.

Tables, Sidebars, and Maps

About the Authors

Richard Boyer writes both fiction and nonfiction. In addition to co-authoring *Places Rated Almanac* and *Retirement Places Rated,* he is the creator of the award-winning Doc Adams mysteries published by Houghton Mifflin Company. Formerly of Chicago and Boston, Mr. Boyer, upon completion of *Places Rated Almanac,* followed the book's advice for selecting good places to live and now resides in Asheville, North Carolina.

David Savageau is principal-in-charge of PreLOCATION, a personal relocation consulting firm. Over the previous 15 years, he and his wife, Karyl, have lived successively in Denver, St. Louis, Indianapolis, and Boston. They now make their home in Gloucester, Massachusetts.